FIT NATION

Fit Nation

THE GAINS AND PAINS OF AMERICA'S EXERCISE OBSESSION

Natalia Mehlman Petrzela

The University of Chicago Press

Chicago and London

The University of Chicago Press, Chicago 60637
The University of Chicago Press, Ltd., London
© 2022 by Natalia Mehlman Petrzela

Published 2022
Paperback edition 2024
Printed in the United States of America

33 32 31 30 29 28 27 26 25 24   1 2 3 4 5

ISBN-13: 978-0-226-65110-1 (cloth)
ISBN-13: 978-0-226-83336-1 (paper)
ISBN-13: 978-0-226-65124-8 (e-book)
DOI: https://doi.org/10.7208
/chicago/9780226651248.001.0001

Library of Congress Cataloging-in-Publication Data

Names: Petrzela, Natalia Mehlman, author.
Title: Fit nation : the gains and pains of America's
exercise obsession / Natalia Mehlman Petrzela.
Description: Chicago : University of Chicago Press, 2022. |
Includes bibliographical references and index.
Identifiers: LCCN 2022014513 | ISBN 9780226651101
(cloth) | ISBN 9780226651248 (ebook)
Subjects: LCSH: Exercise—Social aspects—United
States. | Physical fitness—Social aspects—United States. |
Physical fitness centers—United States. | Well-being—
United States.
Classification: LCC GV471.U6 P48 2022 |
DDC 306.4/6130973—dc23/eng/20220406
LC record available at https://lccn.loc.gov/2022014513

♾ This paper meets the requirements of ANSI/NISO
Z39.48-1992 (Permanence of Paper)

In memory of Patricia Moreno, who taught me that the most powerful lessons we learn in the gym are those we take into the world.

Contents

Author's Note

This book was born at the gym, or—to be more exact—just outside it, on a crisp evening in 2011. Hair and tank top still damp from the exercise class I had just taught at Equinox, a high-end New York City fitness chain, I was reflecting on a breathless conversation with a student. As I was packing up, she ran over, words spilling forth. "Thanks to this class, I don't even need therapy anymore! And I am having the best sex!" she gushed with an abandon that, five years into teaching fitness, had become strangely familiar. In emails, on social media, or after class, students shared predictable triumphs such as fitting into their jeans or completing a marathon, but also disclosed surprisingly, and even troublingly, private details about their pregnancies, mental health, and sexual experiences. The intensity of the authority and intimacy these people—attorneys and account managers and editors and executives—projected onto me was unexpected and a bit unsettling. After all, I knew most of them only by first name, and I had only the most basic fitness credentials. But who was I to judge anyone for getting a little starry-eyed thanks to an inspiring sweat? My own experience of exercise, after all, had been so transformative that I had embarked on a shadow fitness career alongside my job as a history professor, teaching exercise classes before and after work several days a week.

I was ruminating on whether some students were unhealthily invested in their workouts as I traversed Union Square, a neighborhood some would soon dub "FitDi"—"fitness district"—thanks to the concentration of yoga studios, juice bars, and athleisure shops that signaled the affluence of its population. A group of mostly Black and Latino teenagers talked and laughed as they strode past the stalls spilling over with bunches of kale and artisanal sourdough loaves, heading for the increasingly anomalous McDonald's (it has since shut). They were almost certainly students at Washington Irving (also since shuttered), an enormous but under-resourced high school one block east, which was a relic of the early-twentieth-century faith in large public institutions to transform the lives of the poor. Washington Irving students were about as unlikely to be members of Equinox as to attend the private, four-year liberal arts college where I taught, also only blocks away. As the scene vividly revealed, bodies—like homes, bank accounts, neighborhoods, and the number of diplomas on the wall—are yet another marker of socio-economic inequality.[1]

My passion for fitness had, up until that evening, existed largely apart from my jobs as a middle-school Spanish teacher and then as a historian of education. For the first time, a few months later, I brought these pursuits together, co-founding with food-justice activist Ellen Gustafson HealthClass2.0, an experiential partnership between the New School and the Washington Irving Educational Complex. Over five years, we expanded to collaborate with principals, teachers, health educators, students, and local businesses to serve over five thousand youth in three boroughs. My college students, Ellen, and I would drag our stereo and boxes of snacks to physical education classes and after-school programs, co-creating a curriculum that enabled engaged, even pleasurable, experiences of healthful food and exercise, as well as strategies to integrate these practices into daily life independently and affordably. Many "wellness education" programs already existed—and even more do today—but our key contribution was to set common advice about "making healthy choices" in the context of the structural factors that can make fast food more economical than healthier alternatives, and access to the time and space to exercise a privilege. This book emerged from that activism, a quest to understand how "fitness" has evolved to represent far more than physical exertion, to be connected to a set of values that privileges the individualistic, disciplined pursuit of health—or at least its outward appearance—as a virtue, and to transpire in spaces not universally accessible, challenging some inequalities and intensifying others.

I did not arrive at this project naturally. I grew up in the Boston suburbs in the 1980s and 90s, and I felt intimated by, averse to, and apathetic about the exercise activities available to me—sports and dance. All seemed to require talent and technique I lacked, and in auditions and tryouts where other kids shone, I only envisioned embarrassment. Short-lived, lackluster forays into ballet and lacrosse only affirmed my antipathy, but the activity I most despised was the required one: physical education. As a bookish kid unfailingly last on the rope climb and mile run—and even at hopping up on the bleachers before class began—I invented every excuse to escape this obligation. My salvation came when I learned I could obtain course credit for participating in an unspecified "supervised physical activity." Annoyed, the department head reproached me, "That does *not* include team sports." No problem!

In 1994, my options were hiring a personal trainer (*That's for rich people*, my parents rebuffed) or participating in an activity included with our family membership to the Jewish Community Center: group fitness class. I suited up in lime-green Umbro shorts and an oversized T-shirt decorated with dancing Grateful Dead bears, and tentatively walked into Step Aerobics. The youngest by at least a decade, I hung in the back, marveling at the synchronized movement of the men and (mostly) women. Before long, I was at the front, my reflection a version of myself I barely recognized: spinning around the molded-rubber-and-plastic Reebok Step, purple risers stacked ever higher, new muscles visible under the tight bike shorts and sports bra I'd bought at the mall. After class I felt breathless, strong, and ready for anything, or at least for my homework and high school social drama. I had discovered fitness—not sport— and its codes, rituals, and hierarchies, which I somehow felt more capable of navigating.

I didn't yet know the vocabulary of "self-care" or "wellness," but I knew I was hooked on the exhilarating feeling that overtook me when the thirty-two-count workout music piped up and I focused only on mastering choreography. I also didn't realize that I had entered that studio at a moment when the fitness industry was expanding dramatically, both in market size and in the ever-loftier promises it made to a clientele increasingly encompassing more than bodybuilders and "gym rats." Over the coming years, I experienced that expansion firsthand. In order to take free classes while in college, I worked the reception desk at a World Gym. Handing out towels and swiping cards, I observed the twin spectacles of New Yorkers sculpting their bodies and of a franchise frantically attempting to compete with the sleek new health clubs that featured aerobics classes, cardio machines, and yoga mats rather than iron barbells. I moved to California and found a recreational running culture more inclusive than anything I had seen back east, and the presence of people of all ages and sizes paired with the opportunity to fundraise for leukemia and lymphoma research—and warm weather—inspired me to run my first marathon. I became certified to teach intenSati, a fitness class that combined aspects of martial arts, dance, and yoga, and was hired at Equinox, an expensive chain with a self-serious motto: "It's not fitness. It's life." When my classes filled, I was chosen as a brand ambassador for yoga-inspired retailer Lululemon Athletica, a huge poster of my pregnant body swathed in expensive stretchy fabric hanging on the store wall, a reminder that spending on exercise (and its accoutrements) was a socially acceptable form of conspicuous consumption during the Great Recession. My students often asked how I could smile so broadly while teaching such hard classes so early in the morning, and I would truthfully say that I was in disbelief, given my anxieties about my insufficient athleticism, that rooms full of people regularly showed up to exercise with me.

But I was also a scholar, and my personal satisfaction at my participation in the fitness world didn't explain *how* fitness had become so central to the American ideal of self-fashioning, yet remained, in so many ways, undeniably exclusive. My enthusiasm for fitness always coexisted with a profound unease about the destructive dynamics present in essentially every exercise activity; access was far from the only problem. Step may have saved me from the humiliations of PE, but it was in those mirrored studios that I learned to scrutinize and name every inch of my body—thunder thighs, muffin top—as a present or potential "problem area" to be slimmed, or more violently, "blasted," especially after enjoying rich food I came to moralize as a "guilty pleasure," especially in advance of "bikini season," which I used simply to call "summer." I still don't know whether my joy derived from the sweaty exhilaration of class or from meeting the internalized expectation to constantly work on myself, but I sometimes took classes back-to-back-to-back around dinnertime, marveling at how my hunger would dissipate after the first couple of songs, the bass drowning out the growl of my stomach. I also noticed how, as I raised money for various charitable causes through road races, the difference between nondisabled runners and the recipients of their fundraising was often depicted as troublingly stark: the runners altruistic, athletic heroes and the disabled or ill forlorn, frail charity cases. At Lululemon, I was compensated only with literal "exposure": borne of the snug leggings and sports bras I earned for teaching free classes among the rolling racks or for storefront window demonstrations, a living mannequin sweating behind glass pasted with Ayn Rand quotes and platitudes about "upgrading your outlook." Many other brands soon also sold stretchy pants alongside an uncritical embrace of individualist "fitspo" that conveniently ignored the obstacles that prevent many from pursuing physical fitness, and the elusiveness of the standard of "thriving, not just surviving." So much of this whole world was blindingly white, and even if women figured prominently as workers and consumers, the owners, investors, and managers were overwhelmingly men. I knew the gym could germinate collective and individual transformation, but it could just as powerfully reproduce the many inequalities of American life outside the gym—and create new ones.

I have spent the last decade figuring out how we got here, and this book traces processes that originated more than a century ago. Yet it was the coronavirus pandemic, which came late in this project, that has both posed the biggest challenges to contemporary fitness culture and revealed how embedded its assumptions and practices have become in American life. Almost overnight, thousands of brick-and-mortar fitness establishments went dark in March 2020, and in those last days before the shutdowns, going to the gym had morphed from a virtuous act to a narcissistic one that actually threatened public health. On the September day when New York City gyms reopened, I lined up around the block at 5:45 a.m. with other Equinox members who also radiated excitement at returning to what had once been an ordinary ritual but now felt almost exotic. After temperature checks, we streamed, masked, into a fitness funhouse filled not only with strangers but with long-unused, hulking equipment: squat racks, treadmills, Pilates reformers, a solid-wood barre drilled into a mirrored wall.

Given the far more momentous tragedy, participating in such sweaty spectacle felt indulgent, not least because just months before, freezer trucks had lined the sidewalk in front of the hospital across the way. Countless small studios operating on thin margins had closed during the pandemic, while Equinox, with its private-equity funding, had endured. The fitness industry nationwide lost 44 percent of its jobs, with 17 percent of its businesses permanently shuttering by the end of 2020. The crisis brought together cosmopolitan entrepreneurs and suburban gym owners.[2] "There is no curbside pickup for fitness," IHRSA (International Health, Racquet and Sportsclub Association), the industry's trade organization, pled in support of a federal bill that requested thirty billion dollars of relief appropriations.

I called and tweeted in support of this measure, the Gyms Mitigation and Survival Act, as well as the related Personal Health Investment Today Act, which allows Americans to use pre-tax dollars for "physical-activity related expenses" such as gym memberships, fitness equipment, and youth sports fees. But their framing reveals a fundamental weakness: they fail to even recognize, much less redress, the lack of *public* investment in physical education and recreational fitness. Couldn't bipartisan support for the importance of exercise be an opportunity to consider a new framework for the provision of fitness?

Members of a high-end gym typically had access to online alternatives, proximity to safe outdoor space, and more room to exercise at home, as well as relative control over their schedules. In many cities, however, public basketball courts, parks, playgrounds, and beaches, not to mention schools and children's sports leagues, were closed. People who skirted regulations to enjoy the sun and sand, play Frisbee at the park, organize children's sports, or go for a run, were often condemned for their irresponsible disregard for health. Giving a seminar for physical educators gearing up for another pandemic school year, I learned that despite the boom in digital fitness, it was becoming harder than ever to convince people that physical education in even a constrained form—online, masked, distanced, or without balls passed between children—was worth the effort or risk.

The existence of that excited predawn lineup outside Equinox revealed how encoded exercise had become as essential. Yet the collective failure to fight for its public provision only underscored that fitness is seen primarily as a consumer good, rather than a human right. Exercise is no longer just "working out" in the narrow physical sense, but neither is it "working out" as the collective public project it might be. Charting how and why these histories have unfolded is imperative to imagining, and making, a more equal future.

I hope you are experiencing this author's note as a sort of warm-up—even if that phrasing makes me seem too invested in exercise. No pursuit of truth is ever perfectly unbiased, and certainly, I am "that person" always up for a workout, and I do believe that a world in which more people have more opportunities to exercise on their own terms is one worth fighting for. I am also a white-presenting woman in a straight-sized, nondisabled body, which absolutely affects my interactions with the world, in and out of the gym. My expertise in American political culture equips me with the credentials to write this book, but my intimate connection to this subject has pushed me to reflect more deeply than ever on how my experience and identities shape my scholarship, and has given me an appreciation of nuance and emotion that more clinical analyses can lack. Because I—like any reader—have not been personally subject to every sort of discrimination rampant in our culture in general and in fitness spaces in particular, I have labored to emphasize how these biases have been constructed and perpetuated. Furthermore, my experiences working out and in fitness environments—from school gyms to store windows to locker rooms to fancy studios to community centers—have led me to interviews and archives publicly unavailable, a boon to this project, but also a circumstance that means I explore more deeply certain topics, individuals, and phenomena to the exclusion of others. No history that spans a huge nation over more than a century can be exhaustive, and I believe this in-depth approach is more intellectually satisfying than a sprawling, but ultimately shallow, alternative. I hope that this chronicle of how we became a nation obsessed with exercise but insensible to the power of both its oppressive dimensions—pains—and life-changing joys—gains—can help make these processes and underlying assumptions visible, and thus strengthen us to fight for a better path forward, at the gym and in the world.

Introduction

WHAT IS THE FIT NATION?

When Justin Pritchett finally decided to call the cops on an October evening in 2017, the manager of a Skokie, Illinois, XSport Fitness franchise had had enough. No matter how vigilantly he watched the reception area, securing every entrance and exit, that kid *just kept showing up*, running the length of the basketball court with his friends, or pumping weights on the gym floor. "Almost like a magic show," Pritchett later told the press, fifteen-year-old Vincent Gonzalez "would just randomly appear, not walking past the front desk." Veteran police officer Mario Valenti answered Pritchett's frustrated call reporting trespassing, but he didn't arrest, fine, or remove Gonzalez, who had been an XSport member until he could no longer afford the fees. Noting Gonzalez's "gentle nature," Valenti offered the teenager one hundred fifty dollars of his own money to put toward a membership. XSport executives were charmed, and they supplemented Valenti's gift to cover a two-year membership for Gonzalez, valued at around seven hundred dollars. Thanks to this generosity, Gonzalez's mother gushed, Vincent could focus on his studies at his charter high school, free to work out without worrying about the cost or, for that matter, a police record.

Most news-making incidents that involve calling the cops on young men of color take a different turn, and the internet thrilled at this "unbelievably positive" story. But the XSport story raises crucial questions about fitness in the twenty-first-century United States. One, why does Vincent's committed quest to exercise—to the point of lawbreaking—so pull at our heartstrings? And two, if it resonates because we believe that exercise is integral to everyday life, why are we satisfied with—and even celebrating—the fact that it is seen as a private good, with access to it resting on the arbitrary altruism of a good-humored police officer or health-club executive?

The answers to both of these questions lie in the history of the last seventy-five years, during which an astonishingly expansive consensus about the importance of exercise has emerged in America. Working out evolved from a strange, even suspicious, pursuit to a social imperative, embraced as crucial by Americans otherwise increasingly divided by identity and ideology. Today, it's almost impossible to open one's inbox or walk a few city blocks without experiencing some exhortation to exercise: Walk 5K to cure cancer! Ignite your inner sex kitten at pole-dancing class! Sweat like a celebrity at SoulCycle! Even *resisting* these fitness trends often involves embracing others: "harden the f*ck up" at a CrossFit "anti-gym," join the defiantly size-inclusive "Fat Kid Dance Party," or breathe deeply into the blissful escape of downward dog. Fitness has become a figurative backdrop for much of contemporary life: an intrepid reporter breaks a story by taking Pilates alongside an inscrutable source; a CEO confides that her hiring secret is observing how applicants perform in spin class; little girls make yoga mats for their American Girl dolls; FitBit data solve a murder. The list goes on. *Exercise is everywhere.*

Except when it's not. As pressure to exercise has ratcheted it up to a moral imperative—while also fueling a $37 billion industry—so too have free or subsidized fitness options failed to keep up. "Fitness" is a slippery concept, but it is hard to deny that the United States is far from physically fit, by any number of measures: only 20 percent of Americans work out consistently, over half of gym members barely use their expensive facilities, and fewer than three out of ten high school students get sixty minutes of exercise a day. Socioeconomic status only intensifies this phenomenon. Eighty percent of Americans live in a "fitness desert," defined as an area without a public park in a half-mile radius. Physical education is often summarily cut from under-resourced schools or taught by an educator without specialized training, yet the field has become so anemic that schools struggle to find physical educators for the few positions that do exist. Even as the United States remains so much the locus of global commercial fitness that Parisian exercise studios market "New York City bootcamps" and "California bodies," this country attracts international attention for its relentlessly rising obesity rates, which are especially pronounced among the poor and people of color. Social critics rightly reject the moral panic over the "obesity epidemic" as driven by fat hatred trussed up as genuine health concerns—especially in perpetuating the idea that fat people are always unfit and that obesity is always the underlying cause of ill health—but it is worth asking whether Americans have the freedom, flexibility, and safe physical spaces to be active in the ways they would choose. The pandemic has worsened the situation, as economic insecurity and the enforced sedentariness of quarantines has made regular exercise an even greater rarity among those with less autonomy over their time and space, and by extension, their bodies.

By contrast, exercise signifies affluence. Gyms—especially in their "boutique studio" form, a super-luxury twenty-first-century invention that was the industry's fastest-growing segment before the pandemic, and that even since has continued to attract private equity investment and spawn IPOs—cluster in wealthy neighborhoods. Many white-collar employees enjoy workplace wellness programs, health-club memberships subsidized by private insurance, and enough control over their work schedules to be able to incorporate exercise into their day. Fitness has become not only a physical pursuit but a ubiquitous accoutrement of an "aspirational lifestyle" promoted by celebrities, online influencers, and the everyday people who emulate them on social media: glistening selfies taken after a waitlist-only spin class, destination marathons, expensive athleisure clothing, a $2,500 stationary bike, or a "fitness concierge" who will plan, book, and accompany you to your workout, actual exercise instruction sold separately.

Money and motivation are necessary but not sufficient for full participation in what I style the "fit nation"; how a person's body is perceived can lock or unlock social benefits and more. One self-described fat, Black, queer woman who is an experienced runner described the patronizing "encouragement" she regularly endures when people in fitness contexts wrongly assume, due to her looks, that she is "just getting started." Wearing pricey technical gear or a T-shirt from a prestigious college, she and other people of color have found, can temper the condescension that greets a body assumed to be an outsider to gyms, race expos, or fitness studios. "The sports bra," a Nike designer gushed to me, "is the new T-shirt," a trend that not only telegraphs a wearer's constant readiness to hit the gym, but also presumes the confidence and desire to display arms and abdominals in a world that harshly judges big bodies. Whiteness and leanness aren't always enough: one writer traded triathlons for lifting and realized that his friends and even his wife were vaguely disgusted by his bulging muscles; members of his professional class were supposed to look like wiry endurance athletes, not hulking laborers.

Despite—or because of—greater attention to inequality, fitness has become a socially acceptable form of conspicuous consumption in a society that celebrates the pursuit of health as practically holy, but not quite enough to make it a public good. This book explains how we arrived here. Over more than a century, activists, entrepreneurs, educators, policymakers, and individuals have created, participated in, and resisted the "fit nation": a society in which exercise infiltrates practically every quarter of American life—in both problematic and promising ways—but in which full, autonomous participation depends on spending power rather than citizenship.

It wasn't always like this. This story of how exercise went from being a peculiar pursuit of the few to a universal preoccupation begins on the stage of the 1893 Chicago World's Fair, where strongman Eugen Sandow preened and flexed, at a time when sculpted muscles and exhibitionism made strongmen and -women "freaks" and even sexual deviants: who else would spend so much time working on their body and immodestly displaying it? But over time, these strongmen and women sold the idea of exercise as a virtuous form of self-discipline, available to anyone willing to send away for a free pamphlet and to do the work it prescribed. Complemented by a generation of physical educators who sought to fortify cerebral university students and office workers—and to discipline the unruly bodies of immigrants and nonwhite minorities—exercise was becoming an everyday activity. By the early 1950s, on Santa Monica's Muscle Beach, crowds of tourists did more than gaze at suntanned acrobats and weight lifters; they began to seriously entertain the idea that exercise might not be the stuff of sideshows, but an activity they might, even *should*, pursue.

It was a White Plains homemaker named Bonnie Prudden, not a strapping bodybuilder, who first sounded the alarm that American children displayed a disturbing lack of fitness, to the peril of the nation. Prudden and others argued that economic abundance was making Americans lazy and weak, too reliant on "push-button luxuries" and the easy, car-and-television-centric life of the suburbs. A generation of white middle-class children was growing up ill equipped to fight should the Cold War get hot, their flabby bodies hardly advertising the supremacy of the American way of life. President Dwight Eisenhower established the Presidential Council on Youth Fitness to take on this issue as one of military preparedness. His handsome, youthful successor, John F. Kennedy, however, proved a better poster boy for exercise, and he amplified Eisenhower's condemnation of corporeally and intellectually "soft Americans" as a national security threat. Unlike Eisenhower, though, he presented fitness as fun, even glamorous, and for everyone.

Such federal efforts at "slimming the soft American" through partnerships with local agencies, celebrities, athletes, and industry powerfully instilled the idea that exercise was a positive, even moral, act. Yet though neither the federal government nor local agencies ever invested sufficiently in infrastructure and antipoverty policies to support this goal, the programs they did support brought about a huge shift in sensibility: transforming the pursuit of physical fitness from a suspicious pastime of narcissistic deviants to a requirement of self-fulfillment and civic life. A generation of exercise entrepreneurs—many hailing from Muscle Beach—profitably commodified this positive new image of exercise, spreading it far and wide through the first chain gyms that sought a clientele beyond male weight lifters and bodybuilders. A far cry from dank weight rooms, many new facilities further sanitized the image of exercise by linking it with affluence, beauty, and science, enticing women and families to join "palaces" with bowling alleys, wall-to-wall carpet, tropical fish tanks, spas, and state-of-the-art equipment.

Of course, many Americans could not afford private memberships, failed the Presidential Fitness Challenge, or outright rejected the Cold War conformism and materialism that was at the heart of both these projects. They too built the fit nation, even as they seemed to be outside it. A surprisingly wide range of people came to embrace two powerfully interlocking ideas:

- One: body and mind are inseparably connected.
- Two: proactively pursuing health is a personal right and responsibility.

In school gyms and health clubs, but also on jogging paths, at yoga retreats, and in activist health centers in the 1970s, these assumptions were embraced and reimagined by groups who were anything but Cold Warriors or striving business owners: environmentalist joggers, yogi seekers, feminist self-defense advocates, and Black Panther martial artists, to name a few. Especially as scientists made clear that exercise could include "aerobics"—what we now call "cardio"—the opportunities for participation only grew. Many of these people did not think of themselves as athletes, but they redefined what exercise meant and who deserved to be physically fit. Exercise, these diverse actors proved, could unmake, rather than uphold, social, political, and cultural orthodoxies about strength, health, beauty, and power.

Not everyone who flexed this new power understood fitness as political. The founder of Jazzercise, for example, specifically distinguished the women in her studio classes from those taking to the streets to protest for equal pay and reproductive rights. A new generation of joggers were as likely to sing the praises of competition and self-discipline as those of communing with nature or achieving a natural high. Bodily autonomy and self-determination were rallying cries of the Left, but they dovetailed surprisingly elegantly with a conservative worldview that prized individualism and personal responsibility. These ideologies together cemented fitness as a priority that transcended politics. By the 1980s, Americans of all political stripes agreed that regular exercise was crucial to a healthy self and society. Feminist Gloria Steinem gushed in 1982 that the locker room after aerobics class engendered a rare environment in which nude female bodies were free from objectification, while gay men saw gyms and studios as "third places" that served as activist centers or just escapist oases. Yet President Ronald Reagan, who reviled feminism and for years refused to acknowledge the AIDS epidemic, posed on a Nautilus machine in 1982, also extolling the virtues of exercise.

Another new consensus was forming, too: that the private sector was the most vital place to pursue fitness, rather than public gymnasiums, recreation centers, or running trails. Indeed, the thinking held, an emphasis on individual empowerment superseded the goal of collective solidarity. A broader climate of austerity that slashed spending on social services only confirmed the sense that private industry offered endless opportunity that the public sector lacked, especially in body-conscious coastal cities and affluent suburbs.

The underlying ideas of the fit nation—that capacity of mind and body are enmeshed, and that individuals have a right and responsibility to exercise—were widely accepted by the final decade of the twentieth century. No space was more powerful in crystalizing these core tenets than yoga classes. While much of the yoga commentariat bemoaned how sacred spiritual traditions had become commercialized and instrumentalized to achieve the sinewy "yoga body" Madonna showed off on late-night TV, yoga just as powerfully reshaped fitness culture too. At the heart of yoga classes was a lofty idiom of enlightenment, imparted by a "guru" figure who made exercise about "something more" than bodily cultivation. This sensibility elevated the experience of exercise and affirmed its importance in people's daily schedules and sense of themselves. Cultivating the body was increasingly understood as a way to achieve "self-esteem" and reduce "stress," buzzwords heard in middle schools and on morning shows. A new focus on "multiculturalism" was equally ubiquitous, easing the mainstream embrace of this Eastern practice and its offshoots, as well as a range of new exercise formats and media that began to challenge the notion that the ideal exerciser was white and slim, and that unapologetic strength was only appropriate for men. These developments were all generally considered culturally liberal, but none of them challenged the notion that self-mastery is the engine of social progress.

It truly began to feel as if a growing swath of Americans could realize their bodily potential and self-worth through exercise. But as the gym rose in collective cultural esteem and apparent accessibility, it became even more ingrained as a consumer product. The "personal trainer" and its elite version, the "celebrity trainer"—a title ambiguously describing both professional and client—were born in these years, normalizing ever more expensive ways to exercise. Home gyms built the commitment to fitness right into the walls of a home, and the trainers who worked in them occupied a newly intimate realm of clients' lives. Entrepreneurs and corporate interests quickly monetized this enthusiasm: branding yoga studios, launching a spate of glossy fitness magazines, and invigorating the new "athleisure" apparel category that defined expensive exercise wear as fashionable.

By the turn of the twenty-first century, the idea that exercise was imperative had become an article of faith. Fitness boosterism was bipartisan: "I'm serious about exercising, and you should be too," Republican president George W. Bush implored the American people in 2002. Six years later, Democratic first lady Michelle Obama launched "Let's Move," a campaign to encourage exercise among working-class people of color. In these years, three seismic events fractured faith in American political, cultural, and economic ascendancy but only served to consolidate the fit nation: the September 11 attacks, the 2008 financial crisis, and the coronavirus pandemic. In the wake of 9/11, yoga and programs that emphasized "the mind-body connection" boomed as many Americans exhibited a growing interest (and willingness to spend) on healing and "wellness." In a very different way, CrossFit and its HTFU ("harden the f*ck up") ethos, inspired by military and law-enforcement workouts, surged in popularity. The Great Recession that began in 2008 clarified how deeply embedded the ideas of the fit nation as both high-end luxury and human right have become. Among the affluent, "boutique fitness" boomed. But the founders of Latin-dance format Zumba, more likely to be found in community centers or inexpensive gyms, were shocked that their enrollments also shot up. The Obamas again made exercise an presidential priority.

The pandemic dealt the fitness industry a body blow, as nearly a quarter of gyms permanently closed. But the fit nation morphed to digital platforms, tricked-out home-exercise setups, and even public spaces. Thanks to social media, the performance of fitness has persisted almost seamlessly, even as many exercised in solitude at home. Despite doomsday predictions, people are now returning to the gym nearly in pre-Covid numbers. Enthusiasm for fitness was sufficiently strong to endure a pandemic, but so too were its fundamental inequalities, as lower-income people who tended to live in smaller, more crowded homes, and to have less access to public recreation spaces, struggled even more mightily to be physically active on their own terms (i.e., outside any physical labor required by their work).

The exercise ideal has become as ambient as the air we breathe but has long had plenty of detractors. Some critics attack specific programs: yoga is pagan, aerobics is anti-feminist, CrossFit is a cult that can debilitate you. But most take issue with the broader social implications of the obsession with exercise. In 1979, historian Christopher Lasch condemned the "culture of narcissism" that defined the age, and pointed his finger squarely at recreational, inclusive fitness that represented a "degradation of sport." A few years later, a cadre of doctors cautioned that although "exercise is sold as the prime panacea of our time . . . almost nothing you have been told about the benefits of exercise is true." (They believed working out was more likely to cause than to prevent heart failure.) In 1987, sociologist Margaret Morse was just as unsparing in her criticism of aerobics videos, which she argued promoted "passive sexuality," isolation, and unattainable beauty standards. Such naysaying had negligible effect on the breakneck growth of the industry, but it did make it all the more difficult for public programs to garner sorely needed support.

Today, most endorse the *idea* of regular exercise even if they fail to engage in it themselves. With the exception of President Donald Trump, who proudly disdained working out as unhealthy, committed dissidents of the fit nation are mostly concentrated in a commentariat disgusted with the "neoliberalism"—market-based ideology that "responsibilizes" individuals to solve structural problems—that has crept even into the intimate realm of the body.[1] "Wellness" and "self-care" may sound like liberation, the argument goes, but they dangerously overemphasize the individual at the expense of the collective. Expecting individuals to improve their health through exercise dangerously sidesteps how issues such as residential segregation, disinvestment in public schools and safe streets, and lack of access to healthful food, all intensify inequality, in fitness and at large. Exercise itself is problematic, social critic Mark Greif argued: the gym is an internalized industrial factory in which narcissists sweat and grunt in a dehumanizing ritual to stave off fat and age. The more expansive "wellness" is a self-serving ideology that lets the fit and privileged feel smugly superior to "the fat unemployed single mother" left to "internalize a sense of worthlessness," Carl Cederström, a CrossFitter himself, opines. The "age of fitness," Jürgen Martschukat writes, feeds the illusion of individual freedom.[2] This book takes seriously those structural critiques but resists their all-encompassing pessimism, which ignores the people who have found genuine empowerment through fitness, by design or otherwise.[3]

So is the rise of the fit nation a story of progress? It is certainly one of expansion. Reams of research and innumerable anecdotes make it incontrovertible that exercise abets many undeniably positive experiences: strong academic outcomes, healthy pregnancy, and longevity, to name just a few. Exercise is the closest thing we have to a "miracle cure," the Academy of Medical Royal Colleges pronounced in 2015. When some critics called that claim hyperbolic, the Academy restated it only slightly less effusively: "Exercise is the best buy for public health." Widespread acknowledgment of fitness as a worthwhile, and even fundamental, pursuit has itself often been a force for positive change over time. Today, many believe health and well-being are a human right, bodily autonomy is recognized as important, and aesthetic ideals are more expansive than ever before. Fitness culture has challenged damaging assumptions about and created opportunities for the women, LGBTQ+ communities, and minorities who have been influential in shaping this field even as it simultaneously marginalized them. The options for exercise are a world away from the one-size-fits-all rope-climbing contests of the Kennedy era, or from the gleaming fitness clubs that only welcomed the already apparently young and fit: adaptive fitness studios, LGBTQ+ CrossFit boxes, Zumba for Orthodox Jews, and "broga" (yoga for men) all now exist. Yet the fit nation can also be oppressive, creating new anxieties and inequalities around wealth, size, and ability at work, the dressing room, school, and of course, the gym. The pressure to constantly contemplate our bodies has become inescapable, in a cheery green poster on my campus instructing us to "burn calories, not electricity, and take the stairs"; in the fashion trend of tight-fitting yoga pants as revealing as Spanx; and in the employer-supplied Fitbits used for colleagues now expected to perform not only in the office, but also on steps and sleep.

In so many ways, the fit nation is not "working out," in any sense. Fitness has morphed from a possibly suspicious physical activity to a pervasive ideal laced into our daily rituals, or at least aspirations, for better, healthier, and happier lives. Far more Americans than the fraction of the population who exercises regularly have thus come to understand dutiful physical activity as their right and responsibility. Some version of "I'm so awful, I don't exercise enough" has been the most common response when people learn I have been writing a book about fitness: an unsolicited, self-flagellating confession only legible in a society where exercise is understood as a moral act. (The next most common reactions are long, vivid descriptions of the traumatizing experience of physical education, or of a current training routine.) This largely unquestioned ideal bestows moral superiority on those who can afford, or who choose, to participate in a largely pay-to-play fitness culture, and it has hardly guaranteed—and even jeopardized—the imperative public investment that might *truly* make America a fit nation. In service of achieving a more just future in which kids like Vincent Gonzalez need not sneak into private gyms, this book explains how the pursuit of fitness—defined in different ways at different historical moments—has simultaneously become a universal ideal and a stark dividing line in a society where exercise can be at once empowering and oppressive, inescapable and unavailable. It could have worked out differently. Perhaps it still can.

Part **One**

WHEN SWEATING WAS STRANGE

I am not a freak of nature.
KATIE SANDWINA, 1911[1]

His defined muscles carefully powdered to more closely resemble the Italian statues that inspired him as a formerly "pale, frail, and delicate" boy, Eugen Sandow perched atop a black velvet box in scanty silk shorts. Posing and preening before awestruck nightly audiences that approached six thousand, the Prussian-born strongman reveled in the enthusiasm of his relatively uninhibited American hosts at the 1893 World's Fair. Especially the women, who lined up to run their gloved hands over his flexed physique. Timid at first, the society ladies who scheduled private viewings with Sandow swooned at his winking invitation to "come feel how hard these muscles are," and were reportedly reduced to "nervous trembling" and even fainting spells upon touching his rippling body.[2]

Promoted as "The World's Most Perfect Man" by famous showman Florenz Ziegfeld, Sandow indeed presented a spectacle for the nearly twenty-six million visitors who streamed through the neoclassical Great White City constructed in fin-de-siècle Chicago. Through the summer and fall of 1893, fairgoers from all over the country gaped at eye-popping installations that showcased the extremes of human capacity. There was the first, 264-foot Ferris wheel; the life-size reproductions of Christopher Columbus's *Nina, Pinta*, and *Santa Maria* ships; the displays of exotic cultures from tens of foreign countries. "Tall, slim, great, little Ziegfeld," as Sandow remembered his indefatigable promoter, had at first booked an esteemed but emotionless German symphony orchestra that failed to impress the throngs seeking intense, sensory attractions. The strongman, however, sold out every seat in the house. Like the Fair's most popular attractions, Sandow inspired a collective awe that appealed across class lines in a moment of socioeconomic strife. Ogling at Sandow's sculpted physique, to Ziegfeld and Sandow's good fortune, proved a universally appealing escape people were willing to pay for.

The spectacle of a strong body flexing onstage was so arresting because the intense physical cultivation it took to arrive at this moment of proud display—and the performance itself—was still sufficiently strange to be a stage attraction. Regular exercise, especially for aesthetic aims, was uncommon for most men and women, who associated girth and leisure with enviable abundance. Weight lifting was so unheard-of, it was only beginning to be integrated into military training regimes.[3] But all that was about to change. Thanks to the efforts of strongmen and women and their entrepreneurial peers, physical educators, the federal government, and the beauty industry, the deliberate pursuit of fitness would start to shed its distant, suspicious cast to become an arena for participation, rather than performance, in American life. But it would take half a century of sweat to get there.

1

Performing Civilization

Exercise was of course no turn-of-the-century invention. The popularity of strength acts in the late nineteenth and early twentieth centuries arose from a growing interest in exercise among everyday people in an industrializing world, but those classical statues that so inspired Sandow and his contemporaries hearkened from a historical moment when developing bodily strength, at least for men, was considered a worthy, and ennobling, pursuit for the self and civic sphere. Daniel Kunitz imagined the physical culture of antiquity as a kind of classical CrossFit; "you don't imagine a physique" like those represented in Greek statuary, he wrote, but "you encounter a hundred versions in the *gymnasium* while watching men wrestle, sprint, lift heavy stones, jump, and do other basic functional movements that build such a lean and well-cut body."[1]

The evidentiary record is clearer in the antebellum United States, when the few boosters of regular exercise were physicians, educators, and social reformers who imported their ideas from Europeans inspired by antiquity. But even those who advocated for "sailing, swinging, and riding in carriages or on horseback" in addition to walking, as salutary forms of exertion, recommended these activities primarily because they brought people from indoors and out of growing cities "forth into the fields" and the "open air."[2] Except for very young children, exercise itself to promote health and beauty was nowhere near as popular as strategies to increase ventilation and prevent "bad air" illnesses like "colds, coughs, and consumption."[3]

A wave of German immigration after the country's 1848 revolution prompted a brief romance with gymnastics and calisthenics, especially among American educators who substantially modified the more "violent" European forms to suit girls' delicate constitutions. They applauded how easily these programs could be completed not only at school but at home, making it more likely participants would form consistent habits that also helped them avoid idleness. Black women physical educators challenged prevailing assumptions that their bodies were built for labor, and emphasized how exercise could be a form of leisure and care.[4] Exercising gently at home also allowed women to escape both the perceived obstacle of their own biological weakness and the dangers of the public sphere. Explaining why white southern women rode horses "only occasionally" as compared to men, despite the salutary effects of a jaunt in the healthy air, for example, a 1931 history of American sport reasoned that this was "because the carriage with its negro coachman was so omnipresent."[5] Indoor exercise presented no such dangers.

Serving God could be one effect of exercise, claimed Protestants who were some of the earliest American exercise enthusiasts, linking a consistent commitment to even gentle calisthenics with a virtuous sensibility that disciplined the flesh more generally. The appearance of the body was understood to be an outward expression of inner spiritual character, so physical exercise was a harbinger of not just health, but morality.[6] This outlook melded well with a secular scientific establishment that embraced phrenology, the idea that one's intelligence was discernible by the shape of one's skull. By the late nineteenth century, "Muscular Christianity" connecting morality, masculinity, and muscles had attained real cultural currency. President Theodore Roosevelt famously linked "the strenuous life" with national strength, ideas to which he was first introduced by his Protestant parents while a sickly child, not robust enough to enact these athletic ideals but apparently readily absorbing the ideology.[7]

But most Americans were resistant to the militarism and rigor of the German programs, and even a calisthenics advocate such as *Godey's Lady's Book* editor Sarah Josepha Hale tempered her endorsement by cautioning readers that "exercise of this sort should never be insisted on once they grow irksome." The limits of enthusiasm for exercise were clear in Massachusetts, home to the country's most elaborate antebellum school system, where in 1842, only 416 children were enrolled in health classes as compared to ten thousand in United States history, two thousand in algebra, and fifteen hundred in bookkeeping.[8] Absent a major sensibility—or policy—shift, regular exercise would remain a preoccupation of the few.

But it didn't. Ironically, an important first step in this process of popularization was to present physical exercise as the *opposite* of a great equalizer. Intentionally cultivating one's strength, Sandow argued, separated men like him from savages. Or so he hoped, given how emphatically he belabored this point with one outlandish anecdote after another, from describing the tailored finery he fancied offstage to the aristocrats who attended his shows and lavished him with luxurious gifts. No story made this distinction between the civilized cultivation of strength and unrefined brute force clearer than a trip Sandow took through Germany, in the course of which he met Karl Westphal, a hulking quarryman with a head "so huge and grotesque as that of any pantomime mask, and a nose as big as [Sandow's] fist." The man's own fists were three times the size of Sandow's, and his boots so enormous that the enterprising and comparatively agile strongman hopped inside one with both feet and "turned entirely round inside." Keenly entrepreneurial, Sandow sensed opportunity in this chance meeting. He hired this man, dubbed him Goliath, and excitedly began planning his career as a strongman in England. Sandow grew even more thrilled about the fortunes that awaited them when he paraded "Goliath" from Charing Cross to Piccadilly after his meaty limbs proved too large to fit into a cab, and thousands of Londoners abandoned their midday work to gape at a sight Sandow could compare only to spotting a "white elephant."[9]

The animal analogy is telling. Before long, Sandow was sorely disappointed with the obtuseness of his would-be protégé. Westphal could hoist enormous loads, but having never deliberately trained his muscles, could do little else, and demonstrated little interest in learning the stunts Sandow knew would please a paying crowd. After seven fruitless weeks under Sandow's tutelage, Westphal had made no progress toward refining his technique, due, Sandow believed, to his idleness. Westphal's apathy may have been despondency due to Sandow's keeping "this rare creature" in captivity, unwilling to let this adult man roam the streets unchaperoned. Ultimately, the two parted ways, but not before they performed together one last time, in a number choreographed by Sandow that unsurprisingly cast Westphal as a hapless lout bested by the more intellectually and corporeally superior Sandow. The show began with Goliath intimidating Sandow but concluded with the relatively slight Sandow lifting Westphal with one hand before dragging him off the stage. The lesson Sandow imparted onstage that night and later in his memoir was that a "strongman" who deliberately trains his body as a form of self-improvement has little in common with a mere "breaker of stones . . . who uses his muscles to earn his daily bread."[10] True strength, he averred, is intentional, impossible without mental acuity, and always trumps brute force.

Sandow took this message across the Atlantic. When he docked in New York Harbor on a blazing hot day on his way to the World's Fair, he immediately found the more socioeconomically fluid and racially diverse United States—"that great country of wonderful records"—a new arena to prove not only his carefully cultivated physical strength, but also the cultural and moral superiority he believed it conferred.[11] It took less than an hour on American shores for Sandow to find his first contest, not on a stage but in the sixteenth-floor stairwell of a Manhattan hotel. After his first-ever elevator ride, Sandow found himself alone with a Black bellhop, a notable circumstance made more so when the man audaciously rolled and lit a cigarette, and took a deep, exaggerated drag right there in Sandow's handsomely appointed quarters. Sandow instructed the bellhop, to whom he referred with a now unprintable slur, to shine his shoes.

"We don't do that in America," replied the bellhop matter-of-factly. Sandow recoiled, unsure he understood correctly. Resolving any confusion but escalating the conflict, the bellhop lit another

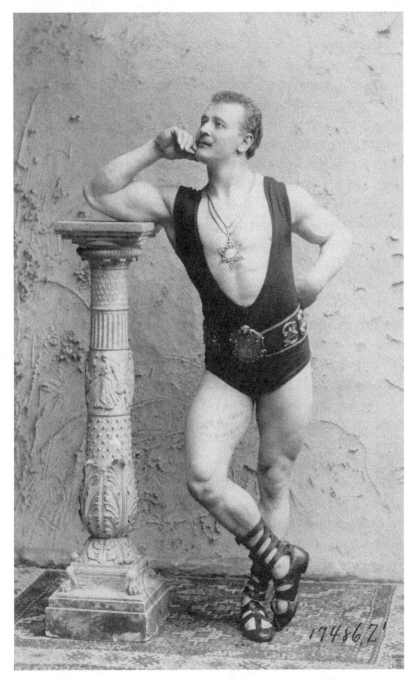

Figure 1. B. J. Falk, *Eugen Sandow, Full-Length Portrait, Standing, Leaning on Column, Facing Left, Wearing Wrestling Leotard, Roman Sandals, and Six Pointed Star Pendant*, ca. 1894. Strongman Eugen Sandow poses in gladiator sandals and a bejeweled belt, standing on an intricately designed rug and leaning on a classical column, a setting designed to present him as civilized rather than as a "mere breaker of stones."

cigarette and sprawled on Sandow's sofa. With a smile, he elaborated: "We (speaking of course for himself and [others] like him) don't clean boots here." In Sandow's esteem, this impudence was "too much for white flesh and blood to bear." He threatened to report the "boy" to the manager, and the bellhop "squared up" for a fight. Enraged, Sandow grabbed him by the lapels and dangled him over the sixteenth-floor banister, "just to give him a view of the depth, which was so tremendous." The "shouts and screams" of the terrified bellhop rang out so loudly that a small crowd gathered. Yet Sandow assures his reader that thanks to his own restraint—he says he had subtly checked that the bellhop's jacket could withstand the strain—tragedy was averted. Once Sandow was satisfied the bellhop would not again challenge European superiority, he pulled him back over the railing and released him unscathed. Sandow warned the shaken man that "if he attempted his impertinences again" he would enjoy no such mercy.[12]

Sandow could have clocked the bellhop in the face, but consciously cultivating strength and wielding it with control was key to how Sandow distinguished himself from, and exercised power over, the louts he so disdained. African Americans, for example, were widely stereotyped as almost superhuman in their strength, but also in their uncontrolled appetites and impulses. In emphasizing that he had developed his strength for self-improvement, and to a lesser extent for looks, rather than as a form of labor; in resisting the urge to let the bellhop plummet to his death; and also in abstaining from most alcohol and tobacco, Sandow linked the cultivation of strength to an enviable capacity for discipline. This was fitness for white civilization.

Such early strongmen are often remembered as the pioneers of contemporary American fitness culture, and in some ways they certainly laid the foundation for the twenty-first-century understanding of exercise as a pursuit of the affluent, disciplined, and attractive. Throughout colorful careers that stretched into the post–World War II era, Sandow and his telegenic, entrepreneurial peers such as Bernarr MacFadden and Charles Atlas spread these ideas through shows, magazines, and consumer products that first displayed fit bodies and later instructed how to achieve them. MacFadden had spotted Sandow at the World's Fair because he had set up shop to sell his own "exerciser" device—akin to today's resistance bands—nearby. But the similarities end there. In this era, most Americans considered the deliberate pursuit of fitness a spectacle to see onstage, rather than an activity in which to engage their own bodies. Crowds lined up to ogle at these strapping exemplars, but it would be decades before any significant proportion of the public would aspire to lift, or look, like them. Indeed, Sandow likely boasts so proudly of his proximity to European aristocrats—and affluent Americans bearing lavish gifts—*because* most strongmen were more likely to be featured alongside bearded ladies and Siamese twins at seedy carnivals and circuses from which Sandow endeavored to distance himself. MacFadden was less successful at avoiding such associations. In 1905, just as the doors to his second annual Physical Culture Exhibition were about to open at Madison Square Garden, the police, summoned by anti-obscenity crusader Anthony Comstock, blocked the doors and tried to turn the crowds away from what he had categorized as an indecent performance. Though the 1904 competition had featured men and women posing onstage in the style of classical statues, such "carnality" was indecent, Comstock and other skeptics insisted.

Just over the bridge in Brooklyn, another European-born strongman was attempting to make his way in America. Born Angelo Siciliano in Calabria, Italy, the scrawny immigrant boy who became Charles Atlas was so bowled over by the beauty of the classical sculptures of Hercules, Apollo, and Zeus at the Brooklyn Museum, he decided he wanted to look like them. In his own telling, young Angelo began lifting weights, and found a job as a sideshow strongman, lying on a bed of nails and daring passersby to walk across his chest. In between shifts, he spent his days flexing on the Coney Island boardwalk in hope of getting noticed for bigger, paying gigs. Those dreams came true when a passing artist spotted him in 1916 and quickly booked him for nude and semi-nude sessions posing for downtown sculptors and painters who reimagined historical figures with Atlas's strapping physique. Before long, New York City statues of the Founding Fathers bore the familiar faces of George Washington and Alexander Hamilton but atop bodies modeled on Atlas's. Subtly, pedestrians strolling through Washington Square Park or Washington, DC, would see a physically fit form attached to the most esteemed Americans, a decidedly different association than that of seeing such a body in a sideshow.[13] Atlas soon broke into another echelon of fame, posing in MacFadden's *Physical Culture* magazine and in 1922 being declared "The World's Most Perfectly Developed Man" by a panel of doctors and artists who analyzed his musculature before a packed Madison Square Garden. Though no longer banned as pornographic, fit bodies were bizarre, extraordinary, entities to be placed on pedestals, rather than emulated by everyday people.

If this fascination with strongmen seems more respectful than rank voyeurism, the experiences of the far fewer strongwomen of the era make crystal clear the limits of such fandom. "Lady Hercules" Katie Brumbach, who later changed her name to "The Great Sandwina" when in 1902 she bested Sandow by single-handedly raising three hundred pounds above her head (he could only reach his chest), is a case in point. Born into a Prussian circus family, Sandwina performed feats of strength as a toddler, and at her father's behest, began taking on wrestling challenges for a price. At the conclusion of one particularly feisty match, she locked eyes with Max Heymann, the slim man she had just pinned to the floor, and they fell in love. The couple immigrated to the United States and struggled to find an audience, performing with tiny vaudeville troupes in small cities like Syracuse and Newport before returning to Europe to try their luck in France and Germany.[14] In 1907, Sandwina got the big break she had been hoping for: circus impresario John Ringling recruited the troupe to join his circus in America, where he knew the public would thrill at a member of the "weaker sex" tossing around her husband and other men half her size.

Sandwina became Ringling's main attraction, performing feats such as hoisting a 1200-pound cannon across her shoulders or letting multiple men lie on a bridge built across her torso. At Ringling's behest, Sandwina stood for a public examination by a dozen doctors under the spotlights in Madison Square Garden, as Atlas would several years later. This spectacle established the bizarre space she occupied in the press as both a superhuman specimen and an ideal type. "In every way, according to her measurements," concluded Dr. Peter Andersen, "she is a perfect woman by all accepted standards."[15] Such glowing estimations abounded. This perfect woman, however, was subjected to analysis of her appearance so intense, and perpetual surprise that a large, muscular woman could be anything but hideous, that much of the praise is better understood as fetishism.

"As she swings gracefully into the arena on supple, slender, silk encased-limbs," one typical profile rhapsodized, "your vision seems to dilate a bit, your eyes adjust to the magnified but perfect womanly proportions and she is more like a new and shining statue of an heroic Venus than the antique knotted and gnarled God of strength."[16] Ostensibly, readers expected a woman who could bend steel bars to be grotesque and even monstrous. Journalist Kate Carew assured readers that Sandwina's arms exhibited "no horrid lumps of muscle, dears—just a little ripple under the skin like mice playing in a mattress."[17] As positive as such descriptions might have been intended, the abundance of nonhuman analogies to describe "the titaness" and her extraordinary body—mice, but also the Sphinx, and panthers, even from a woman journalist who reluctantly made "yet another comparison" of her own sex to "the cat tribe"—highlighted the strangeness of a strong woman. At the same time, the working-class women who participated in the exhibition-boxing subculture inspired no such wonder, and were either ignored or treated like "physical freaks and sexual objects." Historian Wendy L. Rouse noted that journalists always remarked on boxer Gussie Freeman's substantial frame of five feet, ten inches and 180 pounds, for example, but cited these dimensions as evidence for why no man had ever kissed her despite Freeman's wishes to be "more like a woman."[18] By making Sandwina an exception to the rule that muscular women must be unattractively masculine, such glowing characterizations left the dehumanization of other muscular women, and dominant beauty standards, unchallenged.[19]

The acts the "Iron Queen" (among other sobriquets she inspired) performed over the nearly half century she traveled with Barnum and Bailey allowed men and women alike to project their anxieties and fantasies onto Sandwina.[20] The "giantess" would spin her husband around in the air, and scoop him up, along with and like one of their children, on one powerful arm. The topsy-turviness of this spectacle sent crowds speculating in hushed tones about what the Sandwinas' sex life was like, but also sparked fantasies about the larger world. Would a world with women's suffrage, a pressing political issue of the day, mean a society full of Sandwinas, with all men subject to women's mercy? To some women, this was a dream: "If only all women were Sandwinas!" proclaimed the caption of a series of cartoons in which primly appointed ladies spanked their husbands over their knees and gallantly stood on the train so the weaker sex—men—could take a seat. The journalist expressly made the connection to the political debates: "Certainly, if we were all strong as Sandwina, there would be an end to that ancient, reliable, very tiresome argument of the anti-suffragists that women should not have the right to vote because they cannot defend that right, serving on the army, the police force, and all that."[21] To some men who cherished the social order, of course, Sandwina represented a threat.

As much as her physical stature and stunts challenged assumptions about female frailty, Sandwina at times labored to reassure audiences of her normalcy. She often posed in over-the-top frills and ruffles thronged by tuxedoed men, as if to emphasize that her solid, muscular body made her no less a lady. The same *St. Louis Dispatch* journalist who fantasized about an electorate of newly enfranchised women was disappointed to learn of Sandwina's utterly conventional ideas about homemaking. Sandwina delighted in domestic work, and even looked down on "American haus fraus" who "cook too quickly and whose husbands eat too fast." Hardly the voice of the sisterhood this writer had hoped for, Sandwina declared that even though the popularity of her act kept her in the United States, she was unimpressed with the lack of industriousness of the women in her adopted nation: "I have to stay away from American women—They would drive me crazy." Indeed, in this interview, Sandwina barely spoke while her husband, on a break from being batted about by his wife before crowds of thousands, recounted how devoted she was: preparing nourishing homemade meals and doing the laundry daily because "she likes to." Speaking volumes with her silence, at least according to the increasingly crestfallen journalist, "Lady Hercules" only smiled sweetly as her husband hurled a barb at the suffragists and labor organizers fighting the dominant assumption that women didn't belong at the workplace or the polls: "My wife would never appear in public except as she does in her profession. She likes best the family life."[22]

Yet within a year, as the movement for women's suffrage intensified and Sandwina's celebrity grew, she dispensed with the pretense that she disapproved of women participating in public life. In March 1912, she joined a group of acrobats, contortionists, fire-eaters, and strongwomen in convening the inaugural meeting of the Barnum & Bailey Circus Women's Equal Rights Society. The performers had invited famous suffragist and labor lawyer Inez Milholland to Madison Square Garden to address the aspiring activists as they named a baby giraffe, but Milholland had already stood them up twice. Once it was confirmed the esteemed activist was en route to New Haven rather than the giraffe pen, a horseback performer and acrobat marched the few blocks north to the headquarters of the Women's Political Union to inquire if anyone was available to address their politically awakened colleagues. The union activists had no interest in these women whose "daily lot [was] to bound about, blithe and bespangled." Still, one member of the political union agreed to come to the Garden, but only condescended to the circus women, one of whom snatched the microphone away in disgust and announced that as wage earners, and, some of them, property owners, "[we] are not slaves!" Sandwina was elected vice president of the association during that spirited meeting, as her husband silently stood by, unlike the angry man who grabbed his "docile" wife and daughter away from the excited throng. The giraffe was dubbed Miss Suffrage (though he apparently became so agitated that "by nightfall he couldn't abide even the sight of a

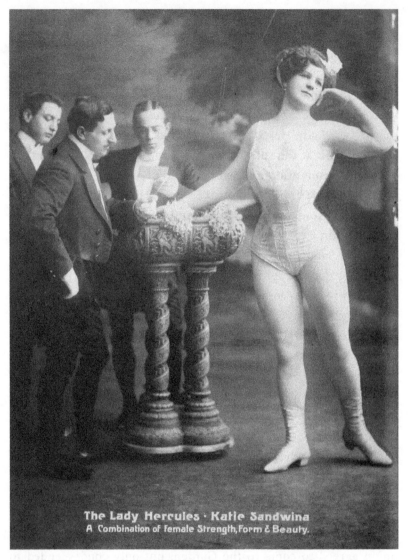

The Lady Hercules · Katie Sandwina
A Combination of Female Strength, Form & Beauty.

Figure 2. *Katie Sandwina, the Lady Hercules*, n.d. Strongwoman Katie Sandwina, known as "Lady Hercules," wears a lacy corseted costume and dainty pointed boots, while striking a graceful pose and modestly looking away from three formally dressed men over whom she towers. Strength and femininity, the scene suggests, can coexist.

suffragette") and Sandwina showed that she could deploy her fortitude to be more than a circus favorite.[23]

Sandwina benefited from, and helped encourage, a growing appreciation among physical culturists that "the frail, delicate, wax-doll standard of beauty in a woman is no longer in vogue," as declared one 1903 article in MacFadden's short-lived women's magazine *Beauty and Health*.[24] Sandwina's unconventional aesthetic made her very existence a challenge to gender norms. She may have been demure and deferential in the presence of her husband and children, but before she was married, in a 1910 interview, she spoke about sexual appetites usually unspeakable for respectable women: "What shall I say? Men are like air to me, you can't live without them. Every now and then I breathe good fresh air, you know."[25] Sandwina's legacy is undeniable, as scholar Patricia Vertinsky reflects, for women who have married strength training with self-possession "on the stage, in the circus, on the pages of advice books, outdoors, and in the gym, reveal a determination to change the order of things, to stare back at the objectifying gaze, refashion femininity, and add a voice to feminist struggles for equality and self-realization."[26]

Even from the vantage point of the nominally "body-positive" twenty-first century, the celebrations of this "Titaness"'s "perfect body" and "ideal form" reflect a surprisingly capacious concept of female beauty. These paeans to her beauty, however, upheld the idea that her aesthetic appeal resided not only in her perfect proportions, "just under a magnifying glass," but also in her whiteness. Hardly a positive article failed to commend her "Bavarian stock," an objective claim that then read as a compliment given that the prevailing racial taxonomy placed whites of Germanic and Nordic extraction atop a biologically determined hierarchy. In general, advocates of women developing their strength presumed that their "weakness" and "nervousness" stemmed from their sloth and slavish dedication to superficial fashion, as opposed to working on the body beneath such finery. *All* these afflictions, however, were thought to affect white, middle-class women whose relative affluence enabled them to lie about, becoming weak and lacing themselves into corsets. The majority of women, who had to work, were rarely even acknowledged in this context, except by contrast. MacFadden emphasized the "duty" of (white) women to train their bodies to achieve "superb womanhood," by contrasting them with "peasants" and "squaws" who were "naturally" much hardier.[27] (Notably, Sandow, who was born to Jewish parents but reportedly converted to Lutheranism, made little of his ethnicity.)

Scholar of physical culture Jan Todd, herself known as the strongest woman in the world for a time in the 1970s, compared the difference between newspaperman Franklin Fyles's description of Sandwina and his estimation of a Japanese tightrope walker who performed with her. Sandwina, of German extraction, was "positively the most commanding beauty I have seen in years . . . in heroic size," in contrast with "a chubby Jap girl with stubby legs, knotted and gnarled muscles, like an old-time ballet premiere's." Black women were almost entirely excluded from American circus labor, and Black men rarely worked onstage, and then only as cooks, waiters, and stable boys. Occasional sideshows like P. T. Barnum's "What Is It?" tent, in which they played "monkey-men," were an exception, since white performers in blackface were greater crowd-pleasers.[28] Echoing many others who evoked the classical era in portraying Sandwina, Fyles styled her a "Venus" who resembled an alabaster sculpture more than she did a human woman.[29] This exoticization is undeniable, but of an entirely different order from the simultaneous dehumanization of African Americans, as the tragic crash of one circus train crystallized. Tallying the fatalities from the destroyed car that had carried horses and Black laborers, the circus owner cruelly bemoaned the losses in the press: "Just think, fourteen of my best horses killed and every one of those darkies saved!"[30]

The case of Strongman Siegmund (to his Yiddish-speaking fans, Zishe) Breitbart, who incorporated his Judaism into his strength act, provides perspective on how such racialist thinking played out in this emerging fitness culture. Selling out shows in Central Europe, his adopted Brooklyn, and American cities from Buffalo to Baltimore, Breitbart bent iron bars into the shape of flowers, let automobiles run over his chest, hoisted a baby elephant up a ladder, and earned the name of "Superman" from his gentile fans; Jews hailed him as Samson. Breitbart invoked the classical ideal, posing as a Greek statue and presenting Roman gladiators as inspiration for Jewish strength. Unapologetic about his religion and race, he connected physical strength to Zionist liberation, aspiring to form an army of Jewish strength enthusiasts to reclaim Palestine.[31] Upper-class Jewish mothers wary of his brash physicality cautioned children "not to be a Breitbart," whereas working-class Jews less ambivalently fantasized about a world in which "a thousand Breitbarts were to arise among the Jews [and] the Jewish people would cease being persecuted."[32] Breitbart both assimilated to and challenged Germanic ideals of strength and beauty in proving a proud Jew could embody them. Building upon his renown and responding to the incipient appetite for mail-order exercise, in 1924 Breitbart launched a mail-order bodybuilding course. The mailing address was "Superman–New York."[33]

2

No More Fat Cats or
Ladies of Leisure

For decades, the regular, deliberate pursuit of exercise outside of organized sports was a marginal, and even suspicious pursuit, while a fat body was widely viewed as a positive sign of affluence.[1] While girth was at times used to signify laziness or lack of dignity, to be, or even look like, a "fat cat" or "lady of leisure" was to project enviable wealth and success.[2] As late as the 1880s, writes scholar Amy Farrell, "fatness was often linked to a generalized sense of prosperity, distinction, and high status. The corpulence itself was not represented as bad, but rather was a sign of how much the rich person had."[3]

Sure enough, gentlemen's clubs for fat men flourished until the 1920s. In 1904, the *Boston Globe* reported on a joyous, regular gathering of one such group founded the year before. The men packed Hale's Tavern "full of bulbous and overhanging abdomens and double chins tonight" while the locals, who ostensibly had less to eat and even less time to spare, were "mostly bony and angular, [staring] with envy at the portly forms and rubicund faces which have arrived on every train."[4] Even one 1870 article arguing *against* such associations was revealing in its critique. The men who paraded through New York City on a ninety-degree summer day on horseback were not objectionable because they were grotesque, but because they excluded those who were not blessed with such formidable physical frames, but who wanted to participate in their "sylvan retreat." Like the slim Julius Caesar, who wished to surround himself with fat men, the journalist wrote, "a well disposed fat man—and few fat men are other than kindly—can dispense happiness and jollity to a hundred of the less fortunate of his fellow-beings, and why should all these reservoirs of cheer be compacted together, in churlish if majestic isolation, while the comparatively fleshless outer world goes sorrowing on?"[5] Fatness, for a time, could be aspirational.

Another, very different, sylvan retreat and its comparatively chilly reception proves the point. When Bernarr MacFadden secured nineteen hundred acres of unspoiled land in Spotswood, New Jersey, to found a colony devoted to outdoor exercise and the consumption of natural foods, he imagined a space where his followers—about two hundred—could enjoy a healthy life free from "the saloon, drug store, tobacco shop, and other vices." But in 1905, this apparently modest, even moralistic proposition, inspired intense skepticism among neighboring towns. One problem was MacFadden's distaste for "style," as he called constricting women's fashion, hyperbolically writing that "it has murdered more women, caused more misery, more crime, and more degeneracy than all the wars in human history."[6] Due to this deeply held belief, the residents of Physical Culture City conducted their daily activities in unrestrictive clothing—women even wore shorts—and sometimes even ventured offsite in their bathing costumes. In the neighboring town of Helmetta, two such "girl bathers" were driven into the forest before anyone witnessed the "dangerous sight," but the indecency caused such an uproar that the authorities contemplated reviving a colonial-era statute that mandated the stocks as punishment for "indecorous dress."[7]

Quickly and somewhat ironically, given MacFadden's strict prohibitions on meat, drink, and other vices that would bring about "the moral undoing of man or woman," the outpost gained an inaccurate reputation as a haven for nudists and sexual impropriety, suggesting how strange MacFadden's commitment to a life centered around exercise was perceived to be. "Beefsteak Eaters Beat Vegetarians!" a 1907 *New York Times* headline read, gleefully pointing out that the Rutgers College football team, which subsisted on steak, had trounced the vegetarian Spotsville squad. The team had showed up to the recreational match in a "hay wagon, accompanied by a flock of pretty young girls in bloomers" studying under "MacFadden"—a surname apparently so familiar it required no introduction.[8] A decade later, saddled with debt due to his legal woes and stripped of his right to use the federal mail for having published a story on venereal disease, MacFadden was in dire financial straits. He sold, at a loss, several health-food restaurants he had opened nationwide, as well as the Spotswood compound, and soon after moved to England, though the courts continued to dog him—and the papers to mock his "so called Physical Culture City"—well into the 1920s.[9]

Even in the days when fatness was seen more favorably than today, being *too* fat still made one a laughingstock. In 1877, the *New York Times* mocked these socially maladjusted "auxiliary fat men" and their ill-begotten attempts at socializing as a function of the fact that "the fat man is a mystery to himself, and his vague gropings after his correct solution are shown by his practice of associating himself with other fat men in clubs, and performing herculean feats of public overeating." The *Times*, tongue-in-cheek, had found a cruel solution to make "life no longer a fat and foolish mockery." Grouped together six at a time, men of more than three hundred pounds could comprise an "auxiliary fat-men wave-motor" whose collective power would exceed that of a thousand horses and power ships to sail even on still days.[10] A century later, as the national fascination with jogging, yoga, and dance-exercise had solidly entrenched a slim, fit, ideal for men and women, the *New York Times* reminisced nostalgically about the days when "fat was in fashion"—mostly—rather than a blight to be burned off at the health club. A "hilly and lustrous landscape of flesh" had for centuries symbolized, in physical form, the "almost limitless possibilities of human mind and body."[11]

Industrialization began to change that. Cities attracted rural migrants and immigrants in unprecedented numbers, rendering the United States an urban nation by 1920. Modernization expanded access to food, transportation, and labor-saving technologies, increasing the number of sedentary desk jobs that would become a defining aspect of middle and upper-class identities. Gaining weight was no longer so difficult, and the social meaning of the fat body changed accordingly: by the 1920s, corpulence signaled an inability to resist a range of newly accessible pleasures rather than exclusive access to them. New Year's resolutions increasingly focused, as one 1922 *Los Angeles Times* headline declared, on "CARE OF THE BODY," which, for women, meant weight loss. "Making a hog of yourself," or even "swallowing a mouthful" within two hours of waking up, was as serious a betrayal of the Christmas spirit as greed or flashy gift-giving, one column aimed at women sternly advised. Though "thin was in," according to best-selling diet authority Lulu Hunt Peters, slimness wasn't only about looking pretty: the stakes were moral and civic. During World War I, Peters recommended establishing "Watch Your Weight Anti-Kaiser Clubs" to demonstrate the self-control to resist indulging while others starved. Still, this "care" was largely about food restriction rather than exercise, still rare for women interested in "reducing." A supposedly wise resolution for young girls aiming to be more virtuous in the new year was to steer clear of "overindulgence in physical exercises and games," which might stress their delicate constitution. That "the flesh is weak" was assumed; what was not yet obvious was that deliberately sculpting that flesh with intense exercise would become a quintessential commitment of women within a few decades.[12]

The white, middle-class men who constituted the overwhelming majority of a newly white-collar workforce that had the privilege of working with the mind—at a desk all day—rather than the body, faced a new pressure to make a deliberate effort at physical exertion. (If exercise was understood as unladylike, dieting was defined as effete). On the one hand, not having to exert themselves at work conferred class status that differentiated such men from the mere "breaker of stones" from whom Sandow also took great pains to distinguish himself. On the other hand, this newly created "clerking class" found that the sense of superiority afforded by cerebral work could not compensate for the toll their jobs took on their bodies, known as "desk diseases."[13] Nikil Saval, in his history of American office life, contrasted the finery these new salaries afforded with the atrophied bodies it cloaked, which might be emaciated or bloated, but were certainly deconditioned: "They had sharp pen-manship and bad eyes, extravagant clothes but shrunken, unused bodies, backs cramped from poor posture, fingers callused by con-stant writing. When they were not thin, angular, and sallow, they were ruddy and soft: their paunches sagged onto their thighs."[14] While this clerking class would become the market, albeit a modest one, for the first real commercial gyms, they still viewed muscular bodies suspiciously, for such bodies were associated with the deval-ued work of the immigrant and minority laborers "who literally do the heavy lifting."[15] Taking time to cultivate one's body evoked an almost worse stereotype: that of the effeminate man excessively preoccupied with outward appearance.

Learning Fitness

Embodying restraint and bodily discipline became identifying traits of an elite class, but these tendencies had to be learned. It was on college campuses, arenas of elite formation, that a culture of deliberate exercise—as bound up with class status and moral virtue—took hold. "Sedentary habits predispose to every kind of outbreak, especially in youth," psychologist G. Stanley Hall warned in 1904, and he commended Amherst, Princeton, and Yale, and the athletic movement in particular, for advancing college gymnasi-ums from their "feeble beginnings a few decades ago" to "the best safety-valve and aid to college discipline."[16] As early as the 1850s, college students had organized "recreational" cricket, football, and baseball teams meant to engage those who might, perhaps wisely, shy away from participating in the brutal football of the time, which involved "savage blows that drew blood, and falls that seemed as if they must crack all the bones and drive the life from those who sustained them," as one Princeton student described matches.[17]

On that same campus in 1870, the athletic director had attracted attention by scheduling a one-time track meet open to any student, regardless of ability. Formal intramural sports programs managed by a dedicated administrator were introduced at the University of Michigan and Ohio State in 1913, and the University of Texas in

1916, reflecting and encouraging a desire among college men who weren't quite varsity material to engage in sport nonetheless, for fun and for what were becoming more widely acknowledged as the greater social and salutary benefits of regular exercise.[18] That the university was dedicating space and money to create these opportunities marked one important step in the entrenchment of a commitment to fitness in American life. Meaningfully, though college was a place of privilege, attendance expanded dramatically in the 1920s. By 1939, Elmer D. Mitchell, who was director of intramural sports and professor of physical education at the University of Michigan, highlighted the urgency of pushing for such programs (which were then still exceptional): "Today our schools graduate a man specialized for a particular vocation but they do not show him the way to health and happiness by keeping the play spirit alive."[19]

"Man" was the normative word, but Mitchell's boosterish book also featured photos of "activity-minded" college women playing field hockey and swimming, and he heartily endorsed the new understanding that "healthful and recreative" outlets were good and appropriate for women. Barring "combative" sports like football, boxing, wrestling, and ice hockey, which required physical contact and "violent or prolonged effort," colleges began to offer group dance and other noncompetitive activities "for the game's sake." Fieldball, field hockey, archery, basketball, and even light forms of boxing—emphasizing sparring and shadowboxing, and lacking any semblance of roughness—were popular with college women across the country.[20] At Tulane University in 1915, Sayers McDonald, "a leading society girl of Mississippi" who also happened to be reigning champion of a women's boxing contest, reassured critics who tried to cancel the competition that boxing was "a splendid form of exercise" that fostered "grace and self-reliance."[21]

Anxiety that white women lacked vitality and fortitude meant that on relatively sheltered and racially segregated college campuses, female students inspired by "New Woman" ideal were often enthusiastically welcomed, even by conservative administrations. Sports like golf, which "curbed a woman's impetuosity because she stood, still, walked slowly, and was deliberate in action," were a way for women's sports advocates to make inroads on college campuses as well, for such activities were seen to cultivate proper ladyhood, rather than challenge it.[22] The "character building and social values of sports" became embedded in school curricula, with girls engaging in more sport than ever before, but only to assimilate the deliberately measured lessons that excellence should be pursued only for the team, and that "belonging and togetherness" were more important than individual glory. Chewing gum or questioning athletic officials were as strictly forbidden as acting "a lady at all times" was categorically required.[23] In such programs, colleges sent the message that intrinsic to a full education, and personhood, was strengthening the body, since the "natural" course of daily life would not, by dint of their class position, necessarily include much physical exertion. And healthy white men and women, after all, ensured the propagation of the race.

The importance of educational institutions imparting this message, and not only to men, is undeniable. But these programs promoted this sensibility and its attendant practices to a swath of society that by design almost entirely excluded immigrants, the formerly enslaved and their offspring, and anyone who could not afford college: most of America. Also, while the establishment of these programs signaled the rising social value among elites of exercising for health, character, and beauty, college students had to pay to participate in the programs, signaling that recreational exercise was still considered more a form of leisure, or part of a kind of finishing curriculum, than a fundamental aspect of education or life.

In the less rarefied realms of public schools, the idea of regular exercise stood to get its strongest grip on society. All fifty states had adopted compulsory education laws by 1890, and school was becoming a more integral institution in the lives of all American youth. As massive immigration transformed the nation's demographics, educators, reformers, and—more ambivalently—parents invested public schools with the responsibility to teach children not only academic skills but also how to care for their bodies. Some such curriculum was practical, if prosaic: memorizing for how many minutes and with how much soap one should scrub one's hands. Others were outright offensive, such as teachers instructing Mexican students that the frijoles their parents prepared were unhealthy, Lithuanian women learning to swap out their bean dishes for "American" salads, Mexican American girls having to prove they appreciated the importance of "clean and durable underwear," or children who read the 1918 federal *Student's Textbook* and had to prove they appreciated what a toothbrush was, how to use it, and that visiting the dentist annually was a requirement of clean American living.[24] All such lessons imparted the idea that intimate choices about managing one's body bore upon one's civic identity and degree of "civilization," a word often used to contrast the United States with the countries from which immigrants arrived.

Exercise was an important part of this educational project, which transcended the schoolhouse walls. Public initiatives such as the 1919 "Keeping Fit" and "Youth and Life" poster series recommended moderate exercise for girls and boys alike; a complementary series that emphasized fitness for agricultural labor and the bodily discipline of Frederick Douglass and Booker T. Washington targeted African Americans. By 1920, most states required physical education in the public schools, and these classes represented both the liberatory and limiting sensibilities of this growing commitment to exercise. On the one hand, some educators took up educational philosopher John Dewey's impassioned call in 1916 "to develop the mind especially by exercise of the muscles of the body" and to dispense with the damaging idea that "bodily activity [is] an intruder . . . an evil to be contended with" that "lead[s] the pupil away from the lesson with which his 'mind' ought to be occupied."[25] In Dewey's framework, intellectual progress was inextricable from the engagement of the body in children's education. His philosophy of progressive education influenced some educators to integrate not only physical play but also gardening, construction, and community exploration into school days otherwise defined by sitting at desks.

On the other hand, broader concerns about which bodies were appropriate for which activities constrained physical-education efforts. Many Americans worried that building muscular strength and competitive spirit would masculinize girls.[26] Popular beliefs held that girls were ill-suited for running, weight lifting or even vigorous calisthenics, all of which were feared to cultivate excessive individualism, build bulky muscles, and even compromise fertility. These advocates often found that group dance—which became a staple in public schools and on college campuses, and remains today a core element of women's fitness—represented a workable compromise between physical culturists and a conservative medical establishment that clung tenaciously to the idea that women and girls were constitutionally weaker than men.

Paradoxically, exercise advocates found common cause with some physicians who subscribed to a belief that girls were intrinsically weak and thus in need of specific activities to redress "enfeeblement, lack of luster, debility, squeamishness about food, lack of interest in life, languid confidence, lack of incentive, and clammy hands." White, middle-class girls who needed to be robust mothers and wives should not be idle but would benefit from moderate athletic activities such as "romping, ball, beanbags, battledore, hoops, running, golf, tennis, bicycling, self-bathing in cold-water, [and] deep breathing exercises once or twice a day." Group dance satisfied both groups. Stanley Hall wrote that better than modifying established sports to "sedulously reduce" the competitive element, "dancing of many forms should be the most prominent of indoor exercises . . . as dance cadences the soul; the stately minuet gives poise; the figure dances train the mind." Importantly, however, this opinion hardly envisioned such exercises as part of a project of self-actualization. On the contrary, they recommended to schools that light athletics could be a useful avenue to limit girls' intellectual aspirations: "The development of ideal lawn-tennis girls would be a better goal for modern institutions than scholars made at such a cost."[27]

African American and immigrant children experienced physical education primarily as a form of discipline, for their bodies were understood by many whites to be inherently unruly. Whereas Hall expressly recommended intense, even "savage" physical activity as "a necessary ingredient of everything which captivates a boy's soul" for young men at risk of being feminized by the "gentle, give-and-take style" of doting mothers, teachers, and even emasculated fathers, he quite obviously meant white, middle-class boys. They could be the victims of the "social instincts of girls . . . in danger of too wide irradiation." Fears of feminization and "race suicide" were closely enmeshed. Hall reminisced about a time when classrooms and church groups were unadulterated by "girly" influences, and when a white middle-class man's "racial forbears at the stage he represents were rollicking, fighting, hunting, courting, as they roved with wild freedom on a quest for adventure."[28] Emboldening nonwhite children would endanger the social order that Hall, Roosevelt, and other advocates of a rugged, hardy, "strenuous life" strove to uphold. Especially during World War I, as public messaging about fitness for citizenship and military service proliferated, physical education became a relatively high public priority, even as its provision reflected society's underlying racist and sexist ideologies. Institutions that could afford it, like college campuses, mixed institutional funding with student fees to consolidate offerings in recreation and fitness. Even when the Depression stripped back public-school programs, a new department remained entrenched in normal schools (schools of education): physical education.[29]

The whistles and drills of school gymnasiums filled with sweaty children could seem a world away from the onstage whimsy of circus strongmen, but they converged in promoting self-possession through the cultivation of strength—even for the very young. Indeed, Sandwina's child, known in the press as "the superbaby"—he weighed fifty pounds as a two-year-old and went on to become a renowned professional boxer—was named after Roosevelt, who had personally commended her for the positive example she set for all Americans, whom he believed should exercise for personal health and moral development. Sandow also recommended that even babies should have "light wooden dumbbells as playthings" at their disposal. Those who bought his book, *Strength and How to Obtain It*, could learn daily exercises described as "Children's and Ladies," "Men's," "Athletes,'" and "Athletes' Extra Heavy." At almost the same time, MacFadden marketed his own "Exerciser" bands, each of which could be attached to a door frame, as respectively appropriate for "strongmen," "ladies," and a "child." These performers parlayed their fame in intentional and unwitting ways to encourage the ideal of exercise for *everyone*. That exercise was a way to ennoble self and society, if not always an exactly democratic one, was slowly becoming a mainstream truth.

3

Sanitizing—and
Selling—Fitness

This growing interest in fitness in the first decades of the twentieth century paradoxically both upheld and began to erode dominant assumptions about gender and exercise. On the one hand, the popularity of muscular Christianity, military readiness for two world wars, and a significant government investment in boosting up the bodies of American men and boys invigorated traditional ideas about male strength that could be newly expressed in sculpted physiques. Similarly, group dance classes emphasizing grace, as well as new, clunky reducing gadgets that amplified messages about women's weakness—and their duty to spend time and money to achieve an ideal modern, feminine figure—could in important ways entrench the idea that women were made to be passive and pretty. Yet these body projects introduced thousands to the idea that deliberate cultivation of their bodies was a meaningful, wholesome pursuit worth spending money on—a departure from an older way of life, when working out had been the domain of circus performers.[1]

A majority of states required some form of physical education by the 1920s, but the Depression scaled back many such costly efforts. Yet soon, the New Deal promoted physical fitness in compelling new ways, specifically for young men. The federal Civilian Conservation Corps (CCC) put three million unmarried young men to work on land conservation projects between 1933 and 1942. Enjoying one hundred times the funding of the Children's Bureau, which focused on schools and other youth-educational outreach, the CCC's

$300 million budget allowed it to promote the idea that an ideal adult male body was muscular and able to do physically challenging labor.[2] This fit-male ideal was strikingly different from many men's physiques of the time: the scrawny, impoverished bodies of the poor or the even larger group afflicted by influenza; the veterans who lost limbs or were otherwise disfigured in World War I; the effete, slender office workers who were suspicious for their over-developed brains and underdeveloped muscles; and, of course, the corpulent capitalist whose girth no longer signaled enviable luxury but decadence. Importantly, that new ideal was also white. For a few initial months, the CCC was racially integrated, but southern Democrats put an end to that by 1935; two hundred thousand African Americans who served worked in segregated camps. Similarly, an Indian Division employed eighty-five thousand Native Americans on reservation-development projects, but minorities were not allowed into leadership positions, nor were their bodies featured in the CCC's extensive publicity campaigns, affirming the whiteness of what one scholar later styled "musculinity."[3]

Playgrounds, recreation pavilions, skiing areas, swimming pools, and campgrounds were just a few of the thousands of federally funded sites that promoted democratic participation in fitness and recreation. A celebratory 1965 retrospective on the rise of "the sportswoman" looked back fondly on the 1930s as an era when women, "whether school girls or graduates," could enjoy such facilities.[4] By the end of 1930s, however, the United States had largely settled into what historian Rachel Louise Moran calls an "advisory" role in promoting the bodily health of its citizens, encouraging Americans to get fit, but stopping short of investing in the expensive infrastructure, education, and enforcement necessary to ensure they did so.[5]

The federal government had also commissioned unemployed artists to design vivid, brightly colored posters that promoted the CCC, featuring toned men hard at work revivifying the American economy and their own virility in the process. These paper images, hung in public buildings like post offices and train stations, spread this ideal. Yet a controversy over one mural commissioned by another federal initiative, the Public Works Administration (PWA), revealed that the New Deal reimagination of physical exertion as positive was hardly complete. In 1934, the gay artist Paul Cadmus completed "Fleet's In," a PWA-funded mural depicting strapping sailors drinking, laughing, and otherwise carousing with women in tight-fitting, attention-grabbing dresses and high heels. The subjects were getting "too friendly with each other," Navy Admiral Hugh Rodman charged with outrage before demanding that the "sordid" and "depraved" tableau—which included men draped over one another, and a well-dressed male civilian lighting a cigarette for a male sailor—be removed from the Corcoran Gallery of Art.[6] Cadmus, in intimating the homoerotic charge of muscular male bodies, had struck a nerve in a society grappling with just how to define masculinity and, secondarily, its relationship to bodily cultivation.

Notably, a painting Cadmus completed for the Treasury Relief Art Project the next year was also deemed "unsuitable" for display in a federal building. "Golf" showed a young, muscular caddy laboring for a group of paunchy old men in expensive-looking clothes chomping on cigars and more interested in leering at their employee than engaging in sport. Cadmus promoted what was becoming a dominant set of assumptions about the male body: muscles that showed work were more attractive than flabbiness that conveyed laziness and dissipation. But his suggestion that these newly attractive bodies might attract male attention, and that the moral failings of the rich might be sexual, was too much for the public to bear, or at least for the federal government to fund. As art historian Josep Armegnol has pointed out, Cadmus was fired for doing exactly what he was hired to do, "for even if the (official) discourse of the Roosevelt administration asked the publicly hired artists to record, paint, and write about what they saw, it is clear now that they always expected some things to be kept hidden, some red lines not to be trespassed."[7]

Physical education, public health policy, and popular culture introduced and established the attitudes that laid the foundation for the modern fit nation and gave rise to a market for fitness. Charles Atlas took the prize money for his two consecutive "World's Most

Perfectly Developed Man" wins—MacFadden canceled the contest after 1922, declaring no man could ever overtake Atlas—and tried to establish a business selling fitness devices. But the business foundered until, ironically, 1929: the year the economy crashed. The "Dynamic Tension" devices Atlas sold with his savvy marketing partner, Charles Roman, built strength by "pitting one muscle against another," a technique that had occurred to him as scrawny boy observing the enormous strength of a lion, who never lifted a weight in its life, loping powerfully through the newly opened Bronx Zoo.

Atlas had to sell the relatively new idea that a strong body was attractive and desirable enough to merit investing time and money in it. He brilliantly targeted teenagers and young men through comic strips that showed a now-iconic "97-pound weakling" whose silhouette was embarrassingly similar to that of his slender girlfriend, powerless to defend himself against a brawnier figure with designs on his date. The message, though its claims were untested and ultimately inspired a lawsuit, resonated with young men coming of age in the Depression era, unsure of their ability to fulfill the most basic responsibility of a real man: to get a job to provide for his family.[8] Moreover, selling a program that required no equipment to manufacture or ship made the product an affordable novelty. "I Can Make This New Man of You," Atlas promised in boldfaced type, and the initial commitment was only sending away for his free book. The invitation proved so enticing that by the 1940s two dozen women worked in his Manhattan headquarters, fielding inquiries from as far as England and India. Under different ownership, the business still operates.

Mail-order businesses, which often promised that the results of physical exercise could be attained at home in just minutes a day, without the inconvenience and potential embarrassment of going to a gym, proved more lucrative than building brick-and-mortar facilities. Physical Culture City had foundered in a few years, due not only to outside opposition, but to the relatively few people keen to devote their whole lives to physical culture. Even less-demanding gymnasiums struggled to survive in a culture in which spending time and money to exercise, and in an unfamiliar and semi-public group, was a foreign concept. In the first three decades of the twentieth century, MacFadden, Atlas, and another bodybuilder named Jack LaLanne all struggled to find a clientele for their gyms.[9] Other challenges loomed, from finding investors to infrastructure; when LaLanne opened a gym in Oakland, California, in 1936, he had to hire a blacksmith to custom-build his equipment. Far more effective were the media and mail-order regimes that these men—and others, like York Barbell founder Bob Hoffman—used to spread the precepts of the fit nation to a public that was still diffuse and undefined.

Exercise was *still* considered strange, and the men who frequented "sweaty dungeons" to lift weights were often considered unintelligent or effete. The cultural association of male muscularity, the gyms where it was cultivated, and "deviant" masculinity wasn't only abstract. In an era defined by what historian of sexuality George Chauncey calls "the exclusion of homosexuality in the public sphere," physique culture provided cover, and sometimes solace, for gay men who lacked places to safely meet one another.[10] Magazines such as Bernarr MacFadden's *Physical Culture*, with their near-naked models inspired by ancient Greece, labored hard to prop up traditional notions of gender *because* these associations with deviance were so strong. Advertisements in the booklet *Muscular Manhood* contained odd language intended to dispel the idea that such publications were for gay men (or perhaps to attract that very audience): publicity for a six-book "Personal Problem Library" that included a "PROFUSELY ILLUSTRATED" title, *Sex Physique Averages*, clarified that the books were written by physicians and "not for curiosity seekers or minors. They are intended strictly for grownups. The sale is limited to adults over the age of 21, to married couples, and those intending to get married."[11]

MacFadden celebrated those who beat up men he considered excessively effeminate and openly reviled those whose prurience led them to associate his magazine with homosexuality: "Those who possess such vulgar minds are the enemies of everything clean, wholesome, and elevating." Chauncey argues that MacFadden was so strident because he so acutely feared being perceived as harboring "the depraved sexual desires of a degenerate."[12] Sandow, the ambassador of bodybuilding, mostly kept quiet about his sexuality, but the press wrote about how his "great and inseparable friend" Martin Sieveking crossed the Atlantic with him, and they "took up housekeeping" together on West 38th Street in New York, a fact that leads some contemporary scholars to identify Sandow as bisexual.[13] Much as Sandwina had performed her "normalcy" by wearing frills and proclaiming her love of laundry, Atlas and his fellow male entrepreneurs played up an exaggerated heterosexuality, most notably when the 97-pound weakling makes clear he invested in Dynamic Tension to impress his girlfriend *and* to punch out, rather than cozy up to, a bigger, more muscular male suitor.

These new enterprises thus had to sell bodily cultivation as refined but also red-blooded and virile. Brawny bodies suggested working-class brutishness, but deconditioned clerks' bodies were also unattractive. Working on one's body might now be necessary, but the places where that labor took place were considered louche. A new physique, toned by products and practices pitched specifically at white-collar workers, emerged. Simon Kehoe, a Brit who imported "Indian Clubs" to the United States, lamented that gymnasiums were few and far between, and that those that existed were rarely "acquainted with the manifold graceful and artistic evolutions" possible via use of the clubs that the British army had first seen among Indians during colonial occupation.[14] The clubs, Kehoe claimed, were perfect for professional men who were not necessarily athletes: "Merchants, bankers, clerks, and those engaged in daily business pursuits, who need some available means of exercise to counteract the ills arising from their sedentary occupations, are many of them becoming experts with the Clubs, and reaping everlasting benefits." Their bodies were changing the city's landscape, Kehoe effused. In stark contrast to the neighborhoods populated by "the shoals of painted, perfumed, Kohl-eyed lisping, mincing youths that at night swarm Broadway in the Tenderloin section," or "haunt the parks on Fifth Avenue, ogling every man that passes," as MacFadden had in 1904 denounced neighborhoods known to be frequented by gay men, Kehoe wrote approvingly of a different scene emerging: "Note in the crowded thoroughfare of Broadway now and then and occasional passer-by, with well-knit and shapely form, firm and elastic step, broad-chested and full-blooded, and you may mark him down as one of Kehoe's converts. The names of these well-known New Yorkers are too numerous for mention here."[15]

Ironically, despite intense anxieties about women engaging in sport or developing strength, fitness had in some ways been since the nineteenth century an easier sell to them than to men—if its pursuit was about beauty. Ads targeting men buried any indication that the reader might be purchasing a beauty product beneath layers of unctuous appeals to masculine strength and virility. At the bottom of Atlas's earliest print ads, he promised aesthetic results in fine print: "Banishing such ailments as . . . pimples, skin blotches, and the others that do you out of the good things and good times in life."[16] Clear skin and a small waist were results promised to both men and women taking up regular exercise routines, but antebellum reformer Catherine Beecher was early to link exercise with these aesthetic results. Beecher detested how sartorial presentation had become "the ruling thought" of many young girls' lives, distracting them from more important pursuits and crippling their self-regard, spirit, and sometimes quite literally their bodies. The "protracted agonies" of deformed bones, palpitations, and a constant nervous, anxious state, Beecher pleaded with a reader she assumed to be white, were more damaging than "horrible torments inflicted by savage Indians or cruel inquisitors" that would be rightly recognized as unjust.[17] Redefining beauty was needed, Beecher wrote, because "the war of fashion," waged with whalebone stays and corset strings, disfigured the very bodies it was meant to beautify. Physical attractiveness *was* a paramount virtue, Beecher explained, but it was rooted in teaching a girl to "realize the skill and beauty of construction shown in her earthly frame," as the more she does so, "the more she will feel the obligation to protect it from injury and abuse" through salutary pursuits like moderate exercise, healthy food, useful work, and sensible dress—not by worshipping at the false idols of fashion.

Beecher was not alone in reimagining beauty standards to celebrate the robust frames and flushed cheeks that showed the effects of exercise as opposed to store-bought style, but this line of thinking did not always lead to liberatory ends. Nearly thirty years later, MacFadden's perspective on the matter made clear the limits of his career-long campaign against the "grotesque deformity" of the bone-crushing corset. According to MacFadden, "woman's universal desire" for a small waist was beyond question and only worth challenging because the popularity among white women of the corset as the means to achieve it threatened to "deteriorate the race." In his 1901 text on "superb womanhood," MacFadden quotes Professor O. S. Fowler, a fellow combatant in the war against corsets, who makes clear that the well-being of women is totally beside the point:

If it were merely a female folly, or its ravages were confined to its perpetrators, it might be passed unrebuked; but it strikes a deadly blow at the very life of the race. By girding in the lungs, stomach, heart, diaphragm, etc., it cripples every one of the life-manufacturing functions, impairs circulation, impedes muscular action, and lays siege to the child-bearing citadel itself. By the value of abundance of maternal vitality, air, exercise, and digestion, is this practice murderous to both. It often destroys germinal life before birth, or soon after, by most effectually cramping, inflaming, and weakening the vital apparatus, and stopping the flow of life at its fountain-head. It takes the lives of tens of thousands before they marry, and so effectually weakens and diseases as ultimately to cause the deaths of millions more. No tongue can tell, no finite mind conceive, the misery it has occasioned; besides those millions on millions it has caused to drag out a short but wretched existence. If this murderous practice continues another generation it will bury all the middle and upper class of women and children, and leave propagation to the coarse-grained but healthy lower classes. Most alarmingly has it already deteriorated our race in physical strength, power of constitution, energy, and talents. Reader, how many of YOUR weaknesses, pains, headaches, nervous affections, internal difficulties, and wretched feelings were caused by your own or mother's corset-strings? Such mothers deserve execration.[18]

Execration! Slowly but surely, even those with deeply conservative ideas about women were becoming comfortable with the notion that exercise, if appropriate for the female constitution, could enhance traditional femininity rather than erode it. Sure enough, the most powerful growth in women's fitness in the early twentieth century came not from federal investment or from athletics. Rather, tending to the body for beauty became a powerful way that a nascent industry sold "figure control" and "slenderizing" at first through "passive exercise" to women who wouldn't go for sports, self-defense, or more intense activities. The sensibility shift was widespread, and often at the grass roots. Black women established "rolling clubs" in the first decade of the twentieth century to "literally roll off excess weight," as the *Savannah Tribune* reported in 1910. The fourteen Oklahoma women who gathered weekly "in a desperate attempt to slim down," had been convened by "one of the stoutest creatures west of the Mississippi." Though mostly made up of relatively affluent "society matrons and buds," the club that put "everything fat and feminine on the roll" was hardly insulated from two simultaneous pressures: the broad popularity of a slim, "hipless" look dictated by the overwhelmingly white aesthetic of the era's fashion magazines and the especially intense pressure for Black women to counteract racist stereotypes that cast them as either obese or masculine; the founder told the journalist that "one might as well be dead to be out of style."[19]

The beauty industry quickly fulfilled this appetite for exercise to enhance appearance through bodywork with new products and spaces such as "slenderizing spas" that employed gentle exercise to help women "reduce" in "luxurious comfort" without disrupting any notions of conventional femininity, and certainly without compelling women to enter gymnasiums, which remained off-puttingly public and often overwhelmingly male spaces. Far from an Oklahoma living room, luxuriously appointed salons established by beauty entrepreneurs like Helena Rubinstein and Elizabeth Arden became popular destinations for those eager for expert intervention on their quest for makeovers that came to include "figure control." The activities in these spaces can barely be described as exercise in the sweaty, breathless, contemporary sense, but these spas created spaces where the idea of women ritually remaking their bodies, together, in service of their femininity, took root.

At the New York City salon that French emigrée Rubinstein established as the "Maison de Beauté Valaze" in 1915, she was careful to tread lightly in transgressing traditional notions of how a woman should act and where it was appropriate for women to congregate. The salon's decor of "deep blue walls, rose baseboards . . . green velvet carpets . . . red tables . . . [and] embroidered pillows" was "reassuringly domestic, somewhat upper crust, and above all respectable," as design scholar Marie Clifford described it, signaling that readers could feel at home there. Rubinstein—who in 1938 married a "supposed" Georgian prince and promptly marketed a "Princess" product line—made the most of her continental connections to attract what she considered a classy clientele. In the advertisements she took out in *Vogue*, as well as multiple features the premiere women's magazine ran over the years, Rubinstein's extensive, richly hued art collection and the salon's intricately wallpapered rooms figured prominently. Effectively conflating the atelier of a Parisian artist, the grand art shows of the surrounding city, and the ballet, Rubinstein did much to elevate the enterprise of cosmetics away from associations with "public women," be they prostitutes or Hollywood celebrities. As her biographers have pointed out, this pretense also served to minimize her Jewishness, which at various points inhibited her professional success, from the real estate discrimination she encountered when renting a studio to the snobbery of prospective WASP clients who took their business elsewhere.[20]

Elizabeth Arden, her primary competitor, operated in the same vein, decorating her modern Fifth Avenue salon with a red door that recalled the chic, bourgeois apartments of her clientele. Arden was earlier to feature an exercise studio as part of these luxurious spaces devoted to bodily renovation. The exercise studio she launched with a ladies' tea was constructed in the same aesthetic; a 1930 *Fortune* magazine piece described it as appointed with opulent satin drapes and chairs covered in an "interlocking pink and green" fabric that evoked Georgia O'Keeffe, whose work would as of 1936 actually adorn the walls of Arden's "Gymnasium Moderne," surrounding women doing rhythmic dance and ballet-inspired toning exercises.[21] Arden and Rubinstein in different ways charted new ground in welcoming "women who could afford it," as one British news segment described it, be they monied Junior League socialites or striving secretaries and stenographers, to spend time and money on the more broadly accepted bodily work of skin and hair care, and increasingly, on still-strange exercise.

The reducing-machine craze went national—"figure control rooms" and "silhouette salons" loosely inspired by Arden and Rubinstein's Manhattan palaces popped up in small towns and suburbs as well as larger cities. By 1957, one city of 750,000 people had twenty-two women-only reducing firms that charged women up to ten dollars for "who-knows-how-many treatments," recounted one skeptical assessment.[22] Catering to women who sought to "soothe the nerves and control the curves," as one 1930s Chicago beauty salon promised of its two programs—one "thorough and scientific" for "the fats" carrying "excess poundage" and a second for "the tired business woman" in less dire need of "curve control"—the relatively affordable salons quickly became popular. Some featured installment plans for as little as a dollar for a fifteen-minute visit—during which you could lose "AS MUCH AS THREE POUNDS OR YOUR MONEY BACK!," as one Milwaukee business advertised in 1956. Located adjacent to beauty salons, or more rarely, given the size and cost of equipment, in private homes, slenderizing outfits were *not* found in gyms, which were still considered the preserve of sweaty, grunting men and entirely inappropriate for ladies who often kept their high heels on during a session.[23]

Scientific legitimacy was key to selling these new services, and such operations consulted with physicians and staffed up with sophisticated-sounding "technicians" to operate machinery ranging from mechanized massagers that primarily vibrated "the right

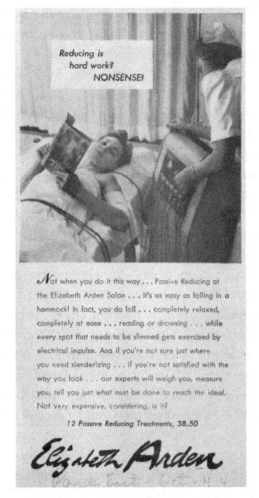

Figure 3. Elizabeth Arden. *Reducing Is Hard Work? Nonsense*, 1944. Beauty entrepreneurs such as Elizabeth Arden sold bodywork as a way to achieve an aesthetic "ideal," but given antipathies to strenuous exercise, were sure to emphasize how passive—and thus appropriately ladylike—fitness could be.

spots" to try to "dissolve fatty tissues" and "eliminate inches" to the full-body "relax-and-reduce" massage that became popular in the late 1940s and 1950s. The effectiveness of these treatments, however, was dubious. Cutting-edge technology supposedly allowed minimal physical activity to be required for weight loss: "Just relax in luxurious comfort. . . . No moving from one machine to another," advertised one early-1940s machine. These "cage-like platforms housing a contraption of coils and metal poles" were billed as so innovative they could increase women's vitality, strength, and beauty without requiring much movement or inducing an unladylike sweat. Safety was also an issue: in 1949, the *Los Angeles Times* reported that one young woman was trapped in a malfunctioning machine and suffered "bone bruises" even after an emergency police squad came to her rescue. Yet women, not faulty machinery or false advertising, were often blamed for patronizing these businesses. One article took aim at delusional women who refused to face their "real problems of overweight" and the work required to redress it, like one "dumpy, middle-aged, old lady who walked into a salon one day recently" and despite carrying "some 25 pounds of dangerous overweight by medical standards," announced, "just get off this roll of fat—right here—and I'll be satisfied."[24]

At-home regimes promised convenient access to the beauty effects of regular exercise. "Exercise for Beauty's Sake," instructed a curlicued two-page headline in *Vogue*. Women who found themselves "fair, forty, and fat," the piece imparted, might understandably be intimidated by the supple, flexible women photographed in backbends and twists, but this was no excuse "not to take action against" the "cumbersome pounds" that stood between so many women and universally desirable "grace of body and courage."[25] Such media coverage was common, subtly normalizing the idea that making time for exercise was something between a right and a requirement of ladyhood. Rare were products that assumed exercises to be suitable for both men and women; a curious 1939 booklet of "West Point Exercises" used by cadets at the United States Military Academy, marketed as "a simple, inexpensive way to achieve a graceful figure," is an exception.[26] Far more common were sales pitches promising minimal work *because* women were still considered ill suited to rigorous exercise. "You exert no effort," promised a 1956 ad for the Relax-a-Cizor. Billed as "the normal, healthy way to pull in inches," the device was marketed to a "busy woman" with no time for gym or salon but with a desire for "real exercise," but not

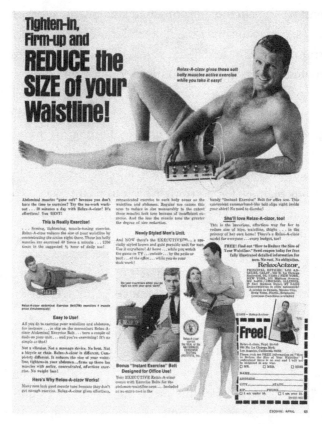

Figure 4. Relax-A-Cizor, *Tighten-In, Firm-Up and* REDUCE *the* SIZE *of your Waistline!*, April 1, 1970. The Relax-A-Cizor marketed passive exercise to women *and* men, by the late 1960s advertising in men's magazines as the "no-work workout" that could be used to burn off abdominal fat, even while users sat at a desk in the office.

ADVERTISEMENT. *ESQUIRE. ESQUIRE* CLASSIC ARCHIVE. HTTPS://CLASSIC.ESQUIRE.COM/ARTICLE /1970/4/1/RELAX-A-CIZOR-RELAXACIZOR.

the sort associated with "bicycles, massage tables, heat, or massage," all of which required a sweat. On the contrary, one could strap this miracle device around one's waist in ten seconds, and with a turn of a dial: "You REST at home. No effort is required. You use it while you read, rest, watch television . . . even while you sleep!"[27]

As ever, women who went in for slenderizing walked a fine line. If prioritizing beauty guarded a woman against becoming too manly, frivolity and excessive vanity were unseemly as well.

Helen McKenna had lived her life "a hopeless prisoner in a ton of flesh," and had been counseled away from reducing regimes by her friends, who somewhat coldheartedly told her about "the horrible things that happen to people who try to reduce," wasting their money and placing misguided hope in faddish salons and equipment. Indeed, McKenna had spent every school vacation subjecting herself to "terrific workouts" of "calisthenics, diet, sports, and massage," dropping as much as thirty pounds one summer but then gaining it all back, "with a little more for good measure." Bored and dispirited, in September 1937 McKenna walked tentatively into a ballet class, her face broadcasting her urge to bolt and avoid the humiliation of being cast out for being too "fat and awkward." She stayed, and as the teacher broke down the steps and even coaxed McKenna into a modified *brisé*, she was entranced. No more able to drop dancing than "to cut her own arm off," McKenna ultimately lost seventy pounds mastering the Pavlova gavotte, the Mexican hat dance, and a Chopin waltz, and was soon wearing "bright, luscious colors," "less old-maidey clothes," and even a "perky, youthful hat."

McKenna was no less obsessed with beauty and appearance than the women who spent their money on dedicated exercise products and places, but her "battle over fat" was won, a feature in *Dance* magazine made clear, *because* she had eschewed superficial reducing regimes and chosen a more elevated, "happy, artistic" pursuit instead.[28] Even one profile of a Chicago silhouette salon that was unquestionably a beauty business, offering manicures, facials, and hair styling, assured readers: "We hope we haven't made all this sound frivolous. It's serious beauty work." The legitimacy had to do with the transactional nature of the experience—"the individual needs of the client are carefully considered"—and its scientific basis: "Some courses are given with the cooperation of a physician."[29] Men might be putting their bodies on the line in war, a British news segment reminded women, but they still had crucial "Battles of the Bulge" to wage on their stubbornly fleshy bodies, quite a different wartime effort than replacing male labor in factories, Rosie the Riveter–style, which women were of course doing too.[30]

By the 1940s, some women passionate about sports, self-defense, and developing their own strength were unapologetically training rigorously, regardless of dominant ideas about how these passions might be perceived by the world at large. But an enduring and powerful cultural expectation that women were not supposed to value their own strength as a virtue kept many from the gym, or at least meaningfully constrained the range of exercises considered appropriate for their supposedly fragile constitutions. Ironically, even as wartime training had demystified regular exercise for a generation of servicemen—especially weight lifting, which had been part of many training regimes—many male civilians still steered clear of the gym for a complementary but contradictory reason: spending so much time on their bodies was thought to *diminish* their virility by distracting them with the effete pursuit of beauty or the blandishments of other men. The point is proven in one 1956 profile of a Washington, DC–area Slenderella salon, where men had expressed curiosity about such mysterious feminine spaces. The company was considering opening men-only salons, "which they will definitely not call Slender-fella!"[31]

4

The California Beach
Body Is Born

More than a half-century after the solitary Sandow flexed at the World's Fair, a very different scene transpired on another stage, on the southern California coast. Santa Monica locals and tourists alike gathered on "Muscle Beach" to watch suntanned strength enthusiasts like Jack LaLanne and Abbye "Pudgy" Stockton—who had been recently crowned "Miss Physical Culture Venus" by MacFadden—throw each other high in the air, sometimes balancing atop one another against the bright blue sky, with hundred-pound barbells held overhead. The men were clad in tight-fitting trunks, and Stockton donned the two-piece she had fashioned from a ripped brassiere to allow her greater range of motion. These exercise enthusiasts had begun gathering at a New Deal–era playground, spreading rugs and tarps right on the sand, to practice and perform gasp-inducing acrobatic feats that drew ever-greater and more enthusiastic crowds.[1] Playground instructor Kate Giroux, with the support of the Works Progress Administration and Santa Monica authorities, had envisioned the modest setup as a space for impoverished children during the Depression, but adults soon flocked to the sandpit, weight-lifting pen, equipment shed, and volleyball and Ping-Pong areas.[2]

The children kept showing up. A typical Fourth of July celebration in the mid-1940s involved acrobats stacked four or five high in human pillars, women dramatically tearing phone books apart or mock-wrestling men for laughs, and apparently effortlessly lifting weights and even young children as part of the act, which would last all afternoon.[3] Muscle Beach was liberating exercise from spaces that had been deliberately discreet—dank, subterranean weight rooms; demure, slenderizing spas; and private living rooms where timid exercisers experimented with mail-order apparatuses or Atlas-approved routines—and bringing it into the bright sunlight. In 1948, filmmaker Joseph Strick released a short movie about Muscle Beach, all smiling children splashing in the waves and licking drippy ice cream cones, and of course, as an accompanying vocalist crooned, tanned "body beautifuls" pumping iron in the summer heat, self-made men in the flesh. Three years later, a spread in *LIFE* magazine on Muscle Beach celebrated the area's strength enthusiasts in a feature on the unique and enviable hardiness of "West Coast Youth." Just as California "tends to produce bigger and better fruits and vegetables, it is producing a healthier and statistically bigger crop of youngsters," *LIFE* effused, integrating photos of flexing Muscle Beach regulars with wholesome images of teenagers surfing, diving into turquoise swimming pools, hanging out at gleaming drive-ins, and sudsing up cars in the sunshine.

Muscle Beach *was* glamorous. Back in those days, remembered regular Les Stockton—Pudgy's husband—"the girl tourists would come by, and the guys would pull them up on stage and throw them up in the air, and they'd go home to Nebraska or Oklahoma or wherever and never forget their day on Muscle Beach."[4] So close to Hollywood, plenty of Muscle Beach regulars were aspiring actors, and casting directors often scouted the stage to find stunt doubles, or occasionally, as with Steve Reeves and *Hercules*, to cast lead roles that would give these strapping bodies a far more prominent stage from which to promote exercise as a way of life. Television gave an even bigger platform to fellow Muscle Beach personality Jack LaLanne, who launched his eponymous fitness program on a local San Francisco channel in 1951, funding the show from his own pocket since no studio executives believed a show about exercise could succeed. Within several months, however, he received heaps of mail from mostly female viewers eager for his expertise on how to improve their shape. "Pudgy" Stockton, one of the few Muscle Beach women who achieved fame, had no television show, but thanks to fawning magazine profiles and the "Barbelles" advice column she wrote for nearly a decade for *Strength and Health* magazine, published by York Barbell Company, she too received hundreds of letters. Some were untoward or obscene "meatballs," but the missives were primarily requests for exercise tips and compliments on her muscular form. Thousands of such letters—often addressed just to "Muscle Beach, USA"—flowed to Santa Monica from those who saw the toned, disciplined acrobats and weight lifters as enviable role models as opposed to freakish outliers.

Still, this transformation was halting. A 1948 *Los Angeles Times* article highlights how embedded was the sense that working out was not just a waste of time, but even a threat to one's economic prospects. The superficially positive report announced the win of the vaunted Mr. America title by twenty-two-year-old George Eiferman of Muscle Beach. The main point of the piece, however, was to emphasize the economic, aesthetic, and intellectual limitations of Eiferman and other "dumbbell boys of the beach." The victor had "hope, tremendous muscles, wavy hair, and no job," and had not even decided on a career path. The journalist pointed out, however, how painstakingly Eiferman had shaved his chest hair. "Mighty Negro from Brooklyn" John Davis, a reigning world-champion lifter, earned even less respect. "Not interested in liftin' that bale," the *Times* described Davis, drawing on stereotypes of Black men as shiftless, writing that he was untroubled by having been unemployed since joining the amateur weight-lifting circuit. "The truth is," the *Times* concluded, "the financial careers of beautiful and weightlifting specimens and weightlifters are sketchy."[5] These West Coast "Tarzans of the sandpile" were characterized as intellectually dim, economically weak, and pathetically vain, all attributes usually associated with women. Ten years later, Ira Wallach's novel *Muscle Beach* reiterates the idea that brains and brawn were distinct: a clever New York City writer becomes fleetingly infatuated with "dumb, divine, Jocie" of Muscle Beach, whom he woos from her strapping beau only to ultimately realize that anyone so fixated on outward appearance lacks an interior life.

As one of the few women weight lifters and acrobats who rose to prominence at Muscle Beach, "Pudgy" Stockton encountered

similar challenges, reflecting the fact that women were largely dissuaded from both strenuous exercise and entrepreneurship. Teased
as "pudgy" in childhood, Stockton found work as a telephone switch-
board operator after high school. She grew restless with the sedentary work—and frustrated with the weight she had gained—and
broke up her shifts by accompanying her boyfriend, Les, to nearby
Muscle Beach. There, she mastered headstands and hand-balances,
and by 1939 was featured in multiple national magazines as well as
flying in the air in a *LIFE* magazine advertisement for the Universal
Camera Company. During World War II, when Les was dispatched to
the Victorville Air Force base, the newlyweds developed the uncommon hobby of practicing Olympic lifts in their backyard for fun.
Back in greater Los Angeles after the war, she organized Los Angeles's Pacific Coast Weightlifting Championships in 1947, the first
such women's contest officially sanctioned by the Amateur Athletic
Union (AAU). By 1950, Stockton had convinced the AAU to sponsor a
national championship, encouraging more women than the nine who
had competed three years earlier to participate in weight lifting, an
activity still considered brutish even for men.[6]

Stockton knew that to appeal to women who had little interest
in heaving iron onstage, she needed to promote the strange pastime of strength training as a way to achieve conventional feminine beauty. In her column, she profiled women weight lifters,
and repeated the advice that "beneath every womanly curve lies a
muscle." Before-and-after photography was not yet a stock feature
of "reducing" marketing, but her nickname and trim frame made
her weight-loss transformation central to her appeal to a public
skeptical of strong women. "Pudgy" signaled to the growing numbers of women who worked in similarly sedentary desk jobs that
a flabby childhood need not seal their fate—if they could muster
the energy to exercise. She both promoted this narrative herself
and never publicly rejected it when it was articulated by others. At
one 1947 weight-lifting event in Nashville, Tennessee, Stockton was
billed as "America's most well-developed woman" and sashayed
onstage in a "royal blue dressing gown" as her measurements—
27-23-34—were recited out loud to the "obvious edification of the

audience." She promptly stripped down to a candy-pink two-piece to perform three Olympic lifts for an audience that might "never have been able to distinguish between a lateral raise or an alternate pullover without help, but were willing to take Pudgy as proof of their efficacy."[7] In 1949, Stockton bestowed a trophy on the new "Queen of Muscle Beach" whom the judges—four gym owners and a wrestler—had expressly chosen "not for muscles but beauty of face and figure." The *Los Angeles Times* reiterated this criterion in its reporting of the event: "Muscles do not count."[8]

Yet something was indeed changing, in part due to these efforts. Physical culture historian Terry Todd remarked to Steve Reeves in a 2000 interview that "people must have seen you walking down the beach and thought you were from a different planet."[9] Certainly, Reeves, who held multiple bodybuilding titles, cut a physically imposing figure even by today's standards. But Pudgy Stockton strove to be not just pretty, but approachable in her self- presentation. Much like "Lady Hercules" Katie Sandwina nearly half a century earlier, Stockton, a.k.a. "the Venus of Muscle Beach," was portrayed as both otherworldly and reassuringly domestic; Stockton "puts aside her barbells and sews a fine seam. She can cook too," a paradigmatic profile reported.[10] Photographs of her sewing and washing dishes at home, and of her slim figure, revealed that her intense exercise regime even enhanced her femininity. Lustrous hair, radiant skin and "miraculous curves" piqued the interest of "America's young men [who] pant with desire, and also pant in their gyms as they try to prove themselves worthy of her," her biographer Jan Todd wrote. In 1949, photographer Max Yavno captured the weekend scene at Muscle Beach—it took him multiple visits before the acrobats and enthusiasts stopped self-consciously posing for his camera—in a telling shot. The action was clearly moving offstage, or maybe, with its irresistible energy, enticing others on. At least eight muscular performers hung on bars in Yavno's tableau, showing off their muscles in an isometric movement that would have impressed Charles Atlas, tossing each other in the air in their signature *adagio* move, and executing backbends and tumbles, their glistening muscles showing their effort and its appeal.

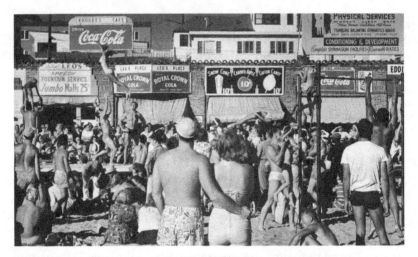

Figure 5. Max Yavno, *Muscle Beach, Los Angeles,* 1949. Photographer Max Yavno captured scenes of street life in California, and by the late 1940s Muscle Beach was a vibrant attraction for tourists, local residents, and—increasingly—those interested in building the strength of their own bodies, not just observing the muscles of those on stage.

GELATIN SILVER PRINT, 10⅞" × 13⅞" (27.7 × 35.3 CM). MAX YAVNO ARCHIVE, © CENTER FOR CREATIVE PHOTOGRAPHY, UNIVERSITY OF ARIZONA FOUNDATION. HTTP://CCP-EMUSEUM.CATNET.ARIZONA.EDU /VIEW/OBJECTS/ASITEM/KEYWORD@RECREATION/19/MEDIUM-DESC.

But far more people milled about the low stage, shielding their eyes to see the action, allowing their children to be hoisted up onto the bars in demonstrations. Many were dressed as revealingly as the performers, making the differences between bodies difficult to ignore. The space between those on the stage and the spectators was narrowing. Just to the right of the stage, a sign that advertised "Physical Services" in "Conditioning and Development" offered spectators an opportunity to bridge that gap, reminding them that if they invested time and money and sweat, they too could become as strong as the performers just feet in front of them, close enough to touch.

Getting gorgeous, healthy, and strong in the sunshine fit seamlessly with the image of an ever more widely marketed California culture, and by the 1940s Muscle Beach and its muscled bodies not only drew crowds of tourists and aspiring hardbodies, but were well entrenched in popular culture, popping up on TV shows like *Tom and Jerry* and as a go-to laugh line, "like Brooklyn," for "wise-cracking comedians of stage, screen, TV, and gossip columns from Coast to Coast."[11] In the late 1950s, Muscle Beach star Bill Pearl would dress up as Sandow, performing the latter's classic stunts in gladiator sandals, loincloth, and a wig, paying homage to early strongmen and also highlighting how much had changed. Vic and Armand Tanny had relocated from icy Rochester, New York, to become Muscle Beach regulars, and by 1958, Vic, who became known as a "gym dandy," owned and operated more than one hundred commercial facilities that catered to those aspiring to some version of the fit figure he cut. No longer just performers, mid-century bodybuilders embodied, and sold, an ideal to which more Americans began to aspire. The audiences that thronged Muscle Beach in its early days were arguably the last who would witness exercise primarily as spectacle without pressure to participate, blissfully free of that familiar twinge of guilt upon seeing someone else sweat: *I should really work out today.*

The fit nation as we now know it was forming, but exercise enthusiasts still faced formidable challenges—including on Muscle Beach itself. Some *LIFE* readers were so repulsed by the country's most mainstream magazine featuring a "vulgar display of brawn" that they wrote letters to the editor recommending that this lifestyle should be "banned and censored," not glamorized.[12] The conservative Santa Monica city council had been opposed for at least five years to the hardy "lads and lasses of Muscle Beach" whom they saw as "sexual athletes" and "queers," "drifters," and "perverts" with "no visible means of support." Enthusiasm for exercise was itself evidence of narcissism and even "perversion"—besides which, more than a few of the men in the "weight-lifting set" had modeled in gay "skin magazines," socialized interracially, or been rumored to be homosexuals.[13] In 1958, when five weight lifters were charged with the sexual assault of two young Black girls in a nearby apartment and motel, city leaders seized upon unassailable evidence that Muscle Beach did "not fit into the city's recreational picture."[14] Claiming that the oceanfront playground was "too expensive to maintain for a few people," Santa Monica recreation director Leonard Bright, police chief Otto Faulkner, and city manager Randall

Dorton argued that these "morals charges"—kryptonite in Cold War southern California—were good reason to shutter the outdoor recreation center and cast out the acrobats and weight lifters who had put it on the map.[15] But there was no way to reverse the transformation already underway in American attitudes about fitness.

Part **Two**

SLIMMING THE SOFT AMERICAN

No one gets cut from the squad of fitness.
PRESIDENTIAL COUNCIL ON YOUTH FITNESS, 1960

Across the country in Westchester County, New York, attitudes about exercise weren't shifting fast enough to counter the troubling transformations Bonnie Prudden was seeing around her. A Broadway dancer reluctantly turned homemaker, who favored calisthenics when the weather prevented her from hiking or skiing in her beloved Shawangunk Mountains, Prudden noticed that though her fellow suburbanites might appreciate the look of the muscled bodies in *LIFE* magazine, or might even order products that promised physique development and commanded readers to "Be healthy!" by way of exercise, their actual fitness was declining rather than improving. The "tyranny of the wheel," as Prudden described the growing dependence on cars and strollers, was making Americans of all ages lazy and deconditioned. Still scarier, children and teenagers who had never known a life before frozen TV dinners and drive-ins stood to suffer most from this normalization of sedentary suburban life.

Prudden's activism around fitness began with her own family but grew quickly as word spread through their bedroom community of Harrison, New York. In the mid-1940s, horrified by a lackluster physical education class she observed, Prudden began offering fitness classes at her daughters' elementary school for the girls and ten of their friends. The sessions combined calisthenics, dance, and stretching, and in the warmer months, outdoor play on obstacle courses, and they soon inspired interest beyond the student body of Pleasant Ridge Elementary. Outgrowing a local Girl Scouts house and then the larger Knights of Columbus Hall, Prudden expanded the classes in the 1950s to include girls, boys, and adults. Attendance spiked, she was bemused to find, when she began charging nominal fees for her services—$2.50 an hour for children and $3.50 for adults, for a thirty-week training program—and officialized her offerings as the "Institute of Physical Fitness" in 1954.[1] Her offerings were apparently *more* attractive to students who felt pride both at their improved strength and the fact that they were investing in an important pursuit like health.

Her students also seemed to be having *fun*, which Prudden, who had grown up climbing trees and frolicking outside until her parents called her in at dusk, knew was crucial if Americans were ever to choose physical exertion over the enticing array of passive entertainment on offer. Housed in a former public school that Prudden renovated with almost seventy thousand dollars of her own funds, the institute eventually included six gymnasiums, locker rooms, a massage room, a snack bar, and, as *Sports Illustrated* described it in a slightly patronizing profile, "a Madison Avenue–type office (which even contains a tilting lounge chair like the one in the movie *The Man in the Gray Flannel Suit*) that seemed an incongruously serious choice for the chipper, curly-haired exercise enthusiast who favored tee shirts, shorts, and generally 'having a wonderful time.'"[2]

But what Prudden witnessed, and presciently addressed, was bigger than her institute or her suburb. After World War II, favorable housing policy, the GI Bill, and overall economic prosperity had expanded access—overwhelmingly to white Americans—to a middle-class, suburban lifestyle taking shape in newly constructed subdivisions outfitted with dishwashers and television sets, and on freshly paved and federally subsidized roads filled with gas-guzzling automobiles manufactured in a booming domestic industry. Prudden had a solution to the challenges all this affluence was creating before her very eyes. But first she had to convince policymakers and everyday people that American prosperity posed any problems at all.

5

White Plains, the White House, and the Paradox of Prosperity

When Prudden and her peers grew up in the Great Depression, they could never have imagined the degree of affluence that would by the 1950s be on display in magazines, catalogs, and multiplying American suburbs. Moreover, American technological innovation had transformed even the most mundane quotidian tasks. Industrial science filled supermarket shelves with quickly prepared frozen foods and just-add-water innovations like Jell-O and infant formula. Drive-in dining and movies were advertised as convenient, affordable leisure pursuits. In the summer of 1959, Vice President Richard Nixon famously debated Soviet premier Nikita Khrushchev in Moscow, and pointed to the kind of dishwasher "built in thousands of units" for "direct installation" in homes affordable to the average steelworker as a symbol of American superiority, wherein "we like to make life easier for our women."[1] Such claims to universalism were overstated: drive-ins were inaccessible to those who lacked a car, as were the suburbs. Only about half of American homes had electricity, making the experience of relaxing in front of a television set as your built-in washing machines and dishwasher whirred in the background still the stuff of fantasy for most. And few of these benefits were available to nonwhite people at all. Prudden was mostly quiet on these concerns, but was early to pipe up that these widely celebrated material comforts meant to show off the superiority of western capitalism might be a source of literal weakness. What was happening to the bodies that would be summoned to battle if the Cold War got hot?

Soon, an international physical-fitness exam, devised by New York physicians Hans Kraus and Sonja Weber, confirmed Prudden's fears about children, but it was Kraus and Weber's adult patients who first raised suspicion. Austrian refugees of the Third Reich, Kraus and Weber had noticed a new ailment in their adopted country: back pain. Unknown in Europe, and in the United States before the late 1940s, back discomfort seemed to be epidemic among the white-collar New Yorkers who visited the Posture Clinic the two physicians had founded at Columbia Presbyterian Hospital in Manhattan. After Kraus treated Prudden for a neck injury, they became mountain-climbing partners, discussing their concerns about the lack of physical fitness they both noticed among their sedentary patients, peers, and children. What, the two friends wondered, could they do to stem this alarming decline that was counterintuitively afflicting the world's most ascendant power? In 1953, Kraus and Prudden wrote up their concerns in the *Journal of the American Association for Health, Physical Education, and Recreation*, but this warning call in an esoteric academic journal attracted little attention.

Undaunted, the two began testing American and European children with what came to be known as the Kraus-Weber Test. Determined to substantiate their mostly anecdotal impressions, Prudden and Kraus administered the exam—six exercises to test back strength and flexibility, administered in just ninety seconds—to 4,400 American schoolchildren ages six to sixteen and to 3,000 of their peers in Switzerland and Austria. The results were as alarming as they had suspected: 57.9 percent of the American children failed at least one of the tests, while only 8.7 percent of Europeans performed as poorly. The children of the world's most prosperous country seemed not to be just weak, but rigid: 44.3 percent failed the flexibility portion of the exam, as compared to just 7.8 percent of Europeans.[2]

The mountain-climbing buddies struggled to bring attention to these findings and their disturbing implications, and as the postwar glow faded and Cold War anxieties intensified, they finally began to find the sort of big audience they sought. In July 1955, surrounded by politicians, business leaders, and athletic luminaries like base-ball star Willie Mays, Prudden and Kraus sat anxiously at a White House luncheon convened by wealthy Philadelphia businessman John B. Kelly Sr., a former national sculling champion and mili-tary officer horrified at the dire situation the study described.[3] As *Sports Illustrated* reported of the mood at the event, "it was one day the stars sat back." The audience digested the fact that nearly 60 per-cent of American children had failed to meet basic fitness stan-dards. It was impossible to ignore; American power was precarious, a fact embodied by the nation's youth.

The statistics were depressing across urban, suburban, and rural areas, as well as across social classes (there was no accounting for race), but it was the children who experienced the effects of what *Sports Illustrated* called "the playpen to the school bus to televi-sion—in short, America's plush standard of living" whose fate most alarmed those at the luncheon. Physical fitness was hardly con-sidered a key component of citizenship in 1955, but Prudden and Kraus began to impress upon the influential group in attendance, and most importantly the president, that its absence undermined national vitality, and even security. The data made it clear that the emergency was not just about personal health; the stakes were civic. A new generation of reformers and policymakers was needed to take up the cause, and urgently.[4] "Dear Dick," scribbled Eisenhower in a worried note to Vice President Richard Nixon, "after what we heard at the luncheon today, I really think we should try to take the lead in doing something."[5] Within a month, Prudden, Kraus, and a collection of advisers traveled to the White House to regroup, this time under Nixon's direction. The group recommended a govern-ment effort focused on youth fitness to begin right away.

Ultimately, it took almost a year for Nixon to gather the group again, this time at the Naval Academy in Annapolis, Maryland. One hundred forty government leaders, educators, youth and civic orga-nizers, members of the media, and health, medicine, and sports pro-fessionals attempted to parse the problem and devise a strategy to fix it.[6] The mood in Annapolis alternated between urgent appeals to stem the weakening of American children and cheery celebrations of the braver, fitter future that awaited the nation if its leaders would just commit to taking responsibility for the well-being of the "astounding" sixty-one million American children, expected to approach seventy-five million, in the coming decade.[7] Conferees such as Katherine McBride, president of Bryn Mawr College and one of only a few women in attendance, traveled to Annapolis at the behest of the president of the American Council on Education, enthusiastic to convince others that "fitness is not entirely a matter of muscles."[8] Rather, it was a matter of national security.

Despite the focus on amenities of the affluent like "the electric saw and power mower," the conference claimed a universalist mission that extended far beyond middle-class suburbs, printed at the very top of the mimeographed fact sheet distributed at the outset of their two days together:

ALL CHILDREN AND YOUTH!

This Conference is concerned with every child in every State and Territory. While the focus is an age-range 5–17 years, the implications for younger children, for older youth, and for adults will not be overlooked.

We hope to keep in mind the special needs of GIRLS AND BOYS:

of all races or creeds

of all socioeconomic levels

in their various stages of development, in urban, suburban, and rural homes

in crowded tenement sections and in well-to-do neighborhoods.[9]

Most states required less than ten years of compulsory public education, yet physical education was gaining greater presence in the school day, and the Bureau of Labor had the statistics to prove it: by 1949, over 75 percent of children took regular physical education, and job opportunities for physical-education majors were growing for both men and women. Less than 1 percent of the nearly five thousand physical-education graduates in 1955 were still seeking employment as teachers just six months after completing their degrees, and the conference's official fact sheets optimistically framed youth fitness not only as a physical state, but as a civic imperative, and as a growth opportunity: enrollments were ballooning, and the only subject matter that enrolled more elementary and high school students was English.[10] Citing a brightly illustrated, eight-page 1955 "career leaflet" titled "Recreation: A New Profession for Our Time," published by the American Association for Health, Physical Education, and Recreation, the conference organizers described promising job opportunities for "trained recreation personnel" not only in schools and municipal parks departments, but also in the thirty thousand companies that had recently created "active employee recreation programs."[11] At the same time, "meager space often remains for play areas," with over 90 percent of elementary schools having no gymnasium, multi-purpose room, medical suite, student showers, or hot and cold running water. The high schools fared far better in terms of infrastructure, but this fact was cold comfort to a nascent profession coalescing around the consensus that the teenage years were too late to form the habits of a healthy life.

"We are not a nation of softies," Nixon told the group, "but we could become one."[12] Nervous about the implications of this potential future for military preparedness in particular, President—and former general—Eisenhower was relatively quick to offer an official institutional response to the goals laid out by the conferees in Annapolis: to raise awareness of the importance of physical fitness for children and adults; to enlist community, civic, and private organizations in providing fitness and recreation opportunities; to enhance the prestige of physical educators and to provide them with greater resources; and to ensure children got regular medical checkups. Not to be forgotten, last was the commitment that "girls should have equal opportunities for physical fitness too."[13] On July 16, 1956, with Executive Order 10673, Eisenhower convened the Presidential Council on Youth Fitness (PCYF) and a Citizens Advisory Committee on the Fitness of American Youth, officially acknowledging that an unintended consequence of postwar prosperity was the atrophying of American bodies.

But the PCYF was designed as a "catalytic agent" meant to "educate and stimulate" the public to make fitness a priority, rather than an agency invested with an extensive budget or any power of enforcement. The athletes, educators, doctors, academics, and industry leaders that the PCYF brought together were tasked only to "sound the alarm" that the American public needed to commit to exercise in government, industry, home, and church.[14] Charged with preparing America's youth "physically as well as mentally and spiritually . . . for citizenship," the first PCYF—with Nixon as its chair and with the support of the several cabinet secretaries and the attorney general—received only minimal funding, deliberately limiting the council's role to that of "a stimulator, a catalyst," as Secretary of the Interior Fred A. Seaton characterized it when he became chair in 1958.[15]

Under Eisenhower, the PCYF was on a public relations mission to change popular ideas about the importance of exercise and fitness. Executive Director Shane MacCarthy traveled around the country, meeting with "communications media," religious leaders, sports associations, educators, and business leaders, imploring them to make fitness and recreation a focus of their work, whether as journalists writing feature stories, real-estate developers clearing shopping-mall parking lots on Sundays for "hardtop activities," or clerics sermonizing about the regenerative power of exercise. MacCarthy was zealous, arriving armed with anecdotes, as well as statistics and directives from the recently formed American College of Sports Medicine. He was looking for firm commitments: at each meeting MacCarthy provided a form which attendees were expected to fill out with their specific promise of how they would integrate fitness into their work.

For all the joy that suffused Prudden's programs back in White Plains, and the PCYF literature's repeated celebrations of "play" being well suited to children's "action-oriented nature," the council's mood under Eisenhower was unmistakably militaristic. When the conferees gathered again in the fall of 1957, at the US Military Academy at West Point, their signal achievement was devising a youth fitness metric based on military evaluation techniques. The military had itself recently reevaluated its approach to physical fitness, given the intensified urgency to "wean" new recruits

from a life that it too found was far more "soft and sedentary"—
and feminine—than that known by previous generations. With the
goal of turning a "boy into a man, and a man into a Marine," the
new approach offered progressions for physically weaker recruits,
emphasized teamwork, and discouraged negative talk. MacCarthy
gushed that it was "the most unique [he had] seen in this country."[16] Much to his delight, the Marine Corps and the JayCees were
soon collaborating on youth fitness programming using this model.
Some veterans and children enthusiastically stepped up in their own
communities, too. "Leadership by Marines in these [youth fitness]
programs is 'natural,'" Captain D. D. Chaplain of the 68th Rifle
Company wrote to the *Marine Corps Gazette* of a 1959 demonstration of Marine training techniques in Camden, New Jersey, that
attracted eight hundred youth and their parents. "Look around your
own community," Chaplain counseled fellow veterans, because fitness initiatives of groups like the Boy Scouts, YMCA, and Park
Commissions, "will be supporting the president and improving the
health of young Americans."[17]

Such an outright, over-the-top campaign was necessary because
Prudden and her peers were pushing physical activity in a moment
when most Americans were still overwhelmingly suspicious of the
virtues of exercise and the credibility of those who espoused it. The
cast of scientific research showcased this conventional wisdom.
One of MacCarthy's favorite studies reflected how slanted public
attitudes were against exercise: researchers examined thousands of
high school and college "lettermen" and assured a skeptical public
that regular physical exertion, particularly if it extended beyond
their years competing, actually enhanced rather than compromised
their health.[18] Forward-thinking doctors repeatedly had to assure
dubious Americans that *lack* of exercise might be more dangerous than exertion. "It's the luxury—not the stress or strain—that
is stopping hearts in this country. Exercise actually aids the heart,"
physician and exercise booster Paul D. White insisted to a generally
disbelieving public.[19] "The unlikely business of selling body conditioning, a commodity that in these comfort-loving times seems as
salable as a covered wagon," was how *Sports Illustrated* described

Prudden's peculiar vocation. Still stranger was her success at it, which the journalist attributed in part to Prudden embodying "the complete opposite of the classic caricature of the unattractive gym teacher," revealing yet another way that those devoted to a life of fitness were perceived as not quite normal, especially in gendered terms.[20]

Tending to one's health through diet or exercise was thought to be especially unseemly for men and boys, particularly when another prong in the Eisenhower administration's Cold War strategy was "cleaning house" of homosexuals, whose supposed loose morals and clandestine sexuality were thought to make them susceptible to blackmail.[21] Prominent figures, such as "wife of a famous senator" Lady Bird Johnson, strove especially hard in this environment to distance fitness from effete associations. In the *Baltimore Sun*, she wrote in 1956 of the "tricks" she had to play to nurse her husband back to health after a heart attack caused by his lifestyle, one typical of accomplished, "on-the-go" men: long hours at work, three packs of cigarettes a day, and meals of coffee and cold hamburgers. Once Johnson convinced her husband that counting calories and fat grams wasn't emasculating, but could be like "following World Series scores," he "fought every pound as if it were a political opponent."[22] When a New York State high school official was presented with the evidence that more than a quarter of "the youngsters in this country can't do one sit-up with the knees bent because they lack sufficient abdominal muscles, the muscles used in childbirth," he was unmoved and refused even more strenuously to administer the Kraus-Weber tests to his district, rejoining with a sneer, "All I can say is that it's a good thing our boys don't have babies."[23] Mocking radio hosts provocatively asked PCYF boosters why any children, but especially boys, should be wasting valuable instructional time on pursuits of the body as opposed to those of the mind.

Eisenhower was aware of such resistance when he established the council and took pains to authorize a logo that framed fitness as a lofty, worthwhile pursuit. But the gold lettering, black torch, and open book illuminated by gold rays of light—to symbolize enlightenment through exercise—was insufficient to offset the idea that fitness was a waste of time and tax dollars.[24] Indeed, the PCYF was at odds with the dominant opinion of educational reformers in the late 1950s, who for decades had criticized what they understood as the outsize influence of child-centered, progressive educational theorist John Dewey. One Department of Education official had in 1937 dismissed schools that focused on hands-on learning and designing curricula in response to the interests and identities of the child as "succumbing to a system of soft pedagogy which makes no demands on anybody anywhere."[25]

This disdain was pervasive: the 1947 Taft-Hartley Act, which severely limited the power of organized labor, effectively communicated that cerebral white-collar work was superior to the physical work associated with unions. Diluting challenging academic content in order to engage the mediocre middle with applied, utilitarian lessons in cooking, crafts, and basic bodily care merely taught students how to "adjust to life" and the world around them rather than analyze, master, or transform it, critics charged. Popular instructional films like *Control Your Emotions* that warned teenagers that both an inability to manage their intense emotions like rage and passion *and* to muster enthusiasm and socially appropriate outgoingness could "lead to a permanently warped personality" had no place in schools, they said.[26] To them, the PCYF and its promotion of fitness-for-all were part of this problem, and MacCarthy and his appointees found themselves engaged in a thankless "process of stimulating, urging, badgering, and cajoling communities, organizations, and individuals" who doubted the community pursuit of physical fitness should be a national priority.[27]

Spending on physical fitness was understood to be especially ill-considered just after the Soviet Union had displayed its technological prowess by launching Sputnik in October 1957. Only a year after the establishment of PCYF, Sputnik and the vision of education it inspired—a "superemphasis on technology and science"— presented a major obstacle to enacting the council's vision of schools as the primary sites to promote fitness.[28] Professionally managed youth programming that began as early as first grade, and district-wide workshops for everyone from administrators to educators to plant engineers, were recommended but unlikely to be implemented in schools under pressure to ramp up their academic offerings. Notably, the famous National Defense Education Act (NDEA) of 1958 didn't even mention physical fitness and narrowly focused on academic training in science and math as key to winning the Cold War.

But *both* the PCYF and NDEA were meant to educate a generation in order to ensure America's global ascendancy. Yet their two goals—intellectual and physical facility—were understood by many to be disconnected, and even at odds. At a "Sports for Fitness" workshop in Chicago in 1960, Rear Admiral Thomas J. Hamilton complained about this zero-sum mentality that fueled "the great competition for time, facilities, personnel, and money." The country's "mad rush for wealth and scientific achievement," however, he characterized as "aimed so that a person will not have to put out any physical exertion to do anything." This worldview affected the educators whom Hamilton believed should know better but who continued to "make derisive statements and recommendations to limit fitness activities." It was maddening, especially since the PCYF and its allies acknowledged "no one can deny the importance of science and mental development, but these should not be achieved at the expense of a healthy, efficient and capable body." Nothing made it clearer that fitness should be a Cold War priority, in fact, than a different Russian victory over the United States, not in space but in the summer Olympics. Using the phrase associated both with detonating a nuclear missile that could destroy the world and the automated home appliances that were killing Americans more slowly through atrophy, Hamilton quipped darkly that Americans were foolish to believe the Russians "are not preparing solely by a push-button."[29]

6

Fitness Makes Us Strong, Not Soft

"FITNESS MAKES U.S. STRONG," declared a 1959 PCYF poster in block letters set against a starry sky, framing a silhouette of a family of four, the son and daughter perfect miniatures of their wasp-waisted mother and slim father. Announcing the first "National Youth Fitness Week" in conjunction with May Day, the poster and its campaign make it difficult to imagine how the Council could be impugned as anything other than totally committed to cultivating Cold Warriors in a society plagued by "the effects of soft living."

Yet in some ways, this concern was understandable. Part of the problem with this "new education," critics such as historian Richard Hofstadter wrote at the time, was a misguided egalitarianism that actually fueled the anti-intellectualism that was a liability in a contest for geopolitical preeminence. Educators in the thrall of this wrongheaded impulse, Hofstadter argued, catered their work to "the dull boy, the defective child," squandering the intellectual resources of the more academically gifted students in favor of a watered-down, insipid curriculum that perpetuated mediocrity.[1] The PCYF pushed back precisely on the sort of elitism that Hofstadter celebrated, disdaining sports leagues, which in the council's esteem, are designed "for the gifted few, who are least in need of the experience, [and] get most of the benefit."[2]

Fitness, by contrast, was a more democratic alternative to sports and stood to include and benefit all Americans. Unwittingly articulating a commitment to exactly the kind of mushy inclusiveness that skeptics feared might undermine American fortitude, MacCarthy proclaimed in a keynote presentation in 1960, "Let's never forget that there is no cutting from the squad of fitness!"[3] That is exactly the problem, his critics must have grumbled. Lack of emphasis on individual excellence could also serve to make the PCYF seem to smack of something scarier: communism, or worse, fascism. Photographs of Hitler Youth and Communist athletic training were often circulated as everything America was *not*, and almost indistinguishable images of state-sponsored calisthenic and athletic youth programming suggested that such activities would enforce ideological conformity rather than individualism.

By contrast, however, promoting exercise as fun and free could go too far in signaling the extreme opposite of an unthinking, regimented militarism. When one boy was asked to define what fitness meant to him, he breezily replied: "Being able to do what you want to do." Interpreting this vague answer as "a paraphrase of the Boy Scouts' 'Be Prepared,'" the PCYF proudly included the apparently charming and laudatory anecdote in a November 1959 report.[4] Yet this sweet story could be construed quite differently: was the council actually, and troublingly, an engine of permissiveness and pleasure-seeking, rather than staunch, individualistic virility? PCYF claims that fitness could cure youth delinquency by "forestalling the sexual impulses from monopolizing and taking priority in the emotional life of the adolescent" proved no more convincing. "Youth wants and admires discipline, and too often adults give them license," one council pamphlet argued in defense of such fitness programming.[5] In a moment when training one's body was more likely to be understood as a distraction from moral and mental development than a worthwhile pursuit, the PCYF still had to tread lightly.

Most of these debates about the appropriateness of teaching fitness transpired at elementary and secondary schools since they were so bound up with national purpose and public financing. But institutes of higher education were also grappling with how physical fitness fit into their offerings. In 1950, a group of intramural directors from eleven historically Black colleges and universities gathered at Dillard University in New Orleans to discuss the value that intramural sports and recreation brought to college students; there, they created the National Intramural Association. In 1957, Purdue University established the country's first university recreation center for students who didn't play on varsity teams, celebrating the role of recreational fitness in a full educational experience. Such initiatives expanded access to "purposive fitness" and further established it as a pastime of the college educated. Universities all over the country evidenced this ethos, even when speaking of other subjects. In a 1952 radio broadcast, the chancellor of New York University announced a plan to expand the campus, using the idiom of physical fitness: "To make sure the university will contribute to the future . . . the university, like any individual, should seek to improve itself. . . . A great university must be dynamic, and keep flexible enough, physically and financially." An announcement about extending the academic mission of the university—"to make knowledge more accessible to everyone"—also meaningfully reflected that democratic sensibility.[6]

If physical-fitness boosters were to sell busy adults on the value of exercise, it was important that colleges impart these values, for the jobs their graduates would hold had the same sorts of harmful physical effects the council sought to combat in children. The office jobs that conferred white-collar respectability on these college graduates also kept them dangerously sedentary, as they sat in cars and trains on long commutes, only to spend the day languishing at a desk. Emergency rooms swelled with patients suffering arterial blockages and heart attacks, and the press frantically reported on a "coronary plague" overwhelmingly affecting men— four hundred thousand in 1956—that threatened the very future of the nation.[7] "Nervous strain" manifested through heart disease was a poorly defined, unquantifiable risk factor that the *New York Times* hazarded was inextricably bound up with modern existence. Men "in the prime of life" were at the greatest risk of fatal heart attack, a condition that had barely existed in the first quarter of the century and raised essential questions about the price of prosperity. Even the pope weighed in on this affliction of the "well-off classes of society and the professions" particularly susceptible to the "agitated pace of modern life and the wear it entails for the (human) organism."[8] Speaking before a delegation to the International Convention of Cardiology, which included President Eisenhower's own heart consultant Paul Dudley White, the pope cast coronary illnesses as a dire threat to the well-being and integrity of "the whole man."[9]

White amplified this message a few months later, emphasizing that doing *any* sort of exercise would stave off increasingly common and potentially fatal thrombosis. The physiological benefit was only the most immediate payoff. "An intense mental worker needs his mind clear," White explained. Evoking the "peripatetic philosophers" of classical Greece, White advised his contemporary counterpart to alternate "mental concentration" with physical movement, or even to do the two simultaneously.[10] An oft-quoted British study compared the far higher instance of ill health and early death among bus drivers than the conductors who circulated about the vehicle and the station, unwittingly getting exercise. It was not a far reach for a generation of office workers to contemplate the comparable dangers of their own thickening midsections. "Wonderful appliances" liberated many women from domestic grunt work endured by their foremothers, but one entreaty to exercise recognized that the constant work of "bending and stooping to pick up after lazy husbands and children" kept women relatively more physically fit than men. Since "obviously, we aren't all going to do household chores to stay physically fit," this public service announcement pronounced, men who needed to be prodded to care about their paunches but could not be bothered to pick up their socks had better start "wearing out their shoe leather instead of shining the seat of their pants."[11]

Because beauty, bodily care, and social survival had long been intertwined for women, inspiring them to commit to exercise for themselves and their families continued to be, in some ways, less challenging. The illnesses of the heart "so much in the news" largely afflicted men, but even *Vogue*, with its female readership, ran a multipage interview with a "Heart Blood Authority" about cultivating heart health for men and women. The editors convened three physicians, who, emphasizing gender, explained in detail scientific research demonstrating the "protective effect of [the] female sex hormone," and discussed the challenge of convincing men to undergo the experimental treatment or even exercise, as some seemed reluctant to "give up their manhood solely to avoid a heart attack." Awkwardly, one of the editors asked the lone woman on the panel, endocrinologist Jessie Marmorston, whether she had ever administered these female hormones to "prevent the look of aging in post-menopausal women." Her answer was a terse no.[12] "Prevention is much more valuable than treatment, surgical or medical," concurred the *New York Times* in describing an emerging scientific consensus in 1957. But convincing a generation unaccustomed to exercise to "establish a regular habit and to maintain it through thick and thin" and to consider this activity "just as essential to good health as eating, sleeping, and working," as White, Eisenhower's own physician did, was no small feat.[13]

Despite Eisenhower's best efforts, somberness and scare tactics were not inspiring Americans to get moving in any measurable way. His successor, John F. Kennedy, amplified Eisenhower's alarmism about the civic dangers posed by what he memorably styled the "soft American." But Kennedy also expanded the definition of exercise and fitness considerably. Fitness programs might still be militaristic, trying to convey seriousness and moral uprightness—like the program at southern California's La Cañada High School, which showcased rows of muscular children and sinewy teenagers performing calisthenics and the like, usually in perfect sync and silence—but it could also be "fun to be fit." Fitness was best understood as a lifelong habit rather than a means to a narrow end like military preparedness, Kennedy ventured.[14] He dropped the "Youth" from the PCYF, reflecting this broader conception, and reframed fitness to be a mark of affluence itself, rather than a punishment to offset its excesses. Deliberately participating in fitness activities signaled that one was sufficiently educated and disciplined both to do cerebral work and to use time off productively.

The youthful, handsome Kennedy (who was treated by Kraus for some of his considerable health issues) proved a far more compelling poster boy for fitness than had the bald, aging, militarily rigid Eisenhower. Under JFK's leadership, this new public commitment redefined fitness as a right—and responsibility—of American citizenship and of a fully actualized selfhood in an age of affluence. Unlike his predecessors, Kennedy and his family were often photographed playing tennis, swimming, and horseback riding at their vacation compound in Hyannis Port, Massachusetts.[15] Their love of the active life—and just as importantly, the *look* of the active life—preceded JFK's presidency, and even the PCYF. Already part of a powerful political dynasty, brothers Robert, John, and Ted Kennedy posed shirtless in the Palm Beach surf for *LOOK* magazine in April 1957, their bodies not quite Muscle Beach material, but undoubtedly fit and unapologetically on display. Most of all, the three smiling brothers looked like they were having fun, and that being physically active was a natural part of being wealthy, attractive, and able to strike an appropriate balance between discipline and leisure.[16]

Kennedy had grown up engaging in what he called the "vigorous life," through private-school sports and summers on Cape Cod. His experiences there and as a member of the Harvard swim team were typical of the upper class, but the youngest president to date was the first to so publicly parlay support for this vigorous life as a form of self-improvement, civic duty, and *pleasure*. Philip J. Kelly made this contrast clear in his 1963 book *How to Grow Old Rebelliously*: "President Eisenhower demonstrated dramatically that regular exercise will make a sick man well . . . [but] don't think that scientific and regular exercise is fun. It isn't intended to be fun. It's work, but it's constructive."[17] Kennedy presented exercise differently, and in a way that made him vulnerable to criticism: scorning the president's "fits of fitness," one essayist contrasted Kennedy's passions for skiing in Aspen and "fitness" in general as inferior to the hardier, "strenuous life" of hunting and boxing advocated by Teddy Roosevelt.[18]

Yet by declaring fitness an honorable, masculine, and healthful pursuit, JFK challenged the ingrained assumption that intellect and exercise were mutually exclusive, framed fitness as an

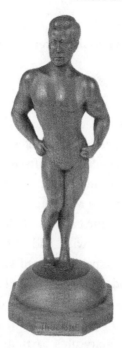

Figure 6. Stephan Swiatek, *Sculpture of John F. Kennedy as Mr. America*, 1963. President John F. Kennedy is depicted by sculptor Stephan Swiatek in a way that signals both his role in encouraging fitness among Americans and the way that agenda made some people perceive him as superficial. He poses as Mr. America upon a base inscribed with the words "Pull In That Gut America."

WOOD SCULPTURE, 12" (30.5 CM). JOHN F. KENNEDY PRESIDENTIAL LIBRARY AND MUSEUM, BOSTON, MA. GIFT OF STEPHAN SWIATEK. MO 74.555. HTTPS://WWW.JFKLIBRARY.ORG/ASSET-VIEWER /MO-74555-JFK-AS-MR-AMERICA.

appropriate leisure activity beyond his elite set, and drew explicit inspiration from Teddy Roosevelt's promotion of ruggedness. In 1908, Roosevelt had challenged the Marines to hike fifty miles in three days.[19] Kennedy raised the stakes to fifty miles in *one* day, and he invited his whole staff to take part. Robert Kennedy took on the task most publicly. Wearing Oxford loafers that were soon soaked by rain, Robert, along with four members of his staff and a rambunctious dog, set out at five o'clock in the morning. Some of the party dropped out, and the team nearly abandoned their mission altogether halfway, but the press continued to photograph the dwindling squad from helicopters. Alone in the snow and slush by mile thirty-five, Kennedy finished the journey and joked that as miserable as he was, he couldn't renege on a physical challenge from his brother.

"Trying to popularize walking in America is like trying to popularize prohibition in Kentucky," journalist James Reston quipped in response to what he dismissed as a mere publicity stunt, and typical of the president's fickleness.[20] Nonetheless, all over the country, and even the world, civilians took up the fifty-mile challenge that the *Baltimore Sun* described as an "instant fad," if an often physically painful one. Washington secretaries and students were trying out the new "craze" that had "jumped the banks of the Potomac," and which one journalist compared to "the twist" and "rock and roll," or less favorably, to the fads of college panty raids or swallowing live goldfish.[21] In Boonsboro, Maryland, at the JFK 50 Mile ultramarathon, only "a couple dozen" aspirants showed at the starting line in its early years.

But by 1973, over two thousand American and Canadian hikers and joggers ages ten to sixty-plus participated in the increasingly popular but brutal event. One fifty-three-year-old man cut his head on the rocky Appalachian terrain, completing the run swathed in "bloody, makeshift bandages," while another spectator wept at the suffering he witnessed: "Some of those guys should have been shot out of mercy."[22] Europeans responded to JFK's entreaty enthusiastically as well. Nearly six decades later, residents of the town of Sittard in the southern Netherlands continue to compete annually in their own local march—as they have since 1963, when four local boys read of Kennedy's challenge and set out to meet it.

Echoing concerns about the perils of the groupthink that state-sanctioned en-masse exercise could engender, others were entirely unimpressed with the challenge and its surprising popularity. White House correspondent Merriman Smith reported on the perception that the "hiking craze brought out the lemming qualities not only of Americans generally, but the Kennedys too."[23] *Town and Country* devoted several pages to criticizing the "personal fetish" Kennedy had made of athletic endeavor, forcing public concern with fitness, even though "like motherhood, what we do about it should be no one's concern but our own." The hike might be useful for military training, the angry article conceded, but "it is as useless for an attorney general or an atomic scientist to do this as it is for a long-distance runner to . . . know quantum theory." Not only were such physical feats futile, but there were no civic benefits either. "Even if every man, woman, and child in the United States managed to walk fifty miles with three copies of the *Congressional Record* on his back it probably wouldn't make us a better nation in any way or help us solve a single problem."[24]

Even exercise boosters took exception to the fad. The PCYF never endorsed the fifty-mile hike, which was so much more intense than the fifteen minutes of daily activity it recommended that even some fitness enthusiasts worried it might scare Americans away from exercising at all, or at least injure those foolhardy enough to undertake it. At the University of Texas, swim coach and youth-camp owner Tex Robertson sniffed that "fifty-mile hikes are fine for Robert Kennedy, Marines, and anyone else who likes them," but emphasized that individuals must "find their own fitness way."[25] Even a Pennsylvania athletic director and physical education teacher who described himself as a "crusader" in the "renaissance of physical fitness" acknowledged that the council never recommended the arduous hike as "the answer to overall conditioning," or even as "physiologically sound," but conceded that it could inspire people to fight against the "apathy and indifference" that had permeated daily life over the last half century.[26]

But the hike was just one example of Kennedy's consistent efforts to underscore the idea that "softness on the part of individual citizens can help to strip and destroy the vitality of a nation," as he wrote in the December 1960 issue of *Sports Illustrated*. "The harsh fact of the matter," the president-elect sternly acknowledged, was that there existed "an increasingly large number of young Americans who are neglecting their bodies—whose physical fitness is not what should be—and who are getting soft." The failures of both adults and children to exercise were equally problematic. Together with the Advertising Council and the Newspaper Executives Association, Kennedy's council ran print campaigns urging parents to help "get the kinks out of the kids" by lobbying their local school boards for more vigorous physical-education programs that would slim them down.[27] In *Sports Illustrated*, the president-elect echoed over a century of health reformers and policymakers who espoused the moral and civic benefits of exercise—but in emphasizing the ugliness of a soft body, he amplified the importance of aesthetics as well.

In 1962, Kennedy pointed out that while Americans were healthier than ever—that is, free from infectious disease—their bodies were less agile and strong. The invention and affordability of new biomedical remedies had diminished the threats of fatal and debilitating diseases of polio and influenza, such that not even children's-health activists advocated especially strenuously to provide medical care at school for children assumed to be generally safe from life-threatening disease—a departure from earlier practice, when many children might *only* receive medical attention there.[28]

No such assumption stood around physical fitness, however. Thousands of letters from children reached the White House, complaining of poor fitness facilities and the fact that teachers often punished the misbehavior of individual children by holding the whole class back from recess or physical education. As one third-grade boy wrote, "since this happens almost every day, we do not have P.E." Perhaps it was because the teachers, overweight themselves, did not understand the importance of exercise, other children speculated. Girls in particular complained about exclusion; one teenager from Oklahoma wrote that though she and her friends tried to follow Kennedy's recommendation to walk to and from school in order to avoid getting "flaby" [sic], the teachers insisted that exercising in public was "unladylike" and that such behavior would "give our school a bad name." Other students, like one fifth grader sore from fifty sit-ups and ten push-ups, complained that the exercises themselves were punishment: "Do you think it is fitness if you end up feeling worse after your [gym] exercises than before you start?"[29]

Children's fitness dictated the future of the republic, and in the minds of Kennedy and his advisers, adults had to be reeducated to proactively change popular attitudes about exercise. That endeavor was intertwined with transforming ideas about parenting: one 1960 pamphlet quoted the American Medical Association's support of the PCYF's pursuit of a "virile brand of young citizenship over the protests of many fathers and mothers who overprotect their own children." Potential injuries like a fractured ankle, the PCYF reported with satisfaction, were likely to "leave less of a scar than a personality frustrated by reasons of parental timidity."[30] This work began with exercise for babies, whose physical *and* psychological health were at stake. In the spring of 1960, in celebration of National Youth Fitness Week, Prudden offered a full fitness program for babies beginning with "diaper gymnastics," which *Sports Illustrated* said was so important "because it puts the responsibility—and the opportunity—for improving children's fitness where it belongs: on the parents."[31]

The idea sold, and as awareness of the salutary effects of exercise caught on, Prudden escalated her rhetoric about the importance of encouraging exercise during childhood. An advertisement for her 1964 book, *How to Keep Your Child Fit from Birth to Six*, proclaimed that "these *first six years* determine your child's future posture, habits, personality, even health." Parents had the power to give their children fit bodies and thus happy lives; a "gift that can't be bought, lasts a lifetime," the bold print exclaimed—or threatened. Should parents *not* head off "today's fatal trend toward the flabby physique," the ad warned, the blame for children's future unhappy lives in ugly bodies rested squarely on them.[32] For all the federal promotion of exercise, the PCYF's own marketing placed more responsibility on individual parents than on institutions. "NOBODY ASKED YOU!" screamed one 1962 headline ostensibly directed at parents who might claim ignorance of the educational program at their kids' schools. "It's time for *you* to take the lead. . . . Find out whether your child's school has an adequate program, and if not, *how come?*"[33]

The idea that parents should enforce a certain level of fitness at home was not entirely new. Bernarr MacFadden and his wife, Marguerite, had coauthored *Physical Culture for Babies* back in 1904, recommending that a mother's physical-culture regime begin as early as fourteen days after birth. The MacFaddens had also conceived of exercise as necessary to save children from the dangerous effects of the modern culture they both loved and feared. Similar to Prudden, who enjoyed a comfortable suburban existence but saw that very ease jeopardizing a generation, the MacFaddens had asked: "Is it too Utopian to dream of a land of sunshine and sand and birds and flowers, where the babes of new generations shall revel untrammeled by housing and clothing and the burdens of the vices of our present civilization, and yet be the recipients of all that same civilization is endeavoring to give childhood . . . ?"[34] Separated by more than fifty years, Prudden and the MacFaddens shared a sense of exercise as ennobling and uniquely able to resolve this tension, and of mothers as responsible stewards of the process. But in the early 1900s, the MacFaddens were outcasts, or at least eccentrics, whereas Prudden relatively quickly had the ear of policymakers, physicians, and even several presidents who helped promote these ideas.

By 1963, the PCYF had dropped the "Youth" in its title to display its commitment to encouraging regular exercise for *all* generations. But it was one thing to push already playful children and babies to more intense forms of physical activity, and another entirely for parents to participate—enthusiastically or at all—in cultivating their own fitness. Ironically, this focus on the playful nature of fitness could make exercise an even harder sell to adults who had grown up in a culture skeptical of its utility. Still, Americans were talking about exercise, and warming to its inherent value, even as they debated the *type* of exercise most appropriate for Americans with differing physical needs. Celebrity spokespeople were key to this ambitious reframing of fitness. In 1961, Kennedy appointed wildly popular football coach Burnham "Bud" Wilkinson as a special consultant on physical fitness. During the 1950s, Wilkinson had been the country's most successful college-football coach, leading the University of Oklahoma to unprecedented victory. Placing a football coach at the helm of a fitness initiative—when Eisenhower's PCYF had worked so hard to distinguish recreational fitness from exclusive athletics—was no accident. Associating exercise with a winning football team burnished its image as a noble, quint-essentially American pursuit.[35]

Even Jack LaLanne, who had distanced himself from his Muscle Beach roots, soon became a spokesperson for the federal initiative. In one 1963 ad, the Presidential Council for Fitness (PCF) promoted isometric contractions as a military-inspired approach to fitness for the whole family. From a technical perspective, this "no-strain exercise" was indistinguishable from Charles Atlas's "dynamic tension" method, which had seemed peculiar just a few decades earlier when it was mostly associated with mail-order advertisements in the back of comic books.[36] By the time of Kennedy's death, the same exercises were promoted by the federal government. And just as LaLanne emphasized how happiness awaited women who took time to train their bodies, Kennedy's PCF began using the term "physical IQ," linking cultivation of the body to the more respectable development of intelligence.[37] Its basic program of fifteen minutes of vigorous daily physical activity similarly promised not only to make children physically "nimble and quick" but also to turn them into "doers" rather than "sitters and spectators," the cost of which was far worse than a flabby waistline.[38]

Eisenhower's efforts had been mostly directed at boys, but this expanded definition of exercise as a path to enjoyment and attractiveness was more palatably pitched to women and girls. Exercise could help women stave off heart disease as it did men, and it could also enhance a woman's beauty. Prudden, whose activism was rooted in a commitment to building strength among a younger generation, and later their parents, had sensed this opportunity early on, repackaging a version of her program in the 1961 title *How to Stay Slender and Fit after 30*. In contrast to the sober tone of her more academic work, Prudden emphasized how *fun* exercise could make life, because it made you attractive and energetic. "There is no area of living that would not be affected by vitality, a strong attractive body, desire, and drive," Prudden wrote. But it took the will to work—"harder even than an Olympic athlete in training" who competes only for medals, while her readers strove for the loftier goal of "a second chance to live as nature intended you to live, and to enjoy the rest of your life to the hilt."[39] Appearance was just as important as health, Prudden made clear, cajoling the complacent woman who might weigh the same 134 pounds as on her wedding day, but who stuffs herself into a girdle only to "move like a hippopotamus" on "a pair of outsized pneumatic legs." Men too must take an honest look at themselves beyond numbers on a scale; an apparently respectable 185-pound weight "won't do a man much good if most of it has run to his stomach." Making male appearance a greater focus than it often was in this era, Prudden pointedly raised an equal-opportunity body criticism: "Would he still look as good in his wedding suit?"[40]

Striking recognizable chords with Helena Rubinstein, Elizabeth Arden, and a generation of slenderizing entrepreneurs who were her contemporaries, Prudden's contribution to this conversation differed because she was first established as a *health*, rather than a beauty, authority. When Rubinstein donned her white coat in the salon to assert vague clinical expertise, it was in the realm of dermatology or cosmetic chemistry. But Prudden traveled in the world of biomechanics experts, public-health reformers, and mental-health professionals, using this authority in a way that would only expand the popularity and power of the emerging imperative to exercise. Anticipating the resistance of some readers of *How to Keep Slender and Fit after Thirty* who might "feel that none of this applies to you, because *your* troubles are 'psychosomatic,'" Prudden reassured them: "There is a fifty-fifty chance that your long-suffering soma is merely taking revenge on your helpless and miserable psyche. Just which comes first is not important—the main thing is that you do something about it." That something was exercise.

Importantly, for all the White House's bold declarations of the "universal" importance of fitness, its concern with the ill effects of suburban life narrowly focused on the white, middle-class people who lived in these leafy, segregated spaces and all but ignored racial minorities, inhabitants of rural and urban areas, and those with disabilities. Moreover, these initiatives were long on inspiring messaging and marketing and short on lasting infrastructure. Indeed, many such programs were born of Eisenhower's "catalytic agency," cobbled together with the support of local districts, community organizations, and celebrity spokespeople, not long-term federal investment.

This lack of enduring investment was not all that was amiss in what was no golden age of physical fitness. The PCYF/PCF programs were bold in celebrating fitness but articulated its value relatively narrowly. The Cold War citizen that the programs prepared was envisioned as male, athletically capable, and white. The girls' curriculum, rarely featured in publicity campaigns, was mostly an afterthought: its anthem, "Chicken Fat (The Youth Fitness Song)," announces, "All right, girls, you're in this too!" in between encouragements to "the flabby guys" who were the real focus. Even as Kennedy, following Prudden's lead, worked to expand the meaning of fitness to be about enjoyment, play, self-fulfillment, and personal development, the constant measurement and ranking of children's fitness by educators and policymakers—activities that were core to the federal initiatives—reminded students exactly which bodies were most valuable to society.

For a time in the late 1950s and early 1960s, private and public sectors collaborated to promote fitness as a civic commitment and, secondarily, a desirable commodity. Under Kennedy's leadership, the federal government worked with states and municipalities to enhance public physical-education and recreation and fitness programs, and partnered with actors and athletes to redefine exercise and recreation as a core personal responsibility and privilege. Even after the shuttering of the Santa Monica public playground that had germinated this mainstream exercise culture, a generation of entrepreneurs—many with Muscle Beach roots—began to promote fitness for all, or at least for women as well as men, and for the young and old alike ("old" meaning over forty). Thanks to the efforts of the PCYF/PCF, these entrepreneurs enjoyed a strong foundation on which to continue to transform Americans' understanding of fitness. Participation in the industry they built was limited to those who could afford it, but people who had little in common with these clean-cut Cold Warriors would also come to embrace exercise as an important part of their identities. Suburban housewives, sinewy bodybuilders, and slick gym impresarios would become the ambassadors of this industry, selling individual empowerment, rather than civic duty, through exercise. "Try to sell it to the kids," is how *Parents* magazine had paraphrased the PCYF's early attempts to "dramatize the importance of fitness," and in the decades to come, Americans with greater purchasing power than children would become ever more willing to spend on sweat.[41]

Part **Three**

FROM MARGINS TO MAINSTREAM

Good health can be merchandised just like automobiles.
VIC TANNY

Back when Bonnie Prudden began to speak out about lack of youth fitness, she was an almost lone voice in connecting exercise to civic health. But pleas of those, who like her, boosted exercise for more than militaristic discipline came to resonate powerfully in a culture that prized individual initiative and self-improvement, at church, in school, and on a growing slate of moralistic television shows. Such ideas, however, were only just beginning to show up at the gym.

Pastor Norman Vincent Peale, who had become a household name with his 1952 bestseller *The Power of Positive Thinking*, which captivated millions with its can-do spirituality and promises of "personal efficiency" in business, romance, and friendship, knew gyms were unlikely places for self-discovery. To emphasize the power of his thesis that *any* environment or interaction could, buoyed by the right attitude, begin the path to spiritual salvation, he set one anecdote in that long-suspicious, unlikely site: the gym. Interviewing Jack Smith, a onetime prizefighter, trucker, and taxi driver whose latest venture was "a health club patronized by many outstanding people," Peale reported that Smith's strategy was to "probe" patrons for both "physical and spiritual flabbiness," for "you can't get a man physically healthy until you get him spiritually healthy." Smith knew few would expect moral regeneration to be on offer at the kind of business that provided "exercise, steam baths, and a rubdown," and he laughed as he recounted a client whose "jaw dropped in astonishment" when he saw the letters penciled on the wall above Smith's desk: APRPBWPRAA, short for "Affirmative Prayers Release Powers By Which Positive Results Are Accomplished." The client collected himself and explained his speechlessness: "Well, I never expected to hear anything like that in a health club."[1]

Indeed. But such anecdotes about finding salvation and self-fulfillment through exercise would become far more common in coming years, thanks not only to the labors of policymakers and health experts who fanned fears of Soviet victory and soft midsections, but to entrepreneurs, intellectuals, and individuals who in the same period promoted and embraced the idea that cultivating the body was not a path to enslaving the mind—rendering one literally muscle-bound, as many had feared—but imperative to its liberation.

7

The Future Belongs to the Fit

"Take a thoughtful look into the future and this much is clear: the future belongs to the fit. The future belongs to those vigorous enough to live it—and shape it!" According to the Presidential Council on Fitness, which penned this declaration in a 1965 advertisement, the pursuit of fitness held providential promise for those engaged in it—and darker ends for those who didn't.[1] Slowly, American children were beginning to show improvements in physical strength, stamina, speed, and coordination.

"What was once superior is now run-of-the-mill," boasted one PCF consultant of rising standards of physical fitness to *Parents* magazine. This typical article assumed a relatively affluent reader: a physically active childhood set Americans up to "become healthier, more productive adults . . . better equipped to enjoy the leisure our society is providing in equal measure."[2] But these visions of a fitter future were no longer restricted to the white, middle-class suburban boys who, as potential future soldiers, had been the focus of its early campaigns. As the sixties wore on and civil rights and antipoverty activists brought attention to the intense inequalities that shaped American life, the growing ranks who were expected to enlist in the project of exercise as self-improvement were found not only in the boys' physical education classes of suburban schools, but across gender, age, race, and geography.

Cracks were also appearing in the postwar suburban idyll, as journalist Betty Friedan activated a generation of dissatisfied suburban women who saw their own lives in her descriptions of the "problem that has no name." Criticism of the bodily effects of suburban life ratcheted up and found a readier audience among those taking a newly critical look at their surroundings. Sedentary comfort was now seen as leading obviously to slothfulness. "Physical fitness, or the lack of it, is not a problem confined to youth alone," a "public interest advertisement" by the American Dairy Association pronounced in 1962. Mr. Joe Citizen, the fictional protagonist of this four-page feature, is a successful office worker who moves from a car with "power-steering, power brakes, power window lifts, and power seat controls" to a cushioned commuter train to a desk where he is delivered lunch ("tycoons" also dine out on "martinis and rich food"). Joe unwinds after work with two drinks, reclining before the TV. Even his weekend recreation—golf—involves an electric golf cart and celebratory cocktails, a routine that renders him "less vigorous than his wife might desire."

The dairy lobby had an agenda in recommending people exercise rather than cut back on cheese and milk, but the parable of Joe Citizen meaningfully defined fitness as more than physically salutary, and not only for kids. Joe needed to *make better choices*, like "walking three miles a day," electing to participate in vigorous sports like cycling or football, or even leaving the car at home. "Fitness," declared the dairy lobbyist loftily, was "a matter of achieving an optimum state of wellbeing that enables us to live and to enjoy living to the maximum extent that our mental development and environment can offer us." The rationale for exercising was simultaneously "patriotic, economic, [and] purely selfish," a formulation whose capaciousness owed thanks to the growing acceptance of the "interrelationship among physical, mental and moral, or spiritual factors in contributing to good health and happiness."[3]

Even in communities that did not fully enjoy the fruits of postwar prosperity, boosters called for the promotion of fitness as fundamental, often by amplifying anxieties that people were not exercising enough. In 1968, the *Milwaukee Star* pleaded with readers to combat lack of fitness among Black urban children, advocating for universal compulsory physical education with an urgency usually reserved for math or science instruction: "We must teach certain things whether our pupils like it or not."[4] Even the few among that cohort who took up exercise, like Black teenage girls, often did so for what were understood to be the wrong reasons: to "look slim, elegant, and hungry—like fashion models"—rather than keeping their "bodies in good condition" for higher aims of civic and personal health, the *Star* complained. Failing to address such misguided ideas and harmful behaviors imperiled individuals and the nation, agreed policymakers, health professionals, parents, and business interests poised to profit from this new fascination. "It may take time to change attitudes, but we cannot afford not to try," the *Star* concluded.

A constant stream of such hand-wringing articles found such a receptive audience in the 1960s because a revolution in ideas and attitudes about exercise was afoot, as many Americans came to recognize exercise as imperative not only to physical health and civic duty, but to social and emotional thriving. A widening variety of actors—not just a loose network of physical education teachers, public health advocates, and gym owners directly involved in the provision of exercise—were beginning to embrace two core ideas that laid the foundation for physical fitness to become a social imperative. The first idea drew on the classical ideal of *mens sana in corpore sano*: mind and body are inseparable, and humans cannot flourish without cultivating both. Health, and even happiness, was unattainable without exercising the body. The second idea was that individuals have a right and responsibility to take control of their own health. These convergent ideas invested new energy into the act of physical fitness—whether doing toe-touches in PE, mail-ordering an Atlas program, or propping up a magazine spread to "stretch for slimness and beauty" on the living-room carpet.

Back when Bonnie Prudden had implored policymakers to make physical fitness a public priority, this emergent consensus was unimaginable. Yet a decade later, it was equally surprising that the federal government, though it had been inspired by those early activists, would not lead this transformation in American ideas about exercise. Nor would city or state governments, despite their many task forces and committees and public service announcements and often loudly professed enthusiasm for physical education and public recreation. Rather, a nascent commercial fitness industry embraced the council's idea that "the future belongs to the fit" with more energy and investment than the state ever had, and it linked this lofty vision with individual fulfillment—and purchasing power—more so than with civic engagement or collective uplift. With no less urgency or grandiosity than the White House in calling citizens to get fit to fight the Cold War, this new cadre of entrepreneurs and health enthusiasts passionately marketed physical fitness as delivering something more than mere physical health: full selfhood and social status.

Taking personal responsibility for cultivating mind and body as an integrated, coherent whole was not a new idea: it originated in the all-male gymnasia of ancient Greece. In the United States, various niche groups of exercise enthusiasts, who were largely mocked as outlandish, had been saying as much since the early twentieth century. Especially in an industrial society where the so-called better men were so disproportionately concentrated in cerebral, sedentary professions, these boosters began to gain traction when they emphasized that exercise was necessary to offset the unhealthy bodies caused by such work, and eventually, to generally improve the self.[5] "We need exercises that require effort, precision and accuracy to discipline the mind and strengthen the will and to give a satisfaction of accomplishment," the *Daily Health Builder* had counseled skeptical readers in 1928. Ahead of its time, the text recommended deliberate exercise as "the method that nature used to make a superior race out of the ruck of the common crowd." The stakes were racial, spiritual, and moral: quick-fix "pills," "massage," or even passive displays of piety were no substitute for physical exertion, for "faith without works is dead."[6]

A broader "therapeutic culture" that optimistically emphasized the positive outcomes of working on individual psychological health encouraged Americans to focus on their interior lives in order to actualize their full potential. New conversations about regulating one's feelings converged with the ethos of military discipline. During

World War II, military doctors had deployed psychological tactics to enhance the performance of the troops, convincing military personnel that even dissatisfaction with external circumstances— like servicewomen "disgruntled" with their assignments to "typically feminine occupations" like cooking and cleaning, or soldiers depressed by having to wait long periods for assignment—was a result of personal maladjustment. Overcoming such malaise, these therapists maintained, was often a matter of mustering individual will. Connecting mental well-being to the completion of particular physical feats became an attractive way for these psychologists to point to concrete proof of the success of their methods, like in the case of a young man who overcame a fear of pole climbing by doing it, and accepting a diagnosis that his overprotective parents had instilled him with irrational fears.[7]

After the war, economic, political, and cultural shifts that would eventually serve to ennoble the pursuit of exercise began to take hold among both individuals and institutions. In addition to higher rates of homeownership and educational attainment and increased average income, the survival struggles of two world wars receded, as did Depression-era privations and the threat of crippling polio that had restricted earlier generations' definition of health, now aided by innovations in biomedicine.[8] A 1948 statement by the World Health Organization codified this crucial foundation for this newly expansive definition of *health*: "a state of complete physical, mental, and social well-being and not merely the absence of disease or infirmity." Personal health, defined in similarly expansive terms but rarely centering exercise, dominated the life-adjustment curricula of the 1950s. Filmstrips and mimeographed worksheets developed by social psychologists and educators instructed children to consider their bodily and moral health as intertwined. From undertaking proper hygiene to resisting the urge to engage in backseat "petting" and striving for "emotional balance," it was up to students to proactively and preventively care for themselves.[9]

Outside schools, this greater confidence borne of rising life expectancy also boosted interest in mental and emotional health.[10]

In psychology departments, on the pages of *Reader's Digest*, and on the office couches of a growing therapeutic profession, ideas like "healthy narcissism" began to gain traction.[11] "The most important challenges to medicine today," even the corporate morality tale of Joe Citizen acknowledged, "are to teach human beings that the human body . . . does require certain minimum standards of care."[12] Individuals, susceptible to the unhealthy temptations of modern life but expected to aspire to thrive rather than merely survive, bore responsibility for upholding these "standards," rather than physicians. It would take until the 1970s for New Age seekers all over the country to flock to "wellness" workshops to learn about a concept of health in which there are "no patients," only individuals who decide to proactively engage in this "active process through which people become aware of, and make choices toward, a more successful existence."[13] But in the years following World War II, the seeds that made this sensibility possible were nurtured by a culture ever more enamored of health as a holistic state that signaled individual virtue.

The notion that mental and physical health were intertwined, and that the steward of this new state of holistic fitness was the individual, was sufficiently novel to require explanation in the 1960s. "The body and mind work together and it is important that they both be maintained in a healthy, wholesome condition," Philip J. Kelly advised readers of his 1963 book, *How to Grow Old Rebelliously*. Aside from women buying beauty products, taking action to stem aging *was* a novel idea, and Kelly strongly recommended that young and middle-aged men "make an effort to maintain this desirable condition" via regular physical exercise.[14] Three years later, in *Your Good Health*, Eleanor Chappell and Kathryn Huss were just as didactic in explaining the importance of exercise to women readers apparently unfamiliar with the idea that "emotional upsets can cause physical problems." If women did not appreciate how peace of mind was indispensable to physical thriving and vice versa, they could hardly be expected to make the "additional effort of self-discipline and self-understanding" required to achieve this state. Especially prone to preoccupation with "imagined slights and vague aches and pains," according to Huss and Chappell, women stood to benefit most from mastering the "marvelous gift" of an integrated human brain and body.[15] Exercise, such boosters emphasized, was not just an avenue to fend off fears of a "blubbery youngster," a heart attack, or unpreparedness to fight the Cold War. It was imperative to a well-rounded life.

8

Training for Life—Body and Mind

In California, a Latvian-born woman who had taken the name Indra Devi was introducing Westerners to this radical idea that exercise and self-actualization could and should go hand in hand.[1] Her medium was an unfamiliar practice to most Americans: yoga. Devi played up the exoticism of the practice that enabled her to perform superhuman feats such as standing on her head for thirty minutes and not suffering a cold for as many years. In her marketing materials, Devi wrote of traveling to "far-off India, primitive civilization of the ancients" in order to study yoga when western medicine had failed to cure a persistent heart ailment. In yoga, she had found "relaxation and refreshment, physical and spiritual."

As Devi characterized it in her 1953 book, *Forever Young, Forever Healthy: Simplified Yoga for Modern Living*, a yogi had no need for pills or surgery to cure ills from over (or under) weight to fatigue to graying hair. Americans who tried it, she promised in an ad, would "exercise [their] mind and body to the full."[2] Most importantly, Devi emphasized to Americans skeptical not only of exercise but of certain religions, that *her* yoga was secular. Even in a 1956 article that described how one of Devi's students moved to Cambodia and became a Buddhist monk, she downplayed any mystical associations, and always asked to be described in the press as a "woman exercise instructor."[3] In 1959, she even insisted on the term "relaxation" rather than "yoga . . . because people will laugh."[4] Framing yoga as secular ironically made the exercise practice more palatable both to God-fearing Americans and the godless Soviet Union. Devi

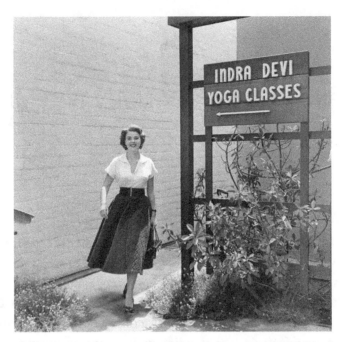

Figure 7. Earl Leaf, *A Student Walks Out of Indra Devi Yoga Studio in Hollywood, California,* 1952. A smiling student exits Indra Devi's Hollywood yoga studio circa 1952. Devi's efforts to demystify yoga for a clientele more interested in health and beauty than spiritual enlightenment proved so successful that she enjoyed international popularity.

PHOTOGRAPH. GETTY IMAGES, MICHAEL OCHS ARCHIVES. EDITORIAL NUMBER 596709037. HTTPS://WWW.GETTYIMAGES.COM/DETAIL/NEWS-PHOTO/STUDENT-WALKS-TO-INDRA-DEVI -YOGA-STUDIO-IN-HOLLYWOOD-NEWS-PHOTO/596709037.

demonstrated yoga at the Kremlin in 1960 and later recalled the minister of foreign affairs barraging her with questions about "whether it was a religion." Not at all, Devi assured him, it was just "a method of physical, mental, and spiritual training," something more and more people could agree was harmless, and even healthful.[5]

Despite the exotic cast of yoga and the "blue silken saris" the silver-haired Devi favored, she strove to position this Eastern practice as an antidote to the woes of "modern living" that troubled Americans. Office workers, housewives, and executives who brought home their work, Devi commented in 1955, stood to benefit from movements such as "the rocking exercise," rolling back and forth on one's rounded back, and arching and flexing "like a cat." Really, "anyone who does sedentary work" could benefit from these and other exercises, she said, but women concerned about aging could particularly profit from the way this practice harnessed the power of the mind. "Mental attitude is very important. You are young as long as you think you are young. Women fear they are old early and that makes them older—the fear of age is more aging than anything else."[6] Notably, Devi not only emphasized the power of deliberate thought to shape the physical body, but maintained that a brow furrowed with worry *literally* caused wrinkles.

Most such "tired-blooded Americans" who sorely needed stretches and breathing would never take a headstand alongside Greta Garbo, Gloria Swanson, or Aldous Huxley, who all frequented Devi's ethereally appointed studio. The effects of this celebrity association, however, reverberated among women and men ever more likely to encounter a version of yoga-for-exercise at their local YMCA or recreation center—or even on the factory floor. In a two-day workshop Devi held for workers at a garment factory, "employees had mats and stretched out near machines, cutting tables, and desks" to practice rhythmic techniques and stretching poses she called out over a microphone. Even a "skeptical male manager" who denied anything could relax him, one newspaper reported, gave her poses a try and dozed off. Six months later, the factory owners reported "physical and mental improvement of their workers" and higher rates of productivity.[7]

"Every week another club has a Yoga program," a glowing *Miami Herald* feature reported, because it's "an ancient do-it-yourself science" that enables practitioners to access "the intuitive knowledge" of themselves that "was supposed to be [theirs] in the first place." Freeing "the mind and body to make them work for you through a specific form of exercise and meditation," as the Corpus Christi YMCA billed its yoga offerings, was an appealing proposition far beyond Devi's California, a region long especially hospitable to countercultural experimentation and out-there body beautification techniques.[8] As early as 1959, the Phoenix, Arizona, YMCA and YWCA cosponsored an evening lecture on yoga, which they explicitly defined as a "major system of Hindu discipline." Yet the ensuing biweekly classes that taught physical movement—separate for men and women—were billed just as expressly as exercise, *not* religion.[9]

The holistic transformation enabled by yoga and its perceived gentleness were both selling points to publics skeptical of certain forms of exercise. In Edmond, Oklahoma, one YMCA launched its first yoga class to a crowd of thirty-two women drawn in by the "deliberate and graceful" moves, so different from the "more violent thrashing about of most calisthenics." Jeanette McElvany, the married, thirty-nine-year-old grandmother and secretary who began teaching these Monday evening classes after two years of study, explained that yoga "brings you to a fuller realization of your full potential, both physical and mental." She did not, however, "subscribe to the religious parts of the rituals . . . just the exercises and the meditation and the concentration."[10] For those who lacked the "get-up and go" to jog or cycle before work, one Dayton, Ohio, advice columnist recommended, yoga was the ideal solution; any "householder, student, sportsman, executive, or street cleaner" needed only "self-discipline" and "self-effort," and perhaps a course at the local YMCA, to get "Physically Fit through Yoga."[11] YMCA classes were inexpensive and often came with childcare, like at one Milwaukee club where adults and children could simultaneously pursue "figure shaping, fitness, and fun."[12]

Some yogis taught both at overtly spiritual sites *and* at the YMCA, like a Canadian swami who directed the Montreal Sivananda Yoga Vedanta Centre and did a residence teaching hatha yoga at Honolulu's Central YMCA.[13] Like Devi, many YMCA yoga teachers were white, possibly a factor that made an unfamiliar practice more palatable to white Americans. These white teachers repackaged and profited from Indian traditions, but they also sparked an interest in yoga that helped create opportunities for South Asians who found a more willing consumer public. Kiku Mehta, a Bombay native who taught yoga while studying international law at the University of Pennsylvania, told the students who "twisted and grunted" through his beginner class at a Camden, New Jersey, YMCA that despite the popularity of his class, he was dismayed that yoga had "acquired a poor image in America." He rejected the same stereotype as Devi:

that of the spiritual fundamentalist who "sleeps on a bed of nails" or the sideshow act that "sticks pins in their bodies." On the contrary, Mehta described the benefits of yoga for busy urbanites. While "cosmic union with the Creator" was an ultimate goal for the most serious practitioners, "control over the body" to lose weight, stop smoking, and sleep better were more reasonable outcomes for committed beginners.[14]

Harnessing the power of the mind through yoga would not encourage practitioners to challenge dominant ideas about the body but enable them to conform to these cultural expectations, media coverage often emphasized. "She Lost 20 Pounds during a Training!" announced the leading caption of a profile on a yogi giving a workshop in Dayton, Ohio, buried several paragraphs below an account of her spiritual journey. Addressing a female reader ostensibly enticed by the slender, white woman on the cover of her 1968 book *Slimming with Yoga*, self-styled "beauty authority" Dodi Schultz explains that, "contrary to the belief of many Westerners, Yoga is not a religion; it is a way of life—both physical and spiritual." Yoga, Schultz reassures, is a means to achieve the goals "that every American woman shares"—"spiritual" in the most liberal sense— "strength and suppleness, grace of movement, and a lovely figure."[15] Yoga-as-fitness introduced Americans to the idea that their body was a (secular) temple.

Across the country, against a backdrop of city streets and back-lit theater marquees rather than palm trees and suburban subdivisions, a very different set of actors were also stripping away the tawdry associations that clung to fitness, and instead promoting the idea that exercise was important to a life fully lived. The most influential missionary of the mind-body connection in this milieu was no sun-bronzed bodybuilder, but a German hospital orderly. Having overcome a frail childhood through gymnastics, skiing, diving, and tussling with his eight siblings, Joseph Pilates moved to England where he worked as a boxer, self-defense trainer, and "living Greek statue" in the circus.

During World War I, Pilates was detained on the Isle of Man and jury-rigged resistance contraptions out of hospital beds and medical equipment to devise a rehabilitative system to strengthen the muscles of prisoners of war. Some swear this regime spared acolytes from the deadly influenza epidemic that ravaged Europe in 1918. Others say these devices were prototypes for the machine that came to be known as the Pilates "Cadillac." Back in Germany after the war, Pilates declined an offer to work with the military and instead trained professional dancers in his evolving technique. In 1926, Pilates emigrated to New York on a second-class ticket and with five hundred dollars in his pocket, and three years later, out of his dark, cramped Studio for Natural Rejuvenation on Eighth Avenue in Manhattan, began offering instruction in a system he called "Contrology."[16] In 1934, he published *Your Health*, a book that championed the importance of "conscious control of all muscular movements of the body" as the way to achieve "the balance of body and mind." Pilates was decades before his time in celebrating this unity and using strength training to achieve it, and he found his first willing audience—that is, not captive prisoners of war—among a niche group especially invested in harnessing the full potential of their physical and mental powers: professional performers who rehearsed near his studio and heard about its strange but effective methods from one another.

In 1940, Romana Kryzanowska was a seventeen-year-old student at the School of American Ballet when she injured her ankle and was certain surgery awaited her. George Balanchine took her by the hand and led her to his friend Pilates's small studio, where the injured ballerina was at first intimidated by the unfamiliar sights of "men with bare chests and a lot of hair sweating all over the place." She called her mother back in Detroit to complain about the awfulness of the place—but soon realized that the bodywork that she did with "Uncle Joe" and his romantic and professional partner Clara on the wooden apparatuses had not just healed her ankle but helped her leap higher than ever.[17] Kryzanowska came back daily long after her injury had healed, becoming an apprentice to defray the ten-dollar session fee, and later Pilates's protégée. She wasn't alone in her enthusiasm. "The petite opera star finds that twisting and stretching her muscles improves her singing," read a profile of singer

Elaine Malbin. The regime involved strengthening exercises for the chest and back, breath control, and torso mobility. The "diminutive soprano," pictured smiling and stretched over one of Pilates's apparatuses, had developed such strength that Pilates, twice her weight at two hundred pounds, could stand on her abdomen without injuring this "toughest diva."[18] Among New York City singers and dancers, Pilates needed little introduction by the 1950s, as profiles of esteemed performers like Metropolitan Opera coloratura soprano Roberta Peters referred to his "special system of strengthening all parts of the body" through breathwork and exercise that enabled the vocal range on display in operas like *The Magic Flute* and *Rigoletto*.[19]

The Eighth Avenue space was near choreographer Martha Graham's studio, a proximity that helped Pilates's credibility as the go-to place for dancers in need of physical rehabilitation. The workshops he ran at the Jacob's Pillow retreat in western Massachusetts, a destination for dancers, only solidified that reputation. And for nearly forty years, performers were the main clients of the muscular, cigar-smoking physical culturalist. Yet as late as the 1960s, strength training was still strange for those who defined themselves as dancers rather than athletes. "None of us [dancers] cared about strength or core training until Pilates came along," professional dancer Elisabeth Halfpapp recalled. "Then it became something all of us did."[20]

But in the 1960s, Pilates's system began to become popular among women who saw the potential for "contrology" to calm their minds and "whittle" their waistlines. "Around the United States," the *New York Herald Tribune* reported in 1964, "hundreds of young students limber up daily with an exercise they know as 'a pilates,' without knowing that the word has a capital P, and a living, right-breathing namesake."[21] Mostly women, these new students had no designs on a professional dance career, but were attracted by Pilates's promise that they could *look* like dancers—not weight lifters. This anxiety, which Pilates and the programs he inspired assuaged, persisted for decades: one journalist who discovered Pilates in the 1990s sang its praises for not making her look like "Sylvester Stallone's separated-at-birth twin

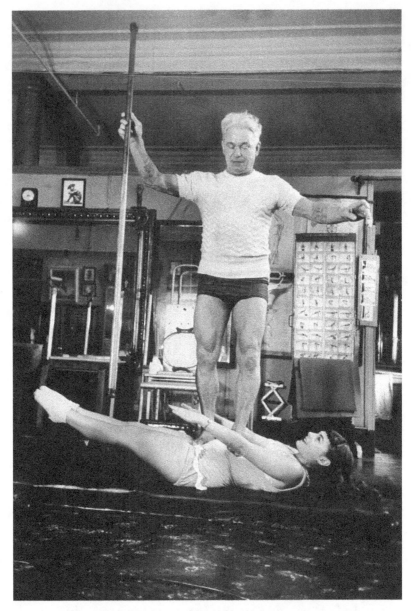

Figure 8. Michael Rougier, *Opera Singer Roberta Peters Balancing Her Trainer, Joseph Pilates, on Her Operatic Breadbasket*, 1951. Joseph Pilates balances on the body of his client, opera singer Roberta Peters, at his Eighth Avenue studio in New York City in February 1951. Pilates's method spread by word of mouth among performers, and then through frequent press coverage, to clients who wanted to look like dancers and singers.

sister."[22] Dance, as opposed to weight lifting or even most sports, was associated with grace, poise, and prestige—traits considered more enticing to the growing numbers of girls and women interested in becoming physically active in the 1960s.

This fusion of dance and exercise in the 1960s also reoriented the geography of the emerging fitness culture beyond California. If the West Coast had always attracted more than its share of health nuts who experimented with strangely colored vegetable concoctions, bodily practices, and alternative medicines, New York City was the capital of the dance and theater world, and it was there that these disciplines elevated the definition of recreational fitness in a new way. Kryzanowska helped the Pilates method evolve to become known by "all the best people in New York and Europe . . . [including] the Vanderbilt family." Jay Grimes, a professional ballet and Broadway dancer, began studying the Pilates method under Romana during the mid-1960s, and he remembered that part of the appeal of Joe's outlook was how he never intended people to be "working out in the gym for hours every day," but *always* to be exercising, just as a dancer's whole life is structured by the discipline: "There comes a point where you become Pilates and Pilates becomes you."[23] Pilates died in 1967, without trademarking his program, but his practice and its offshoots lived on, initially through the efforts of the "first-generation" group of dancers who taught classes and opened their own studios after his death. In 1976, five Pilates studios existed—including Kryzanowska's 57th Street setup in Drago's Gym, run by a former gymnast—and twenty years later, its trademark contested, five hundred did.[24]

The career that a Cuban American ballet and ballroom dancer named Cal Pozo found teaching fitness shows how powerfully Pilates shaped popular understanding of exercise and its relationship to dance. Pozo had moved to New York City from Toledo, Ohio, to dance classical ballet in the early 1960s. Within a decade, however, in space he rented at the dance studio where he rehearsed, he realized he could make more money training women in a Pilates-style format he developed on his own than he could dancing professionally. He was discreet about this work, though, since he considered instructing exercise as a bit déclassé for someone who taught at the esteemed Fred Astaire Studio. "You have to understand," he told me, "I was thinking '*I am a dancer*.' And if teaching jazz is below ballet, teaching exercise is even lower than modern." But his success was undeniable, and he went on to write a fitness book, *Bunnetics*, that garnered attention from the morning talk shows and national press for this "professional dancer [who] has just come out of the closet with his phobia . . . of a fat and sagging derriere."[25] Interestingly, Pozo was gay, and understandably tight-lipped about his sexuality with his clients, though he noticed that something about his affect subtly abetted his success as an instructor. Somehow, he told me, the husbands of his female clients felt "just fine with me spending an hour alone with their wives working on their bodies. . . . Sometimes a man would come in and just announce 'I love what you've done for my wife's ass.'"[26] As opposed to the image of the dangerous "sexual athlete" that stigmatized the men at Muscle Beach, gay men who hailed from the prestigious world of dance and theater could seem less threatening. Pilates was crucial to forging that connection. By the 1990s, *Joe Weider's Shape* magazine commented that "Pilates" was as familiar a brand as Kleenex or Band-Aid, but was "practically synonymous with the dance community," so might be more likely to be taught in a studio than a gym.[27] Both would soon multiply.

9

The "Tanny Touch"

Vic Tanny described himself as "a political as well as physical messiah" to *LIFE* magazine in 1958. But it wasn't exactly clear whether the Muscle Beach bodybuilder-turned-gym-impresario's house of worship was his own body or one of the more than sixty gyms he operated, a significant proportion of the 750 gyms and reducing spas that operated across the country. Especially concentrated in Southern California, brick-and-mortar gyms were becoming popular places where everyday people—five million nationwide—were slowly beginning to adopt the habit of regular exercise in earnest.[1] Every hour spent working on one's fitness at his establishments, Tanny promised, brought members one step closer to a better body, and more importantly, a better *life*.

But exercise-as-actualization, or even as worth the price of a health club membership, was still a tough sell in 1958. It wasn't as bad as 1938, when the Tanny brothers remembered the response to the first gym they had opened in Southern California, on a property for which they paid just thirty-five dollars monthly rent: "Nobody knew anything when we first opened. People would come in and say, 'Are we supposed to pay you to lift those things?'"[2] They hadn't been surprised when no one joined them to lift weights at the gym they had opened a couple of years earlier in their native Rochester, New York, hardly a capital of body culture, but the chilly reception in California came as a shock.[3] It shouldn't have: LaLanne had had a very similar experience opening a club in Oakland, hoping to attract aspiring athletes and health enthusiasts. "People thought I was a charlatan and a nut," he recalled. "The doctors were against me—they said that working out with weights would give people everything from heart attacks to hemorrhoids; that women would look like men."[4] The problem was partly aesthetic—the stereotype of morally suspect, hulking men leaning over rusty weight racks amid clouds of stale sweat and cigar smoke died hard—but it was also existential.[5]

Even in the late 1950s, Tanny later reflected, most men were mortified to "expose their potbelly and desire to get rid of that potbelly in a public gymnasium."[6] The very impulse to exercise, even more so than inhabiting a body that looked like it could be improved by physical exertion, was shameful. Exercise was not just unfamiliar, many assumed, but louche. Anticipating a common stereotype—unquestionably informed by Muscle Beach—the parable of Joe Citizen in one pro-fitness article confronted this assumption head on, acknowledging that many people believed that "physical fitness has been advocated by those people who seem to think that we all need bulging muscles and taut tummies so that we might stand around on the beach in very brief leopard skins to be admired by one and all."[7] In the *Nation*, George A. Silver, chief of social medicine at New York's Montefiore Hospital, went so far as to "ponder the mental health of some of the characters . . . who you see sunning themselves and developing their muscles on the various beaches and gymnasiums."[8]

Tanny gyms were temples that endeavored to elevate exercise to take on a trapping of wealth and health. "The Tanny touch" meant soft lighting, tropical murals on the wall, and equipment for members to take a steam, get a massage, or lift weights while their feet sank into thick red carpet and the calming tune of a waltz wafted through deodorized air.[9] Meaningfully in an era of increasing residential segregation, the fact that Tanny clubs opened in posh neighborhoods solidified the connection between exercise and an exclusive address. Any landlord would be "proud to have a Vic Tanny gym on your property," specified an advertisement seeking Baltimore locations. Reassuring skeptical landlords that a community's best elements would flock to Tanny gyms, he listed his outposts on the "fashionable Miracle Mile on Wilshire Boulevard in Los Angeles, Market Street in San Francisco, and Knobb Hill section of Albuquerque."

Less-coveted locations, one ad unceremoniously announced, would not be considered: "LANDLORDS, PLEASE IF YOUR PROPERTY IS NOT IN THE NUMBER ONE SECTION OF YOUR COMMUNITY, DO NOT TAKE THE TROUBLE OF CONTACT-ING MR. VIC TANNY IN LOS ANGELES."[10] LaLanne followed suit in linking gym-going with a luxurious aesthetic, decorating his chain of European Health Spas with shimmering tile and neo-classical statuary.[11] He hosted Hollywood stars at the openings of Los Angeles clubs, and a Scarsdale location housed a four-hundred-pound caged baby tiger to "symbolize grace, strength, and speed."[12] These entrepreneurs aggressively exploited the new notion that exercise was laudable and worthwhile, but more so as a perfor-mance of individual affluence than of civic commitment.

Operators of these newly sanitized clubs all over the country strove to dispel unseemly associations. Fresh off three years learn-ing the business as manager of five West Coast Tanny clubs, Alex Schwarzkopf opened his own "Mr. Alex Gym" in Boston's Kenmore Square neighborhood. In 1961, a journalist for the *Jewish Advocate* warned readers not to be fooled by the word "gym," which still con-veyed a "dingy, odoriferous, grunt-and-groan palace." Like his men-tor, Schwarzkopf built well-lit, even swank, facilities for men and women that expanded beyond core bodybuilding offerings: tanning beds, gold-plated equipment, wall-to-wall carpeting, rock steam baths, two ten-pin bowling alleys, and masseurs and masseuses were all on offer.[13] In Kansas City, a LaLanne European Health Spa boasted Scandinavian plunge pools, hot springs, "desert-dry heatrooms" engineered to approximate the Arizona climate, and tanning beds.[14] Such amenities inspired some weight lifters and bodybuilders to accuse such entrepreneurs of selling out to the mainstream fitness fad their preferred pastime had helped create.[15]

Paradoxically, as Tanny and fellow fitness entrepreneurs resisted the enduring assumption that fitness was effete, a core aspect of their strategy to upgrade its image was to attract women and children to

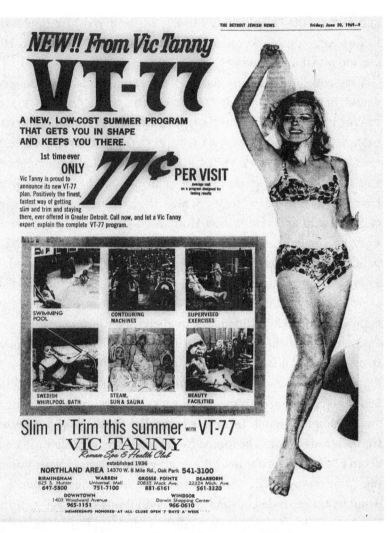

Figure 9. *New!! From Vic Tanny VT-77,* June 20, 1969. By the late 1960s, Tanny gyms were a national chain, famous for their amenities and aggressive membership sales tactics— a strategy copied by facilities all over the country.

their increasingly cosseted clubs. Bowling alleys and tropical fish tanks entertained wide-eyed children while women could exercise on Ladies' Days or relax in the spa. They took inspiration directly from their Muscle Beach peers, Les and "Pudgy" Stockton, who had been early to entice women to weight-lifting gyms, largely because of the example Pudgy set as a beauty queen whose muscles only enhanced her curves. The Stocktons opened a women's gym in a Sunset Boulevard storefront in 1948. The fact that it was primarily a weight-lifting facility was astonishing given that "passive exercise machines"—essentially vibrating belts and tables set up for circulatory massages to reduce cellulite as women "relaxed in luxurious comfort"—were still the types of exercise devices considered appropriately ladylike.

The Stocktons delicately navigated this context, naming the Sunset Boulevard gym the "Salon of Figure Development," and covering the walls in patterned wallpaper and wood paneling. Equipment "made to look more like furniture . . . put women at ease" in an environment that resembled a backdrop for homemaking more than one for heavy lifting.[16] The incongruous juxtaposition of weight racks and delicate floral wallpaper signaled how Stockton played with gendered stereotypes, welcoming women into a space suggesting physical strength could be respectable *and* ladylike. In search of a ritzier crowd, the couple opened side-by-side men's and women's clubs in tony Beverly Hills in 1950, and soon after, inland in Pasadena. Like many former Muscle Beach personalities, they realized that the public was becoming haltingly more appreciative of their commitment to building strength, beauty, and health as laudable.[17] The Stocktons found themselves devoting more time operating their gyms than performing at the beach, and savvy entrepreneurs such as Tanny were inspired by the opportunities their example suggested.

When Stockton gave birth to a baby girl in 1953, she had retired her column and stepped away from the gym business—but her championing of strength training for women had introduced an enduring and important challenge to the no-effort approach dominant in the gym and in products aggressively marketed to women in a largely unregulated market easy to exploit, especially as consumers had begun to equate exercise with health and beauty.[18] "Propagandizing and pamphleteering" for fitness was everywhere, one critic pointed out, placing all physical fitness boosters on a continuum with "the quacks in the field who are milking Americans of huge sums of money for exercise courses, posture and exercise classes and devices supposed to improve muscular efficiency."[19] The ambiguity about what "fitness" meant and ambivalence about those who pursued or promoted it was understandable, as ads for the latest health spas and mail-order products promised similarly improbable miracles of bodily transformation. In the early 1960s, as an enterprising Brooklyn weight-lifter with a BS in civil engineering, Samuel N. Kram developed the "Super Speed System," promising men could build a "giant" chest and arms and "magically reduce" the waist within weeks, working with only their body weight, a towel, and a wooden chair.[20] "Sinkram's Super Speed System" was essentially a booklet of pencil drawings of a muscular man in a bikini bottom executing foundational exercise moves: triceps dips, push-ups, and jackknife leg extensions. Yet Kram, who stood 5'3", had launched his career with a different, impossible product: a "Height Increase System" that promised vertical growth through "the proven principle of interstitial accretions" within twenty weeks (daily growth chart included). "Can an adult add to his height? The answer is an emphatic *yes* as you will now find out," proclaimed advertisements in New York City newspapers and a national network of men's magazines.

Seven thousand people bought that system, and the ensuing 1963 Federal Trade Commission (FTC) lawsuit revealed the blurred line between marketing physical transformation through exercise and peddling pure fantasy. Kram claimed to have grown inches himself, results no one at the Brooklyn YMCA could corroborate. The same caveat went for the fifty-four-year-old witness of "very limited education" who worked as "a porter in work involving the lifting of heavy objects," and who pointed to the two measurements taken by his wife to prove that Kram's system had successfully elongated his 5'7" frame by one and a half inches. The prosecution marshaled the porter's lack of education and manual-labor job to explain why he misinterpreted postural adjustment as a change in stature. Predictably and effectively, FTC lawyers argued that the thirty-year-old Kram, and the collaborators and clients of his "Height Increase Institute," were not credible sources. Such men were easy marks for Kram's patently fake "Institute," which displayed in its marketing materials "an ornate building of considerable size in an apparent park-like setting" that looked nothing like the "one room in a store" out of which Kram and his wife worked. Absent a library or medical staff, the program was based on a handful of popular articles published in the 1930s—some in French and translated by the monolingual Kram with a French-English dictionary. Ultimately, the court decided, no "exercise instruction course or program" could use such "so-called research material" to make false promises of bodily reinvention.[21] The Height Institute was an obvious scam, but the FTC approach made little distinction between such products and those that did so through the more credible endeavor of regular exercise.

Exercise cons were not solely the province of small-time hucksters like Samuel Kram. Bernard Stauffer owned a national chain of 250 reducing salons for "movie stars and housewives alike," and the next year, he faced similar charges for making unfounded claims about the "Posture-Rest Magic Couch," a vibrating seat that allowed women to "posturally reduce through effortless exercise at home." The FTC lawsuit challenged Stauffer's promise to rid women of the inches of fat around their waists, ankles, and thighs. But Stauffer was a formidable defendant, counting over five million women as clients, and operating a factory sprawled over five acres, where six kinds of reducing tables and the Magic Couch were manufactured. By the middle of the 1950s, Stauffer counted clients nationwide and shipped devices as far as Australia and India, where he bragged he counted a princess as a client. Stauffer had begun his career in the vaguely defined "therapeutic field," and touted the credentials of his staff.

On one episode of *Success Story*, a 1950s television show that profiled Southern California businessmen, the host visited Stauffer's research division, where he scrutinized the devices with the precision of an "aircraft inspection"; a visit to the medical section

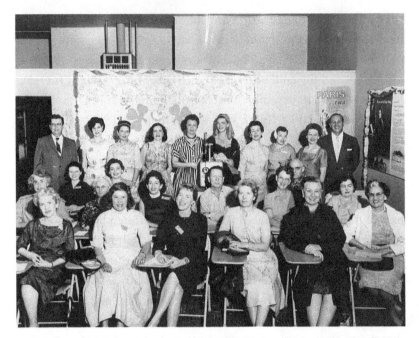

Figure 10. *Help Beauty, Posture at Stauffer Clinic,* 1959. Stauffer "beauty counselors"—who were trained to project an aura of clinical expertise and an optimistic outlook—attend a professional-development clinic at the corporate headquarters in Glendale, California, in 1959.

PHOTOGRAPHIC PRINT, BLACK AND WHITE, 8.27" × 10.24" (21 × 26 CM). *VALLEY TIMES* COLLECTION, LOS ANGELES PUBLIC LIBRARY, LOS ANGELES, CA. ORDER NUMBER 00140283. HTTPS://CALISPHERE.ORG/ITEM /711A48F627C7439CDA782DD68A4C545B/.

yielded a vague conversation about "classified" research on "hypokinetics," a muscular disorder.[22] It was apparently mostly for show. For the FTC case, Stauffer marshaled his own, laughably weak, evidence for the Stauffer Principle: anecdotes submitted by customers aspiring to be featured in the company's "10 Happiest Women" ad campaign, and a study from a general practitioner on the company payroll. The FTC experts, he seethed, didn't understand the business of personal transformation, but were "a bunch of article-writing professors who teach rehabilitation of crippled people, not overweight persons."[23]

Tanny and his contemporaries were no article-writing professors, but they resisted the something-for-nothing proposition, and they mocked those such as Stauffer who marketed "effortless exercise, without work or effort."[24] Tanny's tough-love reminders that "you can't do it by lying on a table and getting bumps and electric shocks," explicitly poked fun at this delicate-flower mentality and signaled new attention to women as capable exercisers. The equal-opportunity, suggestive tagline "Take it off, build it up, make it firm" promised men *and* women that rigorous exercise would allow them to "enjoy every moment and . . . have fun starting a new life."[25] Of course, some such invitations, even as they opened the traditionally male space of the gym, reproduced old assumptions about female frailty and the primacy of beauty as a fitness goal: many clubs promoted weight loss more aggressively to women, were entirely sex-segregated, or—in offering "Ladies Days"—reaffirmed that mixed exercise was improper.[26] At the same time, in enticing women to exercise relatively strenuously, and outside the home, these entrepreneurs unquestionably and self-consciously pushed past their predecessors. Genuine, if ridiculous, confusion about the effect of such novel types of exercise on women's bodies could arise: in 1957, a California woman facing "impending maternity" threatened legal action against Tanny, claiming that despite years of childlessness, she had become pregnant the day she signed her membership contract.[27]

The national empire Tanny imagined was ultimately short lived, but the broad-shouldered, silver-haired crusader and his peers had succeeded in establishing the appeal of a distinctly Californian concept of health, beauty, and happiness that had fitness at its heart and was achieved at the gym, by men and women who paid a membership fee to participate. And it was becoming increasingly clear that it would not be professors, policymakers, or physical educators who most powerfully shaped ideas about fitness and its appropriate place in American life. Midcentury television personalities joined fitness entrepreneurs in promoting, with little regulation, exercise as inextricable from enviable beauty, youth, health, and wealth.

10

Slimming on the Small Screen

Between 1945 and 1959, American home television ownership exploded from fewer than ten thousand sets to over fifty-two million: nearly nine out of ten households had one.[1] More than airy yoga studios, mail-order products, or plush-carpeted health clubs, this was the medium that accelerated exposure to exercise for most Americans. Now, the message that exercise was both enjoyable and integral to a healthy, productive life was reinforced, every mid-morning, in a thirty-minute program led by a former Muscle Beach bodybuilder, at home. Exercise television was ultimately successful, but when Jack LaLanne pitched studio executives a fitness program in 1950, they scoffed at the idea that anyone would tune into a show about exercise, much less follow along in their living room, *especially* when the host had made his name posing at seedy Muscle Beach.[2] Undeterred, he launched his eponymous show out of his own pocket the following year.[3]

Millions of homemakers soon tuned in for LaLanne's folksy fitness advice, which combined exercise instruction with snippets from his personal transformation from a child so sickly he became "psychotic" due to poor diet and idleness into a smiling, suntanned, paragon of physical and emotional health. In LaLanne's telling, exercise had enabled nothing less than a reinvention of the body and soul. Crippled by splitting headaches as a teenager, LaLanne had accompanied his mother, a Seventh-day Adventist, to a packed health seminar led by a man named Paul Bragg, who pointed directly at LaLanne and blamed him for treating himself no better than "a human garbage can." That night, adolescent Jack prayed. "God," he implored, "please give me the strength to exercise when I don't feel like it . . . and the fortitude not to eat dead, lifeless foods" when the urge overcame him.[4] Staring straight into the eyes of viewers at home, undistracted by his dog Happy yapping cheerily around him, LaLanne insisted they too must reinvent themselves through exercise to be better wives and mothers and to just plain *feel* better.

"Come on, get out of your easy chair. . . . Trimnastics time again," LaLanne invited viewers each morning. Metamorphosis would not come from sitting on the sidelines as a spectator to their children's baseball game, or politely listening to their husbands reminisce about time on the front lines of the war. Women had to make time for exercise, for their own sake. "Now if you're going to improve yourself and you're going to make this body of yours over when are you going to do it? Yesterday? Tomorrow? Christmas? There's only one time to start improving yourself and there's only one time in your life and you know when it is? . . . NOW. N-O-W. This can make your life or break it."[5] Looking better was part and parcel of personal transformation. "Which One Watches the Jack LaLanne Show?," a nationally syndicated newspaper advertisement coyly queried. If the side-by-side photos of women's backsides, identical but for their girth, weren't obvious enough, the copy explained that "the woman who follows the Jack LaLanne Show isn't hard to spot. She usually has a lovelier figure, a more youthful looking face than other women her age."[6]

How radical was the *Jack LaLanne Show*? For a generation of women taught that exercise was unladylike and even dangerous, the half-hour, grainy black-and-white program made a radical proposition: exercise was essential to achieving self-assurance. Despite cutesy cues, like instructions to tone the "front and back porch," his words for abdominal work, LaLanne stared intensely into the camera and told women at home, "You're an intelligent person."[7] He reassured viewers that they would not "ruin their figures with exercise"; it would only make them prettier. But *not* exercising paved a sure path to ruin, aesthetic and otherwise. The show was full of such mixed messages, both breaking with received wisdom *and* upholding dominant beauty ideals. Clad in his signature muscle shirt, biceps exposed, LaLanne rejected ageism: "You know what age means? Law of nature is use or lose. If you don't use it, you lose it. Age means absolutely nothing." Such a confident claim might be calming to women marketed countless creams and salves that reminded them of their "horrid age spots" and other telltale signs that "let the world know you're getting old."

But LaLanne also made clear that women who failed to exercise had no one to blame but themselves for looking old and feeling weary.[8] He had little patience for those who prayed to God for a new body, but failed to change their habits: "You say 'Dear God, give me the intestinal fortitude to do something about it.' Then you get your new body. But you have to do it."[9] "You know what happens when you have children," lamented one mother of three about her spreading hips. In a tough-love tone that became typical over the *Jack LaLanne Show*'s thirty-four-year run, he cheerily assured her that in no way was "dumpiness" a foregone conclusion after age forty. Yet he also issued a somber warning: only women's bodily neglect, or "using children as an excuse," stood between his viewers and "the streamlined figure they want so badly."[10] The *work* of exercise, he said, was now a required ritual of ladyhood.

Ratcheting up the stakes of failing to exercise paved the way for more such programming. The assumption that male fitness enthusiasts like LaLanne, who favored slim jumpsuits and soft-soled slippers, were effeminate paradoxically positioned him as a non-threatening voice to offer intimate bodily advice to his mostly female viewership, but women understandably took center stage in this new medium. Debbie Drake, a Corpus Christi secretary plagued by "figure trouble" from her scrawny adolescence to the years after her son's birth, launched a weekly local television show in 1959 in Dallas. By January 1960, "the most gorgeous calisthenics teacher in the country" moved to a daily fifteen-minute format on WISH-TV in Indianapolis and was broadcast nationally on seventy-four stations by the fall, with a syndicated column and book on the way.[11] "Debbie will take you through the wonderful world of exercise, to the land of slim, trim beauty," assured a male announcer over the show's opening music. Beauty and fitness were interchangeable to Drake, and her show moved seamlessly from leg lifts and duck walks to "build up the calves" to neck rolls for double chins, a problem about which many girls wrote to Drake, but which is not solved by muscular conditioning.[12] One 1962 profile acknowledged the increasingly common sense that America's lack of physical fitness was a national security and health issue, while Drake's motto was all aesthetics: "To make America the Beautiful—exercise!"[13]

Drake was just as direct as LaLanne in asserting that exercise was imperative to women's happiness. But she had less pretense of connecting it to self-actualization or strength. Exercise, Drake explained in her trademark leotard, accented by a prim collar that nodded both to propriety and the Playboy Bunny, was a way to please your husband. Her album *How to Keep Your Husband Happy* left little doubt of the importance of exercise—but only because a happy husband was a prerequisite for a woman's well-being. Building strength was only secondary to slimming unsightly thighs that could repulse, embarrass—or worst of all, drive away—a man. In some ways, this *was* progress: in 1918, diet and beauty authority Lulu Hunt Peters had warned women that "jealous dispositions" might make their husbands dissuade them from exercise for fear of attracting the attention of other men. "I almost hate my husband when I think how long he kept me under that delusion," Peters reflected bitterly before advising her reader to "go serenely on her way" and ignore such ill-intentioned acquaintances who shared "cheerful tales of people they have known who reduced, and who went into a decline, and finally died."[14] Attending to your body, Peters advised—even if to discipline it through diet and exercise— reflected a proper sense of self-worth.

By the early 1960s, when Drake published *Debbie Drake's Easy Way to a Perfect Figure and Glowing Health* and recorded albums including *Look Good! Feel Great!*, the idea that exercise could kill women, or that a matronly, unsexy appearance was the fate of a married mother, were beginning to lose credibility. Yet the archetype Drake established was not wholly liberating: the hot wife. This notion dispelled the assumption that marriage and motherhood rendered a woman instantly unsexy, but it created equally damaging pressure to sustain sexual desirability indefinitely. Failing to fight unsightly cellulite could now mean deservedly losing the affection of a man who now expected his wife to exercise to look better. The "matronly Mrs. who had rather be whistle-bait" was the target attendee for a live Drake beauty course at a Birmingham, Alabama, theater.

"The masculine member of the household," the announcement snickered, "would have to do his Drake-watching at home."[15] And he did, as the program was broadcast in many markets at midnight, when some men, much to their wives' dismay, took to watching Drake themselves. One woman complained that such scheduling was indecent—more befitting of a "cheap burlesque show" than exercise programming—for she would find her husband rapt before the television set rather than in bed.[16] "The knowledge that men watch her syndicated program just to ogle," said another profile of the "dear girl," written by a man, "came as a complete surprise" to Drake, who then "set her commercially acute mind" to designing a course of exercises for men.[17] These never took off, though men continued to tune into women's exercise shows and appearances like that on the *Dick Cavett Show*, where Drake got laughs by leading Cavett in a dance that consisted mostly of rubbing her breasts, encased in a bullet bra, against his chest. Exercising, Drake believed, could allow women to become sexy enough to allay their insecurities, but not liberate them from the idea that their self-worth was predicated on their desirability to men.

This idea that exercise was integral, but hardly emancipating, for women, was often shared in advice literature that predicated women's happiness on male satisfaction, amplifying the messages heard on television. *Always Ask a Man: The Key to Femininity* was the unironic title of a 1965 paperback that sold over two hundred thousand copies. As late as 1969, the second printing of Chappell and Huss's women's health book—part of the etiquette authority Amy Vanderbilt's *Success Program for Women*—counseled women, like the thirty-six-year-old Connecticut housewife who rose each morning, even on her birthday, "bored stiff of cleaning and cooking, ironing clothes, and being very lonely," to take a morning walk around the block to "break the spells of restlessness." Though returning to work once their children were grown was possible, the authors reminded women that "on a long-time basis, the best health insurance for a housewife is to stay in love with her husband and work at keeping him in love with her." These books, television programs, and records made much of a woman's responsibility to refuse to wallow and to "pull herself out of the dumps . . . to make a deliberate effort to recover her equilibrium." Five years after Betty Friedan had exploded the fiction that women's contentment lay in marriage, motherhood, and a well-appointed suburban kitchen, these advice texts offered no political or collective solutions. Calm, Chappell and Hull advised, came in a woman gritting her teeth and remembering that if a brisk walk didn't cure her unease, "'this too, shall pass,' and then just wait it out—or sleep it off." But more frequently, happiness resided in "not waiting to be asked to help" in all endeavors, including mustering the effort to exercise.[18]

Nationally, television was also an important medium to diffuse yoga and its attendant message that exercise led to enlightenment. Miami yogi Richard Hittleman became its leading ambassador on the small screen. As early as 1958, Hittleman and his wife put on a "yoga display" at a Jewish singles event at Miami's Alcazar Hotel, where he publicized his paperback book, *Yoga for the Man on the Go*.[19] Actually participating in a mixed-gender hatha class, however, would have been a step too far; to his in-person audience, yoga was a demonstration to observe rather than an activity in which to participate. Hittleman believed himself to be the only yoga teacher in Florida, but his tireless reassurances that yoga was about *exercise* and "the art of relaxation and mental and physical fitness," not some dangerous mystical project, soon helped change that.[20] Building on success writing about yoga and leading workshops of up to six hundred participants in cities like Detroit—"Everybody's Doing It!" one 1960 headline announced—Hittleman released a television program, *Yoga for Health*.[21] The next year, *Yoga for Health* moved into LaLanne's timeslot in the Los Angeles television market, offering yet another form of exercise television, meeting a demand that just a few years earlier executives had doubted even existed.[22]

Reception is notoriously hard to track, but television was unquestionably making exercise difficult to ignore, and not only on prescriptive programming. In 1961, middle-aged comedian Jack Benny, clad in a suit and tie on his eponymous TV show, tried to charm a comely young secretary who, he lamented, only had eyes for "big muscle men" like Rock Hudson and John Wayne. "Maybe if I went to one of those, uh, gymnasiums where they do bodybuilding," Benny surmised, she would change her mind. Inspired, Benny looked up J-I-M in the phone book before calling McGuire's Gym, an outfit where his inquiry for the men's department got the biggest laugh of all. After Benny convinced a similarly staid colleague that he, too, needed to "tighten up," the two businessmen enrolled in a "bodybuilding course," where—clothed in comically baggy shorts and sweaters that showcased their skinny legs—they were mocked for their effeminacy: "riding sidesaddle" on a horse vault and visibly enjoying a vibrating wheel that massaged the behind. The resolution was funny and revealing: Benny sewed shoulder pads into this suit rather than complete the six-week course and earned a compliment on his build from a scrawny passerby, but not from the youthful secretary, who understood that if a muscular aesthetic was newly popular among her generation, it remained ridiculous for respectable men of a certain age and status.[23]

That said, exercise as a salutary habit of daily life was making inroads into even the most buttoned-up institutions—and not just on-screen. In January 1964, a handful of deputy directors at the Central Intelligence Agency received a memo with the subject line "Physical Fitness Room." The coming fall, "on an experimental basis," the agency would be opening a workplace gym: "a comparatively small room with limited equipment" that accommodated up to twenty-five people who paid a thirty-five-cent fee to use it, plus shower, soap, and lockers. While the facility would be open a remarkable twenty-two hours a day, L. K. White, the deputy director for support, was so tentative about this initiative—"because we have no experience as to the extent which the room will be used"—that he didn't even issue an agency-wide announcement and decreed an attendant would be posted once it was clear when the facility got the most foot traffic. Exercise among colleagues looked to be even more awkward than among strangers.

The real sign that working out at work was such a novel concept was that the memo cautioned equally strongly that employees could be disciplined for using the gym *too much*: unless he received multiple levels of clearance for an exception, "regardless of the time of day the employee uses the facility, he will be expected to put in an eight-hour workday." Being too willing to work on one's body, as it long had, signaled suspicious, maybe even malingering, tendencies. First priority was given to male employees who were in medical treatment or whose official duty required "physical conditioning"—why would a man without an affliction or such a job want to work out regularly? Given the federal government's long history of homophobia and the association of gyms with gay culture, this skepticism was pointed.[24] As for women, a decision as to "whether it is practical for the space to be made available to female employees" would come at an undetermined later date.[25] The small minority of women who had penetrated the agency's highly male environment were excluded from this informal space, where working out looked to become a new activity through which to cultivate clubbishness.

Fitness gained more traction than ever in the United States because the notion that exercise was bound up with a positive state of overall health was becoming more widespread among civic leaders, psychological experts, clergy, and, of course, early fitness enthusiasts and entrepreneurs. Brick-and-mortar gyms, mail-order products, a growing body of advice literature, and a new genre of exercise television were the vehicles to spread it.

For all the talk of the universalizing potential of individual exercise, however, the process was halting. Groups like the Adonis Male Club, launched in the summer of 1959 as an offshoot of physique magazine *VIM*, appealed outright to gay male readers who formed an important public for health and fitness media. But that boldness came at a cost: Postmaster General Arthur Summerfield infiltrated the mailing lists of such magazines, raided bodybuilding gyms, and in 1960 even arrested Smith College professor Newton Arvin for buying physique magazines. People panicked as they saw teachers suspended across the Midwest to satisfy a growing public appetite to root out these "sexual deviates," and in 1961 fifty members of the Adonis Club were indicted by the federal government. At least two men attempted suicide due to this persecution: a Harvard undergraduate in his dormitory room and an Indiana University professor who threw himself in front of a car.[26]

Such exclusion could coexist with a rapidly expanding fitness culture because most of the exercise enthusiasts who made fitness a national phenomenon were unwitting revolutionaries, committed merely to selling a product, or more sanguinely, to sharing a practice that had revolutionized *individual* lives. Many of the spaces of fitness, from slenderizing studios to magazine pages, served to reinforce rather than challenge dominant ideas about health, beauty, and the body. Abbye Stockton sold a weight-loss program every time her nickname, "Pudgy," was uttered. LaLanne was remarkable in acknowledging that women deserved to take time for themselves for fitness, but he also solidified the expectation that exercising to look younger was an extension of their domestic duties. Tanny gyms welcomed women clients in addition to "grubby men with barbells," but only to exercise apart from men, reinforcing the idea that it was inappropriate for the sexes to exercise together, or perhaps for women to visibly exert themselves at all. Notably, Tanny was sued for putting African Americans on a suspiciously "long waiting list" when white people were quickly granted memberships.[27] More so than his more apolitical contemporaries, Tanny was unapologetic in seeing his gyms as macho fortresses against communism: "The Russians? Nuts! All our people need is regular workouts at my gyms and they can lick everyone's father."[28]

Building on the federal government's efforts to convince many Americans that exercise was important to both personal and civic health, this generation of enthusiasts successfully further decoupled fitness from narrow associations with military service, athletic competition, or frivolous body modification. Exercise became a crucial way to seek sanity, and even joy, in everyday life, laying the foundation for many more Americans to begin to understand fitness as an avenue of individual liberation. By the time Huss and Chappell advised homemakers on a "course of success" in the late 1960s, they reminded readers, "most of us [women] underestimate our physical resilience and capacity." Exercise could and should be a "pleasurable activity, freely and buoyantly entered into" for its ability to improve cardiovascular and pulmonary function, but more broadly and most importantly, "frame of mind." If their assumption was that this hardier state was desirable in enabling one to find the fortitude to "stick to a diet" or throw oneself more wholeheartedly into motherhood, there was no telling how women—and others—might reimagine the empowering, self-affirming potential of exercise.[29]

Accordingly, more Americans were newly prepared, and at times pressured, to exercise—especially as consumers—throughout the 1960s and beyond. Advertisers quickly rushed in to address, or exploit, concerns about lack of fitness among Americans of all ages. "Most recognize[d] the need for exercise," assumed a 1968 advertisement for the Trimway fitness machine, but had little time for "a complex physical fitness program." Spokesman Andy Livingston, a Chicago Bears running back, promised readers that Trimway could help such busy but otherwise motivated readers to "lose inches" for a "healthier life."[30] A year later, inventor and industrialist Frank Flick realized that while exercise opportunities abounded for those "from high school to 35," few activities existed for "those too young or too old for highly competitive sports, vigorous calisthenics, cycling, running, or jogging." A full-page feature on the Exer-Cor, his creation to meet that growing demand, pictured an elementary school boy and an eighty-one-year-old woman, smiling "on all fours, cycling back and forth in a rhythmic, graceful movement."[31] The preponderance of such devices, whether they worked or not, suggested that the appetite for exercise was growing, and that private industry, not public institutions, would meet this need.

Anxieties about children's flabbiness had galvanized federal concerns about fitness, and they only intensified during the 1960s. But funding for physical education remained effectively static throughout the decade, though after JFK's assassination, even public promotional campaigns, and then enrollment, waned.[32] Instead, children became a target of a growing consumer marketplace that blurred the line between toys and exercise devices. An awareness that "you can't sit and get fit" permeated the public consciousness, and the "push-button luxuries" against which Prudden railed had created a "young boy [who] no longer pushes his dumptruck down an imaginary highway," but was instead reliant on a remote control. "Daddy's little girl" was still no better off in 1972, an ad complained, for she "no longer takes the doll's hands and dances merrily with her," but simply "winds the key and sits and watches her doll pirouette and bow." The answer was to make Christmas an "active holiday season" with gifts that "require physical activity on the part of the recipient," from street hockey to portable hopscotch to an indoor putting green to the "action chair," a "plastic boat-shaped tub chair that rocks, twists, and turns on the floor by body motions of the rider," and that sounded about as effective as Stauffer's Magic Couch. Notably, while a concerned columnist mused that he wished schools would take up more-rigorous forms of physical education, he recommended that since "much of the responsibility for the physical fitness of boys and girls rests with parents," they would do well to make use of such devices—if they could afford them.[33]

Part **Four**

MOVEMENT CULTURE, REDEFINED

We were different from those women marching in the streets.
JUDI SHEPPARD MISSETT, FOUNDER OF JAZZERCISE

On the rocky Northern California coast, Bernard Gunther, a former weight lifter, had found a community as fascinated as he was with psychic and physical individual transformation. Disappointed with how "excessive civilizing" had compromised the "basic sense of being" of Americans in the 1960s, Gunther and his fellow seekers at the Esalen Institute in Big Sur were invested in exploring what they called "human potential," pushing each other to let go of mental and emotional hang-ups in order to fully experience life. The avenues to such self-actualization were sensory and embodied, ranging from peeling an orange to dropping acid to experimental therapies like rolfing or reiki.[1] Gunther arrived at Esalen in 1964, two years after the vast retreat property was founded by two young white men whose studies of Eastern religion and culture had left them dispirited with American approaches to religion, mental health, and daily life. Building on the transcendence he'd glancingly experienced at the gym, in 1972 Gunther explained the methods he had elaborated in a book and film, and at Esalen seminars: "We don't ask them to understand things in their minds . . . we ask them to experience them in their senses and their bodies."[2]

Like "a westernized type of Yoga designed to be integrated more easily into the lives of non-Orientals," Gunther continued, his "body awareness" approach suggested "where the whole new age is moving."[3] By the early 1970s, Gunther was right that such ideas about the desirability of body-mind connectedness, long appreciated by physical culturalists and fitness enthusiasts, were becoming more mainstream. In 1972, *MAD* magazine listed defining "liberal" traits: "taking up yoga," feeding pets organic foods, and "walking around nude in front of the children," in addition to the more expressly politically progressive act of "making it a habit to call Negroes 'blacks.'"[4] But back in 1962, Esalen's commitment to foster "self-actualization, creativity, and human potentiality in general" through experimental—and, to most Americans, unfamiliar—endeavors like Eastern religion, organic food cultivation, psychedelic experimentation, and bodywork had felt radical.[5]

Intentionally cultivating the body was imperative to realizing one's full potential, these seekers emphatically agreed with physical education teachers, health club owners, public health experts, and a new generation of women's sports and fitness leaders—few of whom would ever find themselves in a nude encounter group or a Gestalt-therapy session at the California retreat center. Those who flocked to retreats such as Esalen, the expanding network of New Age bookstores, alternative medicine clinics, and feminist health centers, believed that such mind-body "wholism" was closely linked to social and political liberation from the inauthentic, technocratic, and spiritually bankrupt surrounding world, not just a strategy for individual self-improvement to navigate it more successfully. But these voices could sound remarkably similar: when one administrator commented that Esalen's physical-movement programming was crucial to universalizing the retreat's guiding belief "that the body and mind are so closely related," he unwittingly echoed language one might have heard on the *Jack LaLanne Show*, or increasingly, whispered among women waiting in line for their favorite aerobic dance class or runners stretching before a casual weekend road race, or see stamped on the cover of one of the new best-selling books about exercise.[6] All over the country, Americans were realizing that self-possession through physical cultivation could have revolutionary ends, some connected to formal political projects and others transcending—or deliberately ignoring—them.

11

Yoga and the Counterculture

The Esalen sports center, founded in 1973, was a prime example of this new connection between physical movement and individual emancipation: activities like "yoga-tennis" supplanted traditional contests with an emphasis on "non-competitive organized play and deeper experiences of self-exploration, spiritual community, and transcendence." As such activities attracted a broader public throughout the 1970s, Esalen's founding yoga instructor, Pamela Rainbear Portugal, described how this sort of conscious bodily exertion provided a release that made even bourgeois domestic life tolerable: "Punch a punching bag instead of secretly—even to you—sniping at your mate. Otherwise you might someday 'accidentally' run the family Buick over him."[1] A reporter commented on the spread of this sensibility in new movement programs, noting that "the clout generated by Esalen" could be for sports and exercise "what the storming of the Bastille was to the French Revolution."[2]

Precisely. Gunther and his colleagues perceived these embodied practices as an alternative form of therapy that rejected a western focus on narrowly defined physical fitness, mere absence of illness, and conventional beauty. Portugal advocated unapologetically for embracing one's physicality in order to *challenge* dominant ideas about beauty and modesty. In addition to rapturously describing emptying one's bowels without shame, for example, her memoir diagrams yoga poses with line drawings of a woman whose thick waist, unkempt hair, and protuberant nose are as prominent as her forward flexion.[3] The unorthodox nature of it all was the point: yoga was not a technique to attain slimmer arms or to smooth a furrowed brow, but an embodied openness to questioning western attitudes about aesthetics, religion, medicine, and sexuality.[4] Being "in your body"—a vague phrase circulated more and more, at Esalen and beyond—was key to such self-possession. "As long as you use your senses, you can do whatever *YOU WANT*," Portugal wrote.[5] Of course, not all visitors to Esalen embraced this permissive outlook. One disgusted—if titillated—journalist vividly described a mysterious "yoga girl" with "a fantastic body, completely and beautifully naked, sitting quietly, serenely, on a massage table, facing the ocean and performing yoga exercises," as emblematic of everything morally and culturally awry with the "cold, frightening" retreat.[6]

Nor did this emancipated sensibility apply equally to everybody. Feminist Betty Friedan visited and did not find Esalen much more liberated than the conformist, manicured suburbs that were supposedly its antithesis, noting specifically the "mountain macho men . . . who kept their women barefoot and pregnant . . ." even as they believed themselves "liberated hippies."[7] Indeed, women at Esalen and elsewhere labored to ensure they could fully participate in the enlightenment that yoga—and the counterculture at large— promised. Child-rearing author Jeannine Medvin wrote in her 1974 book *Prenatal Yoga and Natural Childbirth* of a Marin County housewife who traveled to India to learn yoga and was sternly instructed by her male "master" to cease physical asana while pregnant. What foolish but predictable advice, Medvin lamented, for the physical and mental "strength and suppleness" yoga provided were paramount for pregnant women, whose condition was widely misunderstood by the medical establishment *and* yoga masters as a "liability." Medvin had felt similarly alienated by the "hospital regimentation and inhumanities" she faced during childbirth, including being told that a medical incubator provided more effective warmth for her infant than her own body. A "yoga more in tune with the Great Moon Force," Medvin wrote, strengthened women body and mind, a powerful counterweight to such regressive attitudes that threatened woman's essential power, born of her spiritual and bodily communion with a natural environment also under siege by modern society. In a drawing of a woman in labor that blurred the boundaries between her "uterus and the sea . . . the waters of [her] womb flow[ing] out into the expansiveness of the ocean" she wrote, "the oneness was ecstatic."[8]

Developed by a rare lineage of women teachers, Medvin's hatha derivative of prenatal yoga was an avenue to the "sacred pleasures" of motherhood, from knowledge and acceptance of one's own body to achieving orgasm through breastfeeding; Medvin nursed her child until age four.[9] Such unapologetic flouting of social mores was welcome by those wary of yoga-as-fitness they might see on television or in fashion magazines. One enthusiastic reviewer of *Prenatal Yoga* effused at how Medvin's practice contrasted with that of popularizers like Indra Devi, known for gimmicks like demonstrating inversions at Disneyland. Medvin's "point is not to 'exercise' the body, not to look better, not to trouble oneself for the good of the baby."[10]

She wasn't alone in challenging social hierarchies through yoga. In 1975, the Sexual Freedom League championed "Liberated Yoga," explicitly grounding the physical practice in principles of political and cultural emancipation: "Respect for traditional yoga philosophy, except insofar as it tends to be racist, authoritarian . . . or otherwise incompatible with a revolutionary pacifist counter-culture" and "condemnation of sexism."[11] The same year, Ken Keyes's *Handbook of Higher Consciousness* drew on "spiritual traditions such as yoga" in order to "make sex groovier" rather than renounce or regulate it.[12] In 1977, *Yoga Journal* reviewed several titles that argued that yoga allowed practitioners to access their integrated "bodymind" in a way often thwarted by the artifice and consumerism of modern life.[13] The following year, an article on "interpersonal yoga" reiterated how physical postures could unlock "the learning potential" of useless emotions like jealousy born of bourgeois hang-ups, which caused muscular tightness and mental distress.[14]

College students and celebrities alike explored these new ideas and the spaces where they flourished. In Southern California's Topanga Canyon, residents practiced yoga in "encounter groups" and might visit the nudist colony Elysium Fields.[15] In her memoir, singer Carole King recalls relocating to nearby Laurel Canyon to extricate herself from the East Coast's general cultural rigidity and her own oppressive marriage. The "physical grace" and "spiritual peace" she found practicing yoga in an "incense-perfumed room" in the late 1960s allowed her to "live who she really was."[16] For King and her contemporaries, yoga was bound up with her search for "authenticity" achieved by trading "teased, sprayed hair" for "natural ripples," wearing long, clingy dresses, and cooking vegetarian." "Becoming spiritual" at Integral Yoga, King's biographer recounts, enabled "this once-conventional young woman" to "tap a deeper vein of expression."[17] Yet King and her contemporaries were well aware that such new mores could easily reiterate a familiar double standard: "Women wanted to feel free, and men wanted to *be* free."

Self-development through bodily autonomy was especially meaningful to many women who had little connection to these countercultural communities, but who had long been told their bodies were inherently weak. In 1971, the Boston Women's Health Collective released *Our Bodies, Ourselves*, promoting unabashed physical self-knowledge and connecting female nudity to empowerment rather than objectification. The same year, Belita Cowan of the Los Angeles Feminist Women's Health Center taught herself how to use a plastic speculum, flashlight, and mirror to examine her cervix—a practice that she then turned into a public teach-in that inspired demonstrations nationwide.

Campus feminist groups often struck a similar note. In 1972, the Stanford Women's Center published "A Guide for Stanford Women" and spelled out its philosophy in a section headed "MIND AND BODY": Women are fundamentally different from men in their physical and psychological health needs; mental and physical health are inextricably intertwined; and "self-help" can "change women's consciousness about their own bodies," and "provide them with skills to maintain and improve their own health."[18] The movement to link bodily self-determination with social power was coursing through campus, especially once Title IX, the 1972 legislation that helped equalize funding for athletics across gender, was ratified. "Dated Facilities Restrict Women," read a headline in the *Stanford Daily* the same year; college women were protesting the "obvious disadvantage" they faced in exercising their right to be active.[19]

Similarly, rape victims had long been told not to resist their attackers, but in the 1970s, women established and signed up for self-defense classes to challenge this assumption that they should be submissive. Offered first at feminist health centers, these classes became widely popular. In the 1976 film *Stay Hungry*, the instructor of one such class based in martial arts, offered adjacent to a bodybuilding gym, jokes she might have to begin offering "a pink or gold belt" for all the women who were enrolling. But this movement linking bodily health, individual fulfillment, and social transformation was no punchline, and it appealed more intersectionally than fitness pursuits framed either as leisure or merely as a way to offset its aesthetic effects.

Disability rights activists occupied a federal building in San Francisco to demand enforcement of antidiscrimination laws, and in staging a sit-in that lasted nearly a month, made a bold and visible statement of bodily strength.[20] The Black Panther Party founded health clinics staffed by, and serving, Black residents of under-resourced neighborhoods, overtly promoting Black well-being, "body and soul," as a political project.[21] A circuit of recreational martial-arts events sprang up in Black neighborhoods, offering women, men, and children an opportunity to center "friendship first, competition second," and to be agents of their own health and safety.[22] Civil-rights leader Rosa Parks had a robust yoga practice during these years, and by 1973 was demonstrating her yoga at activist gatherings.[23] This culture of Black "movement arts," as historian Maryam Aziz calls it, incorporated dance, yoga, and martial arts, and offered children and adults the opportunity to develop internal strength and find community and "physical release" amid experiences of "trauma, violence, and cultural and spiritual colonization."[24]

This blended faith in social transformation through bodily liberation often rested on assumptions about the connectedness of all humanity, regardless of race. Yoga educator Leslie Kaminoff, who felt "grabbed" by the yoga he discovered at the Sivananda center in

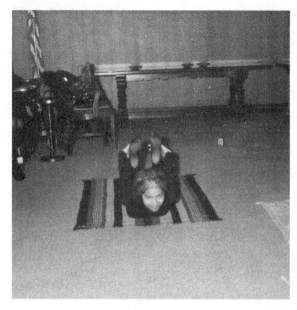

Figure 11. *Rosa Parks Practicing Yoga at an Event*, n.d. Rosa Parks is shown engaging in an activity that was important to her life but long unacknowledged as part of her civil-rights activism.

COLOR PRINT. VISUAL MATERIALS FROM THE ROSA PARKS PAPERS, PRINTS AND PHOTOGRAPHS DIVISION, LIBRARY OF CONGRESS (056.00.00). PHOTO COURTESY OF THE ROSA AND RAYMOND PARKS INSTITUTE FOR SELF DEVELOPMENT. HTTPS://WWW.LOC.GOV/EXHIBITIONS/ROSA-PARKS-IN-HER-OWN-WORDS/ABOUT-THIS-EXHIBITION/DETROIT-1957-AND-BEYOND/ROSA-PRACTICING-YOGA/.

New York before becoming a director of the Los Angeles outpost, reflected positively about the inclusiveness of these communities in the 1970s. "I am not going to say the situation was color-blind," he told me, "but it just wasn't charged the way it is now."[25] The Immigration Act of 1965, which opened American shores to thousands of South Asians including yoga luminaries such as B. K. S. Iyengar and K. Pattabhi Jois, enabled yoga's popularity and dovetailed with domestic civil rights activism, but many white practitioners were enraptured by what they understood as its exoticism.[26]

Such dynamics could be explosive. An early-1970s encounter group at Esalen that brought together Black Panthers and white progressives to explore their shared humanity ended disastrously, with African Americans accusing whites of undermining racial solidarity under the pretense of individual liberation.[27] A *Black Panther* magazine profile of party member and martial-arts instructor Steve McCutchen made that clear: McCutchen had specifically adapted Eastern practices to abet racial liberation—defined by rejecting both the exploitation of Black athletes and the commercialized, culturally appropriated versions of Asian practices used to sell kung fu movies or fitness programs that falsely advertised being able to "turn any 97 pound weakling into a fearsome fighter."[28] Even when pursued as a distinctly countercultural practice, yoga's emphasis on broad cosmic consciousness and individual bodily practice—to the exclusion of collective racial and gender identity—could both legitimately challenge social hierarchies and leave them intact.

Such blind spots are probably why people like Medvin and the Sexual Freedom League spelled out the subversive potential of yoga so explicitly: they witnessed how too-easy appeals to universalism and introspection could devolve into political oblivion, especially as the growing health-and-beauty-focused fitness culture enthusiastically incorporated yoga as offering more than "just exercise"— but still focused primarily on physical health and appearance. Most Americans encountering yoga in the 1970s were less concerned with its politics, however, and more interested in the possibility of transforming their own lives through the mastery of physical postures, an idea that was taking root in magazines, on television, and in suburban subdivisions.

Yoga, *Woman's Day* reported, was a means to satisfy dominant gendered ideals while only gently resisting them. On the one hand, the magazine proposed, in "our car-and-cocktail-party culture," even ten minutes of yoga at home could extend women's "young and trim" years and delay the inexorable social death of being "old and flabby." Yet the same reader might embrace yoga for more liberatory ends, as it "enhanced [women's] sexual pleasure in many ways . . . containing none of the prudishness toward the body and its natural functions that was an integral part of Western culture for so long." At Ina Marx's studio in Roslyn, Long Island, this tension was evident. Due to its "slow and graceful, almost dancelike movements . . . yoga is a natural exercise for women," Marx explained, and she attracted many female clients who thrilled at being active and "in their bodies." Yet Marx also separated couples during class "because men don't like to be put to shame by their wives," who often excelled. Yoga needed not disrupt gendered power relations, after all, or discourage anyone, male or female, from signing up: "If a man keeps at it, he can become better at it than his wife."[29] By 1979, the *Los Angeles Times* recommended yoga for its calming benefits, specifically for stemming sexual anxiety, but not for the transcendence that had thrilled so many: "[Yoga] keeps your mind turned off and engaged only in physical activity."[30]

12

Kenneth Cooper and Aerobics Universalism

Far from such secluded retreats, on an Alabama Air Force base without a yoga mat in sight, a less likely revolutionary was at work on a theory that would just as dramatically transform dominant definitions of physical exercise, and who could and should participate in it. Kenneth Cooper, a Texas physician, had been charged with evaluating the physical-fitness program at the military outpost. Cooper had run three miles daily since 1956, when a heart arrhythmia had terrified him, and he was accustomed to the quizzical looks his ritual attracted: not only was he jogging through the streets alone, but "exercise" was then widely understood as referring to lifting weights or doing military-style calisthenics. Drawing on his personal experience, work with five thousand Air Force members, and the "space-age technology" at his disposal, Cooper realized that "aerobics" or "endurance training"—what we today understand as "cardio"—was actually "the best kind of fitness" to foster "overall health." The positive "training effect" of such activities was undeniable, he proclaimed to anyone who would listen, even on "overweight, over-anxious, chain-smoking slobs."[1]

Cooper often shared a story of three male pilots in their thirties whom he examined in his office: a casual cyclist who biked three miles to the base daily, a sinewy weight lifter who trained five days a week, and a man who was totally inactive. Everyone, he gleefully described, assumed the weight lifter would triumph in any fitness contest. But the cyclist was still pounding away on an inclined treadmill when the weight lifter and the non-exerciser both quit, "completely fatigued within the first five minutes." "Looks are deceitful," he warned readers, as bulging biceps and a slim waist were no "no guarantee" of physical fitness.[2] In 1968, he published the thin volume *Aerobics* to share what he rightly understood as a scientific watershed, but which also became a social one.

Achieving aerobic fitness wasn't about appearance, Cooper made clear, but it *was* about far more than dutifully scoring points on the physical-fitness rubrics that came in the back of his book. "There is a distinction between being fit and being healthy," he wrote nineteen years later. "I exercise for the quality of life I enjoy."[3] The "energy," "desire," and feeling of being "high and creative" got him out on the road each evening after work. More important than "physical rehabilitation" was the "personality rehabilitation" he witnessed and experienced, citing better self-image, confidence, and transformation of introverts into extroverts who wouldn't stop talking about exercise. This improvement in quality of life came in part from attaching moral value, and sometimes harsh judgment, to the "felony of inactivity," in order to discourage it. Not just paunchiness, but lethargy and alienation, were the results of such sloth. The complacent non-exerciser who would insist to Cooper, "Doc, I don't have much need for endurance. I just sit at a desk all day and watch television at night," was well on his way to becoming a "social cripple," each day finding himself "too tired" to do anything, incorrectly and irresponsibly chalking it up to the inexorable process of "getting old."[4]

It didn't have to be that way, Cooper insisted. Fitness was "a desirable state," achievable "for anyone who wants to lead a zestful and productive life."[5] And those who "just couldn't hack" perpetual competition with themselves? They *deserved* derision. An illustrative Cooper anecdote was that of his "seriously deconditioned" friend, at first a reluctant swimmer gasping for air after a few minutes in the pool, but who soon swam forty to fifty laps daily and could barely remember "what the fuss was all about." The best part, though, was his new swagger: "I walk down those crowded New York streets today and sneer at everybody. I look at them and gloat to myself. I'm in better shape than four out of five of you." This was a typical and desirable outcome of regular exercise, Cooper wrote: "first agony, then discouragement, then determination, then progress, then success, then smugness." To those who resisted his block-letter proselytizing—"Scientifically developed and tested! No diets! No willpower tests! No calisthenics!"—Cooper said point blank, "Try it. Then you too can walk down any street and gloat."[6]

Cooper's own passion for exercise and his running were borne of the idea that Eisenhower and Kennedy helped make conventional wisdom: physical fitness was personal but was also a matter of civic commitment, and even national security. There was nothing politically radical about this celebration of military readiness, physical discipline, or male vigor: on the cover of the 1968 edition of *Aerobics*, a woman in a two-piece swimsuit awkwardly posed beneath the wheels of an oblivious male cyclist. Not until 1970 did Cooper release *The New Aerobics*, with "sex-adjusted" charts and a dedication to his wife and daughter. And in the "Mostly About Women" chapter, he began by rejecting his own premise about men: "I tend to disagree with the fellow who says 'beauty is only skin-deep.'" On the contrary, "beauty in a woman is a reflection of her total well-being," and aerobic training, unsurprisingly was the key to "feminine charm."[7] The military doctor was an unlikely purveyor of beauty tips for "age-defying youthfulness," but *The New Aerobics* fit right in with this common, and tepid, definition of empowerment: middle age need not mean physical and social ruin—*if* a woman committed to exercise, rather than "sit before the television set, moping about her lost youth."[8]

Such outdated beliefs hinted at the deep conservatism of Cooper's revolutionary ideas about exercise. He narrated the allegorical film *Run Dick, Run Jane!*, released by Mormon Brigham Young University, decrying "today's American male who gets married, fat, and deconditioned," recounting a "true story" of a "New York state journalist" so depressed that he sets out nightly determined to commit an undetectable suicide: running as fast as he can into the darkness until he goes into cardiac arrest. Six weeks later, he has failed at ending his life, but has cured his depression, rededicated himself to the role of family patriarch, and become a strong, fast runner, smiling and waving as he whizzes past bemused but impressed neighbors.[9]

Christian evangelist Oral Roberts also became a Cooper acolyte. In 1974, Cooper visited the eponymous university founded nine years earlier by the preacher, to speak at the dedication of a two-million-dollar, 114,000-square-foot fitness center named for him. Cooper's preventive approach, he highlighted in his speech, was a way to stem a sprawling American "system" that "provides too much (health) care too late."[10] The Christian institution rolled out an elaborate health program for students based on Cooper's points system and the biblical precept that "the body is the temple of the mind and the strength of the individual is dependent upon the strength of his body, mind, and spirit," as Cooper said, sounding much like the holistic-health advocates at Esalen who'd likely never set foot on, much less approve of, the conservative Tulsa campus. The next year, Cooper received an honorary degree from Oral Roberts University (ORU), but his most lasting legacy was in the "Pounds Off Program," launched in 1976. In addition to requiring participation in physical education and sports, Pounds Off mandated fat students to lose weight or be sent home, under the pretense that fat was an outward sign of sin.[11] Cooper's work fit right into ORU's commitment to "develop[ing] the whole person: mind, body, and spirit."[12]

But the way the small Christian college's fitness program came on the national radar reflects the bizarre moment in which evangelical Christians and countercultural seekers spoke in the same idiom of mind-body holism. During the spring semester of 1977, ORU junior Debbie Padgett faced suspension due to "insufficient weight loss": she had to lose thirty pounds or leave campus. Her protests were repeatedly brushed off until she transferred to a nearby college, found common cause with other students who had experienced similar discrimination, and teamed up with the American Civil Liberties Union and the National Association to Aid Fat Americans, both left-wing activist organizations. As historian Jonathan Root has written, this unlikely cooperation highlights "the fluidity of U.S. society on the eve of the culture wars." *Especially* in terms of ideas about the body: Roberts had founded ORU specifically as an alternative to the radicalism associated with college campuses nationwide, yet his signature program—and commitment to "make the world whole again, beginning with individual "lifestyle"—made him sound much like the very hippies he was training trim, pure, Christian warriors to resist. Padgett and her allies ultimately dropped the case, but the chorus of agreement with the university—the *Wall Street Journal* called fat people "medical criminals"—*and* the claims of critics who insisted that bodily self-acceptance was crucial to their dignity spoke to a shared sense that the body was at the center of selfhood and social value.[13]

Cooper's coziness with ORU's conservative mission spoke to this widespread embrace of fitness-as-wellness in the 1970s. But it's also remarkable because his research gave way to a more radical reimagination of exercise. Beyond cycling, walking, jogging, and swimming, Cooper's work inspired—and legitimized—a much wider range of exercises for Americans who increasingly understood exercise to be imperative, but also fun. Thanks to Cooper, those who had shied away from cavernous weight rooms, the humiliation of trying out for an exclusive sports team, or the tedium of military-style calisthenics, would realize working out need not involve any of those. Eventually, Cooper's "aerobics" would fuel programs, such as Jazzercise and Spinning, first popular among women and in sweaty coastal clubs and studios—pursuits and places that this former military doctor likely never imagined.

13

Run for Your Lives!

But first there was running, or jogging, terms that would become contested as more Americans headed out to huff and puff through the streets in rubber-soled sneakers. By any name, the late twentieth-century version of the pastime with primal origins brought together the popularization of aerobics science, countercultural exploration about the transformative potential of embodied practices, and the affections of a nation thoroughly convinced of the moral and social value of athletic training, but still deeply skeptical of recreational fitness.

The American jogging craze started with sports, specifically via an Oregon track coach. Two years before Cooper published *Aerobics*, running coach William J. Bowerman and heart specialist W. E. Harris released their own mass-market paperback promoting "an exercise program of relaxed walking and running that will improve the level of fitness of nearly anyone from seven to seventy."[1] *Jogging* made grand universalist claims; "RUN FOR YOUR LIVES" was stamped in bright red across its 1967 reissue. Yet *Jogging* is significant for how much it *downplays* the very activity it promotes. Its prescriptions relied on Bowerman's favorable impression of New Zealand joggers, his own experiences as a runner and a college coach, scant data correlating regular walking and decreased instance of heart attacks in men (no research existed on women), and common sense: "the accepted principle that regular exercise in moderate amounts is good for most people."[2]

Right-thinking, thrifty folks were in luck. "JOG ANYWHERE—
OPEN YOUR DOOR AND YOU'RE IN BUSINESS" instructed
one chapter dismissing the need for clunky contraptions or health
club memberships. Nor was specialized, expensive clothing required: "You don't need to be a fashion plate . . . nearly any comfortable, informal outfit that you already own is appropriate," though
a dedicated ensemble could "help the spirit." Rubber-soled shoes
were the only imperative, but their treatment in *Jogging* highlights
the immaturity of the marketplace for such accoutrements. Bowerman was the co-founder of Blue Ribbon Sports, but rather than
push his own product, a training shoe imported from Japan, the
book features runners wearing lace-up Converse high tops (with
belted khaki shorts) and a vague recommendation to purchase supportive footwear from "a number of firms specializing in sporting
goods . . . or get by nicely with what you have at home."[3] When Blue
Ribbon co-founder Phil Knight, who idolized Bowerman, read these
words, his stomach dropped. "Maybe he thought this was true for
the casual jogger, as opposed to the trained athlete," he later wrote,
"but by God did he have to say so in print?"[4] Blue Ribbon survived
the slight—and rebranded under its current name, Nike, in 1972.

Emphasizing the simplicity, accessibility, and commonsense
appeal of jogging was a smart strategy when the idea of regularly
exercising (and in public!) was still strange. But jogging also gained
legitimacy from its association with an established sport. How to
sell the plodding task of keeping a schedule of jogs? "World class
runners" do it. A detailed distance and pace regime? Modeled on
the program of a "long list of international track and field champions at the University of Oregon." Consuming strange snacks
like hot bouillon, even in summer? A typical hydration technique
of elite athletes.[5] This approach was of the moment: the federal
government, which for a decade had endeavored to distinguish
inclusive "fitness" from competitive sport, had changed tacks. In
1968, President Nixon expanded the name of the council he had
first chaired under Eisenhower to the "Presidential Council on
Physical Fitness and Sports." Two years later, another executive
order further strengthened this connection, and in 1977 the council

ranked jogging higher than any other sport in terms of "contribution to physical well-being," but meaningfully ranked recreational
fitness activities and sports—like jogging for fitness and running—
together in a single category.[6]

Not everyone embraced such easy interchangeability between
running and jogging. Inspired by New Zealand coach Arthur Lyd-
iard, Bowerman, Harris, and Cooper had popularized the term to
present the activity as less intense and intimidating, and to distinguish its recreational form from the "roadwork" done by athletes in training. While shoe companies, sports announcers, and
advice literature conflated the two—one sub-three-hour marathoner
was described as "jogging" the 26.2-mile race—others vehemently
insisted on the distinction. "The meaning's not the same," explained
one longtime, self-styled runner in the *Honolulu Advertiser*. "Running
is in our genes, while jogging is 'in' like jeans," he said, echoing many
who disparaged what they thought of as a fad.[7] Kathrine Switzer,
who went on to make history in 1967 as the first woman to officially
complete the Boston Marathon, would correct a moody boyfriend
who would goad her by asking her "How's the *jogging* going?" by
reminding herself "No matter how slow I was, I was a *runner*, dam-
mit, not a jogger."[8] To Mike Spino, the director of sports programming at Esalen, the difference was sensibility: jogging was plodding,
conformist drudgery—"one-dimensional, like working on an assem-
bly line"—whereas what he, a former cross-country star, did, was
running: "a way in which to evoke a spirit and sense of possibility."[9]
Simple speed could be a deciding factor, though Jim Fixx, author of
The Complete Book of Running, denied any "particular speed at which
jogging turns into running," and preferred to dismiss the former term
entirely in favor of a kind of equal-opportunity athleticism: "If you
feel that you're running, no matter how slow you're going no one can
say you're not."[10]

Beyond Jogging: The Innerspaces of Running was the title of Spino's 1976 book, and in it he made a strenuous case for embracing
running for its resistance to the soul-deadening forces of modern
life. At Esalen and in four-day workshops, Spino offered "a new
approach to body-mind fitness" that combined yoga and meditation

with more conventional goals of physical fitness.[11] His approach might have seemed airy-fairy to Cooper and his buttoned-up peers in cardiology and the armed forces, but they resonated with those seeking liberation through embodied practice and individual achievement. Indeed, running was anti-authoritarian. In 1962, the film *The Loneliness of the Long Distance Runner* chronicled a young working-class protagonist who worked out his frustrations by running for miles, a curious habit then, of a piece with his outsider status. When the juvenile facility to which he was remanded expected him to represent it in an organized race, he easily surpassed the competition only to stop short of the finish line, allowing the other runners to win. His talent, the message was, would not be tamed, especially not by his oppressor.[12]

Running was well suited to outsiders, who often clashed with more staid athletic institutions. Vincent Chiappetta, who began running in 1948, trained with the midtown New York Athletic Club team until the mid-1960s, but when he started wearing a beard, they threw him out. "So many younger, faster runners grew their beards and long hair after college," he recalled, "the clubs had to choose between long hair and no runners."[13] In 1972, the winner of the New York City marathon, an urban-affairs major at the University of Maryland, told the *New York Times* that he refused to run for his school because the athletic department had insisted he change his "lifestyle" by giving up beer and dressing neatly.[14] To young adults who chafed at the wasteful consumerism of car-centric suburbia, running was an easy way to display such distaste, especially during the gas crises of the 1970s. They got high off it, too; running offered a purer pathway than drugs to unleashing psychedelic potential. The endorphin-fueled natural "runner's high" was vaunted by those who embraced running for its "zen" and "psychic power" rather than its ability to ward off clogged arteries and heart attacks.[15]

But by 1977, jogging was no longer the province of outsiders but a genuine national "craze," with a cast of celebrity enthusiasts that included actress Farrah Fawcett, Senator Strom Thurmond, a thirtysomething anchorman named Tom Brokaw, and the first Jewish Miss America, Bess Myerson, who would trot across Central

Park on errands.[16] Spino himself, though he tried to infuse a greater degree of mindfulness into what was becoming a form of mass leisure, did not completely avoid the mainstream. In 1978, he held a four-day workshop at the Bahamian Princess Tower, a resort hotel patronized by a "sedentary clientele" more likely to don "plain polyester slacks than striped running suits," remarked one journalist (and jogger) who attended. Given the surroundings, Spino's approach seemed strange: "the Pied Piper" abandoned the casino hotel's newly built track and led guests through sandy beaches and shaded palm groves in a series of "fresh swing, good swing, shake-up, surge, and sprint" that felt "more a dance class than a jogging clinic." The final move, which the journalist incorporated into his jogs back in New York City, involved wildly throwing up one's arms, connecting the fingertips, and shouting "Ping!" during a final sprint, gawking onlookers like the "startled sunbathers" at the resort be damned.[17]

14

Title IX and Its Limits

For all this celebration of equality of opportunity represented by jogging, in the sport of running women still faced massive barriers to entry. Cyndy Poor grew up a Navy brat on the East Coast in the early 1960s, seeking out every chance to "run and play sports," whether joining in a game of tag or hiding her long hair in a stocking cap beneath a helmet in order to sneak into her brother's football scrimmages. "I really felt I had to make a choice," she told me: "Either be an athlete or feminine." And because "they didn't have shoes or athletic wear for girls, and I wore boys' stuff . . . I was a tomboy." Not that a serious running career was an option: only when she watched the 1964 Olympics did she first think of running as a sport in its own right, much less one a woman could pursue. When her family relocated to Saratoga, California, the high school had no girls' track team. But Poor found the San Jose Cindergals: a club that allowed women to train and compete, as long as they could rustle up dues through raffles and bake sales.

Less than twenty miles away, a trim, blonde aspiring runner named Lynda Huey resisted the jock-sweetheart dichotomy but faced similar obstacles that shaped her life on and off the track. Miss Van Pelt, the high-school physical education teacher who had first encouraged Huey to run competitively—which she also did with a club team—warned her that cheerleading should be her top priority. At the boys' sports banquet, which Huey and other cheerleaders attended to support their boyfriends, the local newspaper reported that Huey took home the "Prettiest Statistician" award for her service to the baseball team, but that at the sparsely attended girls' athletics banquet, she had also won "Outstanding Basketball Player and Track Athlete."[1] When Huey invited a similarly fast classmate to train with her Amateur Athletic Union (AAU) club team, the classmate demurred: "My calves are getting too big already. They might get bigger." Even once Huey enrolled at San Jose State University and inquired about running in a 1968 invitational race, the athletic director sneered at her. "Can you really run?" Aside from chasing cute boys, he snickered. She established herself as a national-caliber sprinter in that race, but the paper articulated her ambitions differently: "To erase the image of the . . . big burly Russian shot-putter, which still hangs over track and field." Reading loud and clear these messages from leering athletic directors and even other women, Huey quit running—but not for long.

Ultimately, the inimitable thrill of yelling "Track!" as she whizzed by weekend joggers, the total expression of body and mind she felt on the course, was too exhilarating for Huey's hiatus to last. She decided to prove wrong the coaches and classmates and competitors who doubted her. But rather than simply rejecting the idea that her self-worth was tied up in her ability to catch a man, Huey set about proving she could train alongside *and* be sexually attractive to male athletes. At San Jose State, she trained with elite runners such as Tommie Smith, who became internationally famous for raising his fist in the Black Power salute on the medal stand at the 1968 Olympics. She taught physical education and coached women's track, at times spending her own money to put up the team in accommodations like those covered for the men's team. She also unapologetically dated Smith and others she met through training with men, ignoring the disapproval of colleagues aghast at both her brazen athletic ambition and her interracial relationships.

Huey strove to show that being a female athlete need not mean second-class status or social ostracism. Rereading a draft of her 1976 memoir, Huey first bristled at how her editor's "feminist viewpoint" made her sound "militant"—she was no "griper."[2] But eventually, remembering bringing bag lunches to tournaments where boys were served buffets, saving up for spikes only to be told girls couldn't use them, and the steady stream of discouragement her gender afforded her, Huey began to warm to the idea that her life as a woman and a runner might be a story of feminism, though she had not before understood it in those terms.[3]

Poor, an evangelical Christian, wasn't trying to make a point about women's liberation either. A few years younger than Huey, she graduated from Saratoga High School in 1971, where athletic opportunities for girls were scant. Even after 1972, many schools and colleges had "not embraced Title IX," as she diplomatically described the evasion of federal law. And even those that did, reported one Stanford swimmer, often employed physical-education teachers rather than professional coaches to guide women's teams, left female athletes to wear "hand-me-down sweats from the P.E. department that were returned at the end of the season," and even adopted a "play day" approach of mixing up women from different colleges on different teams so as not to encourage unladylike rivalry or competition.[4] Such come-one, come-all programs whose only objective was "a good educational experience" denied the fact, as she saw it, that "intercollegiate athletics is not a welfare institution . . . you earn [places on a team] with fast times and hard work." Denying women this opportunity was, she felt, a form of condescension.[5] Clubs such as the Cindergals, run by the Amateur Athletic Union, continued to be the one of the few places girls and women could compete seriously.

On the one hand, having grown up without school athletics, Poor recalled feeling "just happy to be out there." But her awareness of gender disparities became more acute as she advanced to the Olympic trials at the University of Oregon in June 1976, where for the first time, men and women competed alongside one another.[6] Poor qualified in the 800- and 1500-meter events, but she remembers that the women's trials felt like a "a tea party," complete with a folded, turquoise invitation she showed me. Poor went on to be the first female staff member of Athletes in Action, the sports division of Campus Crusade for Christ, where she also became the first coordinator of women's track, and eventually met her husband, Ron Jensen. This work was pioneering, she acknowledged, but she did not see it as political: "I was never much of a feminist. I was able to do what I wanted to do. . . . It's not about politics. . . . There was nothing stopping *me*."[7] She might not have "really been paying attention" to how her work resonated with that of women's liberation, but she began to notice more women exercising in general and jogging in particular. In the late 1970s, she felt more like an inspiration than an outlier: "*I'm* on track, everyone else is starting to figure it out."

Indeed. At the 1967 Boston Marathon, Syracuse University student Kathrine Switzer, who like Huey and Poor had patched together a training program with men's teams and an AAU club, registered for the storied race under the ambiguous initials "K. V." A kid who had "lived for the annual President's Council on Physical Fitness and Sports fitness day" when she bested the boys at sit-ups and sprints, Switzer had managed to ignore warnings of her friends' parents that running would give her big legs and a mustache, as well as genuinely concerned inquiries from the milkman and mailman— running in circles around the yard was not considered normal for a teenage girl in suburban Virginia.[8] So too did she resist the derision of catcallers who assumed she was a lesbian, and the skepticism of her male coach at Syracuse, who had been certain "no woman can run the Boston Marathon!" (After a thirty-one-mile practice run, he passed out, gray in the face, but awoke convinced of her abilities.)

On race day, Switzer remembers a light mood, as runners asked for snapshots with this peculiar creature, a female marathoner in freshly applied lipstick, and for tips to get their wives running. Around mile four, however, Switzer was alarmed to hear "the scraping noise of leather shoes . . . amid the muted thump of rubber-soled running shoes." Frightened, she turned to find "the most vicious face I'd ever seen. A big man, a huge man, with bared teeth was set to pounce, and . . . grabbed my shoulder and flung me back, screaming, 'Get the hell out of my race and give me those numbers!,'" swiping at her bib. Her assailant was race manager Jock Semple, who was ultimately tossed out of the way by three men flanking Switzer: her coach, a fellow cross-country runner, and her boyfriend, a beefy former football player and nationally ranked hammer thrower. So shaken by "the physical power and swiftness of the attack," Switzer "wet her pants a little" but kept running. A few miles later, her boyfriend realized that attacking a race official would likely disqualify him from the Olympics and lashed out at Switzer. She made history by finishing the race, but not without being dressed down by her boyfriend as "just a girl, a jogger, and a no-talent" who was "running too slow anyway."[9]

In the wake of Switzer's historic performance, the AAU immediately expelled her and upheld its stipulation that women should not run longer than a half-mile.[10] Boston Marathon Committee chair Will Cloney, who had helped Semple ambush Switzer, told the *Boston Globe* he was "hurt to think that an American girl would go where she was not wanted," and as the paper paraphrased sarcastically, "the Boston Marathon is sacred. It cannot progress with the times." Even the lone quoted supporter of "girls running in the marathon," a Yale classics professor, framed his advocacy in terms of the view afforded by running behind Roberta Louise Gibb, an unofficial participant. "For one mile I saw nothing but those beautiful legs. I kept saying to myself, 'I should ask her out to dinner. . . .'"[11]

Switzer herself shrugged off any feminist motivation for her defiance, maintaining she "was just a kid who wanted to run a marathon." Still, she began to ruminate on why it didn't even occur to more women and girls to want this experience for which she had so struggled. Part of it was a pervasive disdain for athletes, that "people who earned their living in physical labor—and that often included pro athletes—were to be pitied because they either didn't have an education or sufficient intellect for an executive kind of job" but it was also because she was a woman. A former beauty-pageant contestant, Switzer later bristled at how "some feminists" tried to appropriate her experience, but conceded that her race experience transformed her worldview: "There was no doubt that I was becoming a very outspoken defender of women's rights."[12]

Switzer wasn't the first woman to run a marathon, but she became a national symbol, appearing on Johnny Carson's *Tonight Show*, in magazines, and at races up and down the East Coast to promote recreational running in general and women's participation in particular. Enthusiasm for the sport as a fitness pastime was growing, most apparent in the road races, usually held on Sundays, where serious runners crossed paths with casual joggers. The Boston Marathon had been around since 1898, but it was the New York City Marathon, established in 1970 as four loops within Central Park, that helped make jogging for fitness a national phenomenon. Mayor John Lindsay had closed parts of Central Park to car traffic in 1968, boosting a modest interest in outdoor jogging and cycling, but in those days, the sinewy runners who took to the roads in skimpy cotton outfits that resembled undergarments were mostly a subculture concentrated in the Bronx. In advance of the race, runners like the New York Road Runners cofounders—ultramarathoner Ted Corbitt and Yeshiva College biologist Vincent Chiappetta— rallied their community, excited for a marquee Manhattan experience and giving it athletic credibility with their presence. Paying a one-dollar registration fee, only 127 runners registered the first year, and less than half crossed the finish line. The one woman who made an unofficial attempt, Long Island homemaker Nina Kuscsik, dropped out after 14.2 miles due to a stomach virus.[13] But the energy was palpable.

Race organizer Fred Lebow, a slight, bearded, Romanian immigrant and obsessive, if not especially fast, runner, sensed the potential mass appeal of a New York City marathon. An inveterate salesman who had honed his skills in the rough-and-tumble Garment District, Lebow channeled these talents toward the race. Even that first year, he commodified every aspect of the event that he could: top ten finishers received wristwatches, and the next thirty-five beer mugs, and all a Statue of Liberty participation trophy.[14] The next year, buoyed in part by President Nixon's National Jogging Day, the race grew. Lebow knew that with further buy-in from brand sponsors, the media, and a city government in sore need of a feel-good event in a time of fiscal crisis and rising crime, the event could be huge.

He was right. Chiappetta was "stunned" at the latitude the race organizers were granted by city officials, given how marginal road-running culture still was.[15] Ensuing years brought Ronzoni pre-race pasta dinners and sponsorship requests so aggressive that four-time winner Bill Rodgers refused to run when Lebow insisted he do so with a Wall Street brokerage firm's name emblazoned across his backside.[16] The city, glad to be associated with such a wholesome event, continued to give race organizers sweetheart deals on security, and in 1976, permitted critical street closures to expand the race to all five boroughs. Growing numbers of elite international runners and thousands of casual exercisers seeking a personal challenge rubbed shoulders at marathon starting lines each year—and not just in New York. By 1978, one hundred thousand Americans had finished marathons.[17] Still, Kathy Smith, who ran the Honolulu Marathon in the mid-1970s, recalled, "You've got to understand how strange it was." At Los Angeles dinner parties, guests would approach her incredulously: "There she is, the woman who ran a marathon . . . so what did it feel like?"[18]

Even so, hostility to women's running was abating. In 1972, the year Title IX passed, the AAU began to allow "separate but equal" races in which men and women ran on separate courses or with staggered start times. Switzer remembers showing up at the starting line at Boston—where women had to make the men's qualifying time of 3:30—feeling a sense of achievement no less momentous than those of her "suffragist foremothers" or of activists for coeducation.[19] Lebow had a reputation as both a supporter of women's running and an incurable womanizer. He balked at planning a full-length women's race in New York City, however, for he agreed with the AAU that only a "handful" of women in New York State could run a full marathon."[20]

But never one to resist an opportunity to promote running, surround himself with women, and attract press attention, Lebow enthusiastically agreed to a "Mini-Marathon": a single 6.2-mile loop of Central Park in June 1972. Switzer and Kuscsik set to work distributing fliers all over the city, even at singles bars.[21] "I was excited and apprehensive," Charlotte Lettis, who took second place, told *Runner's World*. "I thought women were finally being allowed to run distance. We were finally accepted as something more than freaks."[22] But the cause for feminist rejoicing was tempered: "mini" referred not only to the shortened distance of the race, but also to the fashion of miniskirts, which women presumably ran in order to wear. Crazylegs, a shaving cream brand, sponsored the race, on the assumption that smooth, shaven legs were a prerequisite for a short skirt.

The unabashedly sexy miniskirt had been hailed as a feminist milestone by some in the early 1960s, but a decade later—when women were wearing jeans and leaving their underarms and legs unshaven as political statements—it was less obviously empowering for a women's athletic event.[23] Some of the elite runners in the "all-girl" event also chafed at the fact that their numbers were stenciled onto T-shirts stamped with the Crazylegs logo; men were far less likely to find themselves, at the last minute, as unwitting billboards for a beauty product. The presence of Playboy Bunnies at the starting line, circulating among the seventy-eight women runners in their leotards and garnering leers from waiters at nearby Tavern on the Green restaurant, didn't help. Her voice tight, Switzer recalled that she and Nina Kuscsik "had to do photo ops with the Bunnies and we weren't thrilled about it."[24] Lebow was "a male chauvinist who totally supported the women's movement," Switzer explained.[25] Still, the excitement the race generated was undeniable. Jacqueline Dixon, a seventeen-year-old Californian who had trained with the San Jose Cindergals, won.[26] Switzer took sixth, but she was thrilled: the passion for women's running was extending far beyond her East Coast clique.

Three weeks later, Title IX was law, and the intensity of demands for women's and girls' access to sports seemed to be coming from all quarters. Separate "all-gal" races were clearly insufficient, particularly for superior athletes like Switzer, Kuscsik, Poor, and Huey, who had their eye on reforming professional sports and the Olympics. That fall, at the third New York City marathon, six women runners—including Kuscsik, who had won the Boston Marathon earlier that year–sat at the starting line, protesting the AAU "separate but equal" requirement that women start either ten minutes before or after the 272 male competitors. "The AAU is MidEvil" and "The AAU is archaic!" their signs announced to the crowd of

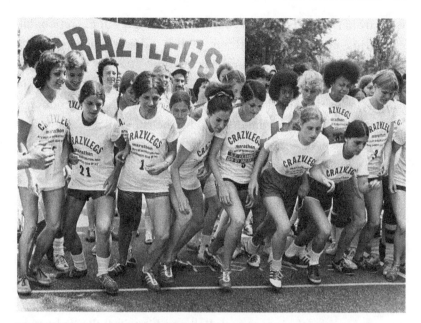

Figure 12. Women compete in the "Mini" marathon in Central Park, with the logo of race sponsor Crazylegs, a shaving cream brand, stamped across their chests.

PHOTOGRAPH. COURTESY OF KATHRINE SWITZER.

five hundred that milled about the start, but that notably didn't join in their chants.[27] (The women eventually did run, and Kuscsik won this time, too.)

There were no protests at the Mini, or at comparable recreational running events that were appealing to young women looking for a fun activity rather than a competitive athletic event. They offered a novel opportunity to socialize, break a sweat, try out some free products, and maybe get a picture in the paper. Such races became a staple of recreational fitness, and inextricable from consumer culture: 1,894 women crossed the Mini finish line in 1977 and more than double that, 4,118, in 1979.[28] Similar races were appearing nationwide. "Maybe sports fans take out their wallets when they learn that a Joe Namath wears Super Seducer Aftershave," Huey had lamented in the mid-1960s, but "no adman saw the possibilities of endorsements by Olympians Wiomia Tyus or Olga Connolly."[29] But by the 1970s, that situation was changing. Women's recreational running went from an oddity, even an outrage, to a largely unobjectionable marketing opportunity. Fittingly, at the starting line of the 1973 Boston Marathon, Switzer and her onetime attacker posed cheek to cheek, smiling. With time, she was coming to understand Semple as "just an over-worked race director. . . . Sure, he was a product of his time and thought women shouldn't be running marathons . . . [but] he gave me the inspiration to create more running opportunities for women."[30] Switzer put her communications degree to work in cultivating brand sponsorships for women's running, such as the one she struck with door-to-door makeup retailer Avon.[31]

Women's consumer brands like L'Eggs, which sold pantyhose in egg-shaped containers, got in on the opportunity. Jess Bell, the CEO of Bonne Bell, an Ohio cosmetic company that since the 1950s had sold young women heavy moisturizers and sunblock creams suited to "the outdoor life," took to sponsoring ten-kilometer women's races with missionary zeal. Bell and his wife Julie had begun running together in 1973, and despite having been married a quarter century, only celebrated the years since they had commenced their daily jogs: he wore a shirt that read "Start Running Around with Your Wife." Their devotion to running was so intense that not only did they credit their daily jog with making them more productive, spiritual, healthy, moral, attractive, and amorous, but they gave extra-long lunch breaks to Bonne Bell employees who exercised at their on-site gym, and encouraged ambition: "Never, ever set short-term goals for yourself. Never say you'll jog a half-hour every day until you can do a mile or until you get in shape or until you lose ten pounds," Julie admonished. "The goal is to run every day for the rest of your life."[32]

In keeping with this extreme approach to exercise, Bonne Bell had first aligned itself with elite athletics, sponsoring the national women's ski team in the 1960s. But reflecting the expansive fitness culture of the 1970s, the marketing for Bonne Bell Runs was far less intimidating, even welcoming. The runs framed exercise and a feminine aesthetic as mutually reinforcing. "This is not just for women who want to win the race, but for everyone who is interested in jogging as well," said Tish Hooker, race director of Nashville's first

Bonne Bell Run, in 1976. Other cities also tried to make the races enticing. In 1979, Horne's, a Pittsburgh department store, took out a full-page ad, inviting women on race day both to clinics by a podiatrist and marathoner and to the beauty counter for a full Bonne Bell makeover.[33] Ottawa's fourth annual Bonne Bell Run began at 10:06 a.m. sharp—a tie-in with the company's Ten-O-Six line of cleansers and creams, billed as a "teenager's password to beautiful skin." Pairing lip gloss and blush with racing might seem patronizing, but the idea that femininity and running were compatible was in itself a challenge to dominant ideas about women and beauty. "It's a challenging course and should separate the ladies from the girls," the race organizer commented about the event, which welcomed eight hundred women, both casual participants and "the competitive side."[34] Meaningfully, these events took place all over the country, in cities like Cleveland, Nashville, Buffalo, Denver, and Atlanta.[35] "It's only very recently that women have become involved in athletics—especially in the South," marveled the First Lady of Tennessee in anticipation of "Bonne Bell 10-K Run Day" in September 1979, when nearly one thousand women registered.[36]

The presence of women runners, and Title IX in general, not only created new marketing opportunities for existing products but opportunities for essential new ones, like the sports bra. A vast women's-fashion industry did not provide sufficiently supportive bras for teen girls and women to participate, and the stretchy tights and leotards sold in dance shops didn't do the trick either. Switzer remembers that even when she was a college field-hockey player, her teammates wore hot, latex "long-line triple-zip panty girdles," intended to keep them looking slim (and to communicate their chasteness) even if it constrained their movement while playing and "turned a pee into a ten-minute ordeal." Even Switzer's cotton garter belt, or the men's shorts she repurposed for running, were far from ideal athletic apparel.[37]

When two sisters, Lisa Lindahl and Victoria Woodrow, were commiserating about exactly this problem, Victoria quipped, "Why isn't there a jock strap for women?" It was a joke, though not without precedent: Brooks Brothers had begun offering women's business suits, and feminists were fighting for the Equal Rights Amendment. When her husband joined in on the joke and stretched one of his jockstraps over his head, Lindahl and a childhood friend, Polly Palmer Smith, realized amid their laughter that sewing together two of the elastic-fabric garments would work to bind women's breasts. Lindahl sketched this "jock bra," and in the summer of 1977, Smith enlisted costume designer Hinda Schreiber to help bring it to life. When the three women confirmed no competitors existed, they prototyped a "brassiere that holds the breasts firmly against the body to minimize any movement that may cause discomfort . . . has perspiration-absorbing properties, and straps that will not slip off the shoulder no matter how vigorous the activity." Realizing that "jock" negatively connoted masculinity, they pivoted and patented the athletic brassiere as the "Jogbra" in November 1979.[38]

"The Great Bra Controversy" merited a paragraph in the best-selling title *The Complete Book of Running*, as Connecticut journalist Jim Fixx remarked that half a decade after the passage of Title IX, women runners were divided on whether a bra was necessary at all. Retailers certainly had doubts. The Jogbra was not an easy sell to lingerie merchandisers who favored lacy, sexy styles or athletic outfitters who perceived the women's market for running clothes as insignificant. Lindahl and Schreiber targeted small sporting-goods shops at a moment when, as Fixx wrote, "practically [no running shorts] are made for women," who "solve the problem by wearing bathing suit bottoms in the summer." Proper shoes were a problem, too, and some women resorted to layering two or three pairs of socks into wide-cut men's shoes, often causing blisters.[39] But marathoner Nina Kuscsik took the commonsense position that a "firm bra, not one of the flimsy, all-elastic ones" was absolutely required to avoid chafing; it was frustrating that without such a garment, "they'll bounce and you'll always be waiting for them to come down before you take the next step." Most women did not run nearly as seriously as Kuscsik but agreed on the need for a "sporting bra," as Lindahl, Smith, and Schreiber soon termed their innovation.

In 1979, the women set up at a booth at a Chicago sporting-goods trade show, intent on convincing wary retailers that they were "not

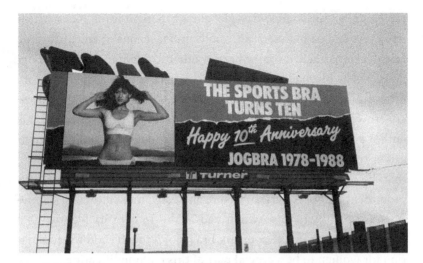

Figure 13. *The Sportsbra Turns Ten*, 1988. A billboard celebrates the Jogbra's tenth anniversary. Over a decade, the "sporting bra" had evolved from a curiosity to a staple in the growing category of women's activewear—and from underwear to a visible fashion statement.

BILLBOARD. JOGBRA, INC. RECORDS, ARCHIVES CENTER, NATIONAL MUSEUM OF AMERICAN HISTORY, SMITHSONIAN INSTITUTION. NMAH-AC1315-0000009. HTTPS://EDAN.SI.EDU/SLIDESHOW/VIEWER /?EADREFID=NMAH.AC.1315_REF39.

lingerie" but also not some threatening contraption: they posted a large photo of a Playboy Bunny wearing a Jogbra.[40] Notably, even as Jogbra got favorable coverage in magazines like *New York* and *Women's Wear Daily*, and described itself with the curious term of "innerwear-outerwear," the brand still offered skeptical sporting-goods stores a "point of purchase display" that "can function like a knowledgeable salesperson, ready to answer the many questions women so often ask about athletic bras." A "detachable poster panel that tells the Jogbra story in detail" was meant to accompany the cardboard box placed beside the register, a location ideal for an item that might be purchased as an afterthought, but that was still too unfamiliar to bring customers through the door.[41]

"A woman who jogs is already explicitly conquering a male domain," the conservative *National Review* scoffed at runners of both genders in 1979, commenting on the glut of "sweatsuits and warm-up clothes striped with gold or silver or scarlet and encrusted with seals, badges, and other virility symbols" that had given way to a market for "jogging brassières; day-glo gloves; perspiration socks; chronometers and pedometers; anti-pollution face masks; and ultrasonic face devices attached somewhere or other to frighten away snapping dogs."[42] The journalist's gripe was with both the self-congratulatory groupthink of joggers and the fact that, "fatally," like "the après-ski crowd," many dressed the part but never actually exercised; his author specified that he would never wear jogging shoes. Judgment aside, this screed against "jog-alongs" was spot-on in identifying that, by the end of the 1970s, jogging, or running, was becoming a prominent part of American leisure and consumer culture. Resourceful startups like Jogbra, which had begun to own its identity as a product "no man-made sporting bra [could] touch" laid the foundation for women to be a crucial part of this commodification.

Once a clear need for women's running apparel was established, big players in sporting goods followed suit. Nike launched a women's running line and adopted a kind of Liberation Lite language in its marketing. "The Liberator Will Fit Only One Woman," trumpeted block text on the arrival of a blue-and-white shoe featuring the trademark waffle sole but "slip-laced," and including a soft, moldable insole to fit a woman's foot. "Put an end to women's suffrage [sic]," a print advertisement for the Aurora shoe awkwardly announced. Deploying an odd mishmash of political buzzwords, the copy did away with the notion of "the gentle sex," for "when it comes to battering the body, women are every bit men's equal." Coyly, the copy announced that yes indeed, "this shoe discriminates on the basis of sex," but the specifically designed narrow last and snug heel were no example of capitulating to women in search of "special favors," but rather evidence of Nike doing its part to ensure women were "on equal footing."[43]

Such branding is more a testament to the growing acceptance of women's athleticism and the larger campaign for equal rights than to Nike's moral bravery.[44] Knight's passion was for supporting women's participation in sports—running, and later basketball—already legitimized by men, not in the emerging "fitness" programs created by women. Impressed with the growth of marathon participation among women throughout the 1970s, Knight profited from this interest and mobilized Nike to lobby the International Olympic Committee to extend the distance of women's events beyond 1500 meters, in advance of the 1984 Olympics. Such efforts, like sponsorship of elite runners like Mary Decker and Joan Benoit Samuelson, combined with manufacturing and marketing products for casual joggers, inspired everyday participation and made athletic women seem normal, and even aspirational.

No one did more to unite plodding joggers looking to slim their waistlines and runners seeking to expand their consciousness than Fixx, who had lost seventy pounds through his daily runs. "No matter how out of shape or fat or old or ungraceful you are," Fixx assured readers of *The Complete Book of Running*, the "special pleasures" of running or jogging, terms he used interchangeably, were accessible. Fixx described his book's contents as "subversive," and claimed that while he had been impressed at his physical transformations, "even more interesting were the changes that had begun to take place in my mind," noting the "sense of quiet power" he was able to summon. This "most perfect exercise" allowed participants to be "more aware of themselves and others and . . . able to participate more fully in all aspects of life, including the sexual." Citing the founder of Esalen, Michael Murphy, Fixx signed on to his idea that runners were "closet mystics," with an ability to experience "paranormal" phenomena while exercising. Considering the number of runners who described their embrace of the sport as a "conversion," Fixx concluded it was no accident that many road races took place on Sunday mornings. The "brain-body connection" enhanced by running, however, was superior to techniques like "Zen, transcendental meditation, assertiveness training, est [self-help seminars]" since the "changes all come from within and are therefore integrated with the total personality."[45]

It was an appealing proposition: Random House had printed thirty-five thousand copies of the book, but in just the first week eighty-five thousand orders were placed. A month later the book hit the *New York Times* bestseller list, which it topped for eleven weeks.[46] Fixx deliberately dispensed with "Kenneth Cooper's forbidding and joyless charts" that emphasized the most mundane

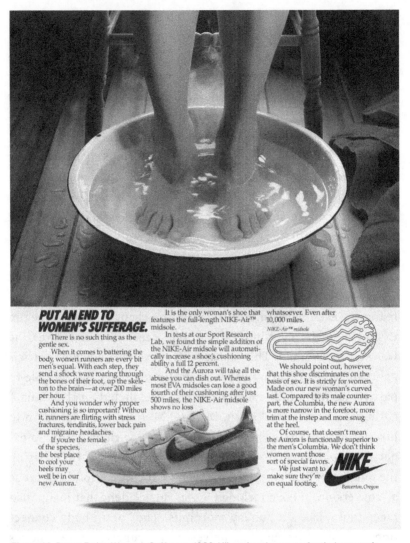

PUT AN END TO WOMEN'S SUFFERAGE.

There is no such thing as the gentle sex.

When it comes to battering the body, women runners are every bit men's equal. With each step, they send a shock wave roaring through the bones of their foot, up the skeleton to the brain—at over 200 miles per hour.

And you wonder why proper cushioning is so important? Without it, runners are flirting with stress fractures, tendinitis, lower back pain and migraine headaches.

If you're the female of the species, the best place to cool your heels may well be in our new Aurora.

It is the only woman's shoe that features the full-length NIKE-Air™ midsole.

In tests at our Sport Research Lab, we found the simple addition of the NIKE-Air midsole will automatically increase a shoe's cushioning ability a full 12 percent.

And the Aurora will take all the abuse you can dish out. Whereas most EVA midsoles can lose a good fourth of their cushioning after just 500 miles, the NIKE-Air midsole shows no loss whatsoever. Even after 10,000 miles.

NIKE-Air™ midsole

We should point out, however, that this shoe discriminates on the basis of sex. It is strictly for women. Made on our new woman's curved last. Compared to its male counterpart, the Columbia, the new Aurora is more narrow in the forefoot, more trim at the instep and more snug at the heel.

Of course, that doesn't mean the Aurora is functionally superior to the men's Columbia. We don't think women want those sort of special favors.

We just want to make sure they're on equal footing.

NIKE

Beaverton, Oregon

Figure 14. *Put an End to Women's Sufferage*, 1980. Nike advertisements for their women's running line capitalized on newly mainstream political discussions about women's empowerment, from voting rights to sexual assault.

ADVERTISEMENT. *RUNNER'S WORLD*. COURTESY OF NIKE, INC., BEAVERTON, OR.

aspects of the potentially life-changing activity. So too were the "effortless exercisers . . . lured by the promise of someday looking like Atlas or a California beach bunny" through "fitness in thirty minutes a week, sweatless exercise" on the wrong track. The "under-exercised, coronary-prone physician" who "sees himself as the authority on health matters" but had no personal experience of running was little help either. Instead, running satisfied "the need to live to our own rhythms" and to make personal choices dictated by "the minute-by-minute requirements of our minds and bodies." While "fear and mistrust" of one's own body was widespread, Fixx wrote that on a basic level, "runners like their bodies" for their impressive abilities and were unselfconscious about bodily functions that are "ordinarily left undiscussed."[47]

Even after a bout of uncontrollable diarrhea, for example, Kuscsik didn't quit the course of the 1972 Boston Marathon, despite shocking spectators with her soiled legs, which she unsuccessfully tried to rinse off at water stations. "After all, what was happening to me happens to everybody at one time or another," she commented nonchalantly at the afterparty. Kuscsik bested her closest rival by nine minutes, but Fixx quoted Spino's understanding of running as a pathway to *question* the competitive, winner-take-all aspect of modern life. When the most enlightened version of running came to "radiate into the remotest corners of everything we do," athletics would change profoundly: "Old concepts of superiority and dominance will subside. Individuals who have prepared for an event will see it as their day to experience something special together. The training buildup will be seen as a preparation rite for a voyage into the physical, spiritual world. And we will have some sense that our bodies belong to us but may be part of a vast oneness, and that each rite we enter takes us closer to our larger potentials." As one acolyte reflected, running allowed one to recapture a childlike state and even resist the passage of time: "You strip away all the chains of civilization. While you're running, you go way back in history."[48]

But such mysticism didn't necessarily suggest radicalism. In some ways, Fixx offered old-school asceticism as the solution to "undisciplined lives." Running enabled self-discipline and could even absolve "secret vices." Abstemiousness could also be a natural side effect, as in the case of one dissipated businessman who discovered jogging and suddenly found he no longer craved a couple of martinis on the way home; he yearned to run instead. Before long, he had given up drinking and smoking *and* become a more productive worker. "Can the federal government help make us fit?" Fixx asked rhetorically, quoting conservative columnist George F. Will on the futility of federal spending on healthcare. Self-reliance, not state support, was the answer, this most widely read book on running made clear: "If neither our doctors nor the government can be expected to bring us good health, to whom can we look? The answer is plain: to ourselves." Not that this ideological affinity meant conservatives necessarily embraced running; William F. Buckley Jr. tried to jog only a few times before declaring it "a miserable form of self-punishment."[49]

Fixx had no explicit feminist agenda to speak of, but in distinct contrast to Cooper or Bowerman, he saw women as capable of fully experiencing the joys and rigors of running for ends other than weight control. Unlike *Jogging*, which contained a stand-alone chapter titled "The Housewife Has Special Problems," Fixx's book integrated reflections of women runners throughout, implicitly emphasizing the shared experience of running. "Running gives me a sense of controlling my own life," he quoted one woman as saying, who logged about thirty miles a week and embraced its ethereal benefits as well: "A good run makes you feel sort of holy." Running could actually erode sexism, as in the case of a group of teen girls self-conscious about the "wisecracks of male bystanders" as they jogged the perimeter of the football field. Echoing the experiences of women like Huey, Switzer, Kuscsik, and Poor, these joggers had gained self-confidence, and the football players "gained respect for their ability and perseverance . . . and even commented that the joggers inspired them to practice harder."[50]

Despite their somewhat awkward engagement with gender, most boosters remained virtually silent on how race shaped the experience of jogging. Cooper and Bowerman's universalist descriptions of running as a *Free! Easy! Relaxing!* activity available to anyone, at any age, who could summon the will to lace up their rubber-soled sneakers and head out the door, overlooked the fact that especially as suburbanization had left inner cities without a vital tax base, many African Americans lived in neighborhoods that lacked safe parks and streets, and faced suspicion if they jogged through majority-white neighborhoods from which they had been deliberately excluded.[51] Tellingly, *Jogging* overwhelmingly featured images of white runners. Fixx, notably, quoted Black elite runner and New York Road Runners founding president Ted Corbitt describing running as "having your own psychiatrist," benefiting "everyone . . . in ways they recognize and in ways they don't."[52] Corbitt was the grandson of enslaved people, and grew up in South Carolina, where running meant racing to do chores on his family cotton farm, and his adolescent running career was always conditioned by the fear of the reception he would receive as a Black teenager. "The color line was drawn," he later remembered, "there were track meets . . . but I was a little reluctant to take part in them, because I did not know . . . what problems I would have getting a place to stay and something to eat."[53] Yet, in a reflection of either his progressivism or obliviousness to the challenges Corbitt faced as a Black man, Fixx didn't mention Corbitt's race when quoting him, identifying him only as "soft-spoken and understated."

Despite this at-times oblivious universalism, or perhaps because of it, the craze caught on, and with it an industry that no longer promoted easy, accessible jogging but instead sold the idea that with the right running gear, personal transformation and even athletic excellence were in reach. More than that, Black publications eagerly promoted the pastime both to combat the heart disease especially prevalent in their readers' communities and to position it as part of an upwardly mobile middle-class lifestyle.[54] But even as recreational running became more popular in the 1970s and 80s, the reality that running was still no equal playing field was too stark for even advertisers to ignore. One 1980 Nike *Runner's World* ad for the women's Odyssey sneaker highlighted the activity's most violent dimension: marathoner Joan Benoit Samuelson gazes out at the camera, a foil heat blanket wrapped around her. Surrounding the lithe runner are three uniformed policemen, arms crossed and staring severely ahead. "Some runners need a little extra protection," the copy reads, explicitly referring to the shoe's cushioning, but alluding to the widely known threat of assault that women faced when they set out alone on the open road.[55] The threat was real, even as the sight of a woman running became less rare: in 1980, the chair of the San Francisco Council on Physical Fitness warned all women of the "extreme danger of jogging in any city during the day," recommending they "jog in groups, preferably on special jogging tracks." Horror stories about women joggers specifically mobilized one activist to fight violence against women, after she described feeling haunted and "wrenched by images of 'long, agonized screams' that went unanswered . . . the screams of all women everywhere."[56] The danger of exercise for women had evolved from the perceived internal threat of bodily ruin to a more pressing possibility of violent attack.

The Safe Space of the Studio

When Kathrine Switzer was repeatedly nearly run off the road by motorists enraged at the sight of a woman runner, she jumped out of the way and continued her daily workouts, hoping for the best. For other women, the myriad barriers to running could feel insurmountable, or just not worth contending with.[57] In 1971, *Cosmopolitan* reported on a passionate convert to yoga who proclaimed it was the first exercise regime that had stuck; Jack LaLanne's eponymous Jumping Jacks were awkward, and jogging outside was just plain "embarrassing" due to getting "cheered along" [catcalled].[58] Others, men and women alike, reported that even in a fancy jogging suit and among supporters, they just couldn't shake traumatic memories of competing in a timed mile in physical-education class. Joan Breibart, who was starting out in the publishing industry, tried running with her husband in Riverside Park but quickly realized that in addition to ruining her carefully coiffed hair, running could wreak more serious damage on her body: "My tits were sagging and my arches were collapsing."[59] She found the more controlled, less sweaty Pilates classes operating out of the Henri Bendel department store, next to the Paul Mitchell hair salon, more to her liking.

Thanks to Cooper, the benefits of exercise other than calisthenics and weight lifting were becoming widely known. Thanks to feminists, physical activity and bodily autonomy were understood as important aspects of liberation, while the beauty and fitness industry assured women that exercise also had anti-aging benefits. Thanks to countercultural seekers and conservatives alike who waxed grandiose about the benefits of cultivating "mind and body," exercise to many felt more important than a narcissistic indulgence, and those uncomfortable on the not-so-open road sought out new studio-exercise programs whose relative privacy afforded a sense of safety.

Iowa native Judi Sheppard Missett was a Northwestern graduate and an accomplished dancer but did not identify as a feminist or especially political, even in the charged environment of Chicago during the late 1960s. But when the former beauty queen went to her local YMCA and took a fitness test modeled on Cooper's, she was confused by the results. The attendant—there were no personal trainers yet—matter-of-factly explained that the exam was geared to male physiology. But he too was perplexed, for she had scored exceptionally well on strength and fitness. "You're only a dancer?" he asked.

Missett thought about this experience while teaching dance at the prestigious Gus Giordano studio, where she had noticed another scene of alienation play out. Mothers sat to the side as their young daughters practiced choreography; the idea of grown women dancing for fitness, or even fun, was totally alien. She sensed an opportunity to solve this problem by bringing together her dance expertise with the diverse exercise modalities she saw emerging around her. Girls and women who were not training as dancers or athletes, Missett surmised, stood to gain from unapologetically "being in their bodies"—for its own sake. How, she wondered, could she design a class that allowed women to enjoy dancing with the same abandon as uninhibited little girls? She soon got her answer. After toning down the technical complexity and turning her often self-conscious students away from the mirror, she found her new adult classes filled. In 1969, Jazzercise—first called Jazz Dance for Fun and Fitness—was born.

Three years later, Missett and her young family relocated to San Diego County, where she found a body-conscious health culture hospitable to her new, high-energy exercise program. She drove all over, papering supermarket bulletin boards with fliers advertising her classes, and reserving unused church basements and school gyms through the city's recreation program, though the spaces never felt quite large enough to accommodate the crowds who showed up to follow the simple, satisfying routines. Missett criss-crossed the southern California freeways with a stack of records and leotards to change in-between classes, sometimes in her car. Military wives in particular packed Missett's classes, but they soon brought their daughters and their friends, sometimes lining up to reserve spots at six o'clock in the morning, overwhelming the municipal workers minding the desk at the Parks Department. This popularity would propel Missett to national celebrity, but teaching so intensely, and without a microphone, took a physical toll; she nearly permanently lost her voice to polyps.

It was the seventies on the Left Coast, but feminist politics had little currency in conservative San Diego County. Missett, with her midwestern roots and blonde-girl-next-door good looks, proved the perfect ambassador to make palatable an unfamiliar exercise pro-gram that might appear of a piece with Title IX activism, which some women feared would lead them on an unappealing path to masculine athleticism. Even on liberal college campuses, some students asked earnestly, "How many girls *really* want to sweat?"[60] When Missett declared her goal was "to help women understand that they can take possession of their lives by being healthy and fit," she might have sounded like a feminist health advocate, but her approach of "culti-vating joy through music" in a "nonthreatening atmosphere" felt less radical, especially when delivered from the lips of a former beauty queen. Moreover, the fact that Jazzercise was rooted in *dance*, a dis-cipline associated with the grace and slim aesthetic of conventional femininity, helped assuage the doubters put off by the unapologetic sweat, muscles, and pro-woman energy of organized sports.

In this sense, Jazzercise was both inspired by feminism and resis-tant to its radicalism. On the one hand, Missett told me that her community was undeniably different from "those women march-ing in the streets" for reproductive rights or against the Vietnam

War. She also distanced her program from the big-city elitism of the health clubs emerging in hip urban neighborhoods, and increasingly understood as playgrounds for the wealthy, sexy, and glamorous. In stark contrast with the singles-bar environment of those gyms, Jazzercise centers were usually suburban, often offered babysitting, and never included the mirrored walls that were standard in most gyms.

The "ordinary women" Jazzercise attracted were "not necessarily changing the world, but they were changing *their* world," Missett told me. Scores of letters she received detailed abusive marriages abandoned, mountains scaled, and—from franchisees—a measure of economic independence achieved.[61] Missett felt these triumphs personally, especially relishing one 1975 victory. One year after the passage of the Equal Credit Opportunity Act, she stood over a sexist Parks and Recreation bureaucrat as he reluctantly wrote her a large check reflecting the business acumen of a woman he had once dismissed as a "little exercise girl." More such success came: when the military husbands of her devoted students were reassigned away from San Diego, Missett created a certification program, and then a franchise system, to keep her fans step-touching and kick-ball-changing worldwide. The changes that Jazzercise was making in women's lives were undeniable, and in step with the pursuit of independence and self-determination at the core of the feminism some hesitated to claim as their own. Jazzercise, it seemed, empowered women to find income and camaraderie in a way that didn't overhaul the patriarchy but softened its hardest edges.

Studio fitness did not explicitly promise political or spiritual transcendence, but it germinated a recreational women's-fitness culture powerful in transforming participants' sense of self. Jazzercise became a household name, but the strikingly simultaneous career of another woman, Jacki Sorensen, across the country from San Diego, suggests how much the idea that the gym could change one's life—*women's* lives—permeated the zeitgeist. In 1969, Sorensen was living on an Air Force base in Puerto Rico with her husband. Trained as a dancer, she was asked by the military to create a fitness television program to be aired at Officer Wives Clubs. The dance-exercise format she named "Aerobic Dancing" became a sensation when she returned to New Jersey and was soon taught by her trained instructors at YMCAs, community centers, and schools. One Aerobic Dancing advertisement signaled how revolutionary the advent of dance-exercise felt to its enthusiasts: "What do Columbus and Sorensen have in common? They discovered a whole new world!" Later, Sorensen joined the Presidential Council on Fitness and designed physical-education curricula based on Aerobic Dancing for use in public schools. In predominantly masculine spaces—the YMCA with its limited metrics or a military base established to prepare *men* for battle—Missett and Sorensen reimagined how those long excluded from exercise might participate in it, redefining both exercise and themselves in the process.

That Sorensen and Missett almost simultaneously piloted such similar programs reveals a crucial moment they were only two of the most prominent to understand and exploit. As greater numbers of Americans appreciated the importance of cardiovascular exercise—and women, in particular, realized that participating would not make their uterus fall out or morph them into muscle-bound jocks—dance-fitness caught on in many communities beyond the coasts. In the *Wichita Times*, a dance therapist counseled such exercise as a fun, life-extending option for older folks whose "culture" prescribed active life to end around thirty; it was time to do away with the outdated idea that only "construction workers, gardeners and farmers are physically fit."[62] In 1978, the Chicago parks program revamped a New Deal–era recreation program to offer "rhythmic exercise programs" based on "synchronized music," in order to "reflect current trends." Attendance tripled over the next four years, with eight thousand women attending at approximately 165 parks throughout the city. As the African American *Chicago Metro News* reported, the demand among women ages twenty to seventy, "with a sprinkling of senior citizen men," was so great that they sometimes turned away as many as they allowed in. "People are much more serious about keeping fit," one of the organizers noted, and at the price of seven dollars for a ten-week membership—about as much as the charge for one class at a private club—the success was understandable. District instructors touted their community classes as "superior to some private and commercial classes," for their accessibility and focus "not only on improving heart and lung efficiency, but on building strength and muscle tone too." Incorporating chairs, hoops, and other props, the routines constantly changed, and instructors handed out Xeroxed pages with additional exercises and nutritional advice for people to follow at home.[63]

Well-Being Is for the Wealthy

Women's desire for their own exercise spaces was a national phenomenon and extended beyond choreographed studio workouts. In New York City, Lucille Roberts, a Soviet Jewish immigrant, opened an eponymous health spa in the early 1970s geared at middle-class women: teachers, secretaries, or policemen's wives who could afford forty-nine cents per week. Her first location was across the street from the Macy's department store, and as its initial name, "The Body Shop," suggested, it made no lofty promises of transcendence. Though she changed the name when people with car trouble kept calling for a mechanic, Roberts maintained that the lofty pursuits of "well-being" or even "health" were upper-class affectations irrelevant to her clients, who aspired primarily to smaller jeans and bigger bras. At Lucille Roberts, the offerings were straightforward: women could enjoy fifteen weekly classes, tanning booths, and the needlepoint shower curtains and broadloom carpeting that distinguished even this discount option from a dank men's gym.

Women were a ready market for weight loss, Roberts knew, but her inspiration to start the club was not only mercenary. Even before launching the chain of gyms—which grew to serve two hundred thousand members—she pushed back against opportunistic men. After graduating from the University of Pennsylvania in 1964, Roberts had taken a sales job at a shoe company, but quit when a male boss denied her a fifty-dollar raise she had earned by surpassing a sales target. Similarly, women she knew personally had spent hard-earned cash joining coed health spas only to be ogled—and often ripped off—from their first interaction with a salesman.[64]

Establishing the gym, and giving it her name, was an assertion of the kind of economic and professional power of which women were so often deprived. It was an appealing promotional tactic that motivated those with less-sincere commitments, such as the male chiropractor who launched the Elaine Powers Figure Salon with an invented name that was purely a sales come-on.[65] Stauffer had marketed his fraudulent couch with a similar appeal to female authority, promising customer "the help and encouragement of another woman"—an ambiguously credentialed "counselor."[66]

At roughly the same time, uptown from the first Lucille Roberts location, the exercise and entrepreneurial ambitions of another European Jewish woman were taking shape and attracting women to a new form of exercise. In London in the early 1960s, professionally trained dancer Lotte Berk, a German-Jewish exile, began designing a combination of ballet, calisthenics, and yoga moves to heal from a back injury. Her strength and vibrancy returned so robustly that people began asking about her secret cure. Berk began giving classes in the method she had devised, filling an L-shaped, carpeted Manchester Street basement studio with women in tight body stockings who pulsed and flexed their pelvises in hourly sessions, and made her a fortune. The format would become known as "barre."

The "models, millionairesses, housewives, and secretaries" who reverently attended Berk's dance-inspired classes were not *only* getting a physical workout.[67] Her exercise regime, she had noticed, not only cured her back injury but improved her sex life, no insignificant benefit for a woman who had embraced the ideology of free love since the 1950s. In her thick German accent, she called out unapologetically erotic instructions to her students, affirming they were deserving of sexual pleasure.[68] "If you can't tuck, you can't fuck," Berk reportedly told students while cueing them through twisting and thrusting movements called "The Sex," "The Prostitute," and "The Naughty Bottoms."[69] In the press, she was more demure about the "possible sexual selling point" of her methods: "If a student is more agile . . . and she feels her body more beautiful . . . her love life with all her other activities will benefit."[70] Women's exercise could communicate a subtly subversive message to clients, and without compromising their femininity. Berk's method in no way challenged the pursuit of the dominant, thin bodily ideal: "The waist can always be made smaller because it doesn't have any bones," she explained matter-of-factly; "the muscles shape the body and should act as a corset." So too did it promote the expectation that women should vigilantly, constantly work on themselves, for the body "goes quickly to pot once you stop," she warned a reporter who aspired to attain Berk's twenty-four-inch waist.[71]

Berk's London studio became a global destination for American celebrities traveling in Europe, akin to the Parisian Cordon Bleu culinary school or the Mayfair florist Pulbrook and Gould. Berk led a fast life, jetting off on lavish vacations, marrying three times, taking lovers she occasionally shared with her daughter, and speeding around in luxurious cars. For all this wealth, the idea that she, a professionally trained dancer, was "just" a "get-fit girl" felt insubstantial to her.[72] But this aura of European glamour dazzled the Americans who encountered it. In 1970, Lydia Bach, a blonde, thirty-year-old former tax lobbyist and schoolteacher from Illinois, capitalized on this dynamic, raising funds to establish a New York City Lotte Berk salon on East 67th Street, and later in the Long Island beach town of Bridgehampton.[73] The infrastructure of the uptown studio that came to be known as the "Lotte Berk Brownstone" was sparse, but it offered a decidedly more upscale experience than Lucille Roberts or the multilevel health clubs that cordoned off special sections for women. About five or six women, from "college girls" to executives, would gather on the hour in the main room, outfitted with a carpet, a ballet barre, and a stretching ladder.[74] Within a few years, Bach had expanded to three floors, hiring five teachers to minister to women who lined up smoking cigarettes and drinking coffee before class began. Men were strictly forbidden and had to wait downstairs for their wives and girlfriends—almost "like a speakeasy," described Fred DeVito, whose wife, Elisabeth Halfpapp, taught there, and who himself became the first male employee in 1984.[75]

Its glamorous European provenance was not all that made the Lotte Berk Method enticing to women. It was suffused by the aura of the prestigious dance world. Halfpapp, who danced with the Hartford Ballet and held a degree in dance education, had a hard time finding work in her field. But in 1980, she replied to an ad for instructors and soon was teaching a full schedule for Bach. This method, she specified, allowed her to be "a teacher, *not* an instructor in a gym, doing the same thing over and over again."[76] At the same time, the barre was more accessible than Pilates, which required clunky machinery and was still primarily considered, in Halfpapp's memory, a form of rehabilitative training for professional dancers rather than an exercise program for women who aspired to resemble them.

Like Berk, Bach tossed ideas about chaste femininity to the wind. "Sex" is the title of the final chapter of her 1973 book *Awake! Aware! Alive! Exercises for a Vital Body*. Through a series of pelvic thrusts, hip circles, and backbends to be performed "seductively, coquettishly," Bach instructs that "well-exercised muscles are sexually responsive." This open acknowledgment of women's sexuality was nothing like the restrained messaging of slenderizing salons, but it was not exactly liberatory either. Clients testified winkingly that "their husbands have never seen them 'exercise' like this before," while "women fifteen or more pounds overweight" were warned to avoid the "Thighs" and "Sex" section, for "if there is too much fat on top of your thighs, it's as if you are working out with weights, and you will overdevelop your thighs!"[77]

But Bach was no Debbie Drake either. "Exercise should never be looked upon as a chore," she held, but as a commitment that "gives pleasure and vitality, instead of pain and a feeling of 'wasted time.'" Pictured on the cover of her book in a purple leotard, tights, and leg warmers, with her gray-blonde hair flowing behind her, Bach was rapturous about the "something very exciting and intriguing about a mature woman who has vitality and an increased capacity for living." The rhetoric was right out of the New Age-y zeitgeist: "Your body should free your mind. . . . Your pelvic area is the source of the movements and energy of your sex life. If you're proud of your body and you feel good, so will your partner." Achieving this enlightened state through exercise was new to some women: in one bit of studio lore, a concerned client implored an instructor about the unfamiliar fluid beading on her arms—sweat. Yet familiarity with bodily training was growing, in gyms and elsewhere. At one point, Bach warned readers attempting a challenging "hollow hold" pose: "If you are not a yogi, professional athlete, or at a very advanced stage of body control and strength, do not attempt this exercise."[78] Women's desire to exercise, for strength, slimness, and self-actualization, was clearly powering innovations of all kinds and transforming assumptions of what women's bodies could and should do.

15

Swap the Fat for Your True Self

A "Sport [that] Contains the Benefits of Jogging with Some Fun," reported the *Los Angeles Times* of "musical fitness" in 1981.[1] Over the previous decade, aerobic dance and a host of other choreographed workouts had become firmly entrenched in fitness culture. That women who flocked to these classes did not often explicitly align them with women's liberation can obscure how much their existence relied upon the feminist idea that women had a right to bodily self-determination. But just as radical was their embrace of the idea that exercise could be not only rigorous, but vigorous. That the joys of exercise could exceed inches lost represented a sharp departure from the dominant messages women had long encountered about their bodies. Still, across all these practices, and even among avowed feminists, condemning fat was an article of faith. Jean Nidetch, a self-described "formerly fat housewife" from Queens who founded Weight Watchers in 1963, makes clear at the outset of her best-selling 1970 memoir of "a successful loser" that her "crusade" to save those "drowning in fat" was *not* "political" or "revolutionary." In acknowledging that women were "killed physically and emotionally" by their girth, she invoked the increasingly hip idiom of mind-body connectedness, but only to reaffirm that fat people deserved humiliation, "to be hurt badly before they do something about themselves." Inflicting this pain publicly—perhaps on the street or in a shared changing room—was imperative. "Looking into a mirror isn't enough," Nidetch said, because lingering on 'how nice my eyes are' makes you forget that your hips are monstrous."[2]

Surprisingly, given its title, *Fat Is a Feminist Issue*, published in 1978, was just as unsparing in framing fat as pathological. Psychoanalyst Susie Orbach led readers through a clothing-optional meditation that sounds straight out of Esalen, enabling women to examine their reflection dispassionately, consciously resisting "flashing to feelings of disgust." Breathing deliberately, the woman is to "feel herself *throughout* her body," acknowledging "the large thighs she may wish to reject are as much a part of her body as the wrist that seems so much more acceptable." Yet the process of attaining a "holistic view of the body" is not one of loving self-acceptance, but rather of separating women's "true selves" from "the fat that surrounds them." Fat was a symptom of patriarchal subjugation, Orbach insisted, and the solution was slimming down. "In giving up the size you are making an exchange—you swap the fat for your own body and that is power." The solution to society's misogyny relied, in her view, on individual restraint at the refrigerator, a refusal to let oppressive media imagery, catcallers, or unequal pay lead to an expanding waistline: "Now we've learned that we have power over ourselves," she offered. "We've made a dent in the thinking of the world."[3]

Born two decades apart, these very different women were shaped by the same generational culture. The self-deprecatory Nidetch never let a single french fry or drop of cold ketchup remain on her children's plates thanks to her mother's reverberating warnings that each wasted morsel meant "somebody in Europe drops dead." She rues, "I sincerely hope the children in Europe benefited—I did so much for them."[4] Orbach somberly tells the story of one overeater similarly haunted by her hovering mother, reminding her at mealtimes of American soldiers risking their lives to prevent her starvation. This scarcity mentality shaped their perspective on weight loss, which felt similarly precarious. "The spectre of hugeness is always around the corner," Orbach warned.[5] Nidetch agreed that one "will never be thoroughly cured of being potentially fat," for "success" meant never feeling "totally safe again" but remaining perpetually vigilant; carrying a "fat picture" at all times was her recommended strategy. Exercise was mostly irrelevant to Nidetch and Orbach, save for Nidetch's memory of realizing that fat girls were never selected for teams, so she spent physical education class hiding out with other girls who had also decided they were not "the athletic type."[6]

Such ignorance of exercise as means of female self-improvement was receding during the 1970s. But both women spoke in an idiom of bodily self-determination that was becoming widespread even in weight-loss circles. When a male radio interviewer in Florida "growled" that Nidetch's lack of medical credentials made her a fraud, she invoked a different kind of authority: "I'm not a politician or a preacher or an evangelist. I'm somebody fat that people can relate to. I'm them, 72 pounds later."[7] Orbach's feminist critique of male experts who sneered at women's self-knowledge was more pointed. The problem was husbands who encouraged their wives to eat heartily, but desired women with a "slim, trim frame." Pediatricians who insisted mothers were uniquely suited to care for children, but just as adamantly disparaged their decisions about birth, nursing, and feeding were also to blame. Doctors who dismissed women earnestly seeking to lose weight, too often had "neither the time nor the interest to examine why this woman got fat in the first place." Her ultimate solution was structural, requiring "a major reorientation of medical and scientific education, organization and practice based on the demands of the women's health movement," but meaningfully began with restraint at the refrigerator.[8]

Sweating in (Semi-) Public, Together

Lady Jayne Seymour Fonda was born in 1937, in the decade between Nidetch and Orbach, and was also raised to believe that weight management was a paramount concern for a young woman. As a teenager, she and her boarding school friends sent away for tapeworms and stuck their fingers down their throats after dinner to stay slim. As Fonda followed in her father's footsteps to acting, a slim body maintained at any cost became even more important to her increasingly glamorous image. The storied liberalism of 1960s Hollywood hardly liberated Fonda and her female peers from these pressures. Despite her involvement in various liberationist struggles—raising money for the Black Panthers, marching for Native American land rights, and (infamously) traveling to North Vietnam to criticize American military involvement—women's liberation was not central to her worldview. In 1969, the year Missett launched Jazzercise, Fonda was flummoxed by a feminist who pointed out how her recent role in the sci-fi film *Barbarella*—all skimpy outfits and sex with questionable consent dynamics—had objectified her: "I did not even know I had been. The burgeoning new women's consciousness had not yet found its way into my mind and heart."[9]

A foot injury Fonda sustained on the set of *The China Syndrome* would be key to developing that feminist identity. In 1978, her stepmother recommended that in order to rehabilitate her foot and get in shape for bikini scenes in an upcoming role, she should visit Body by Gilda, an exercise studio located in a Century City medical building. Fonda had always danced ballet, but Gilda's, which offered strength training and dance exercise and was frequented by actors and celebrities such as Barbra Streisand and Bette Midler, was an entirely different experience.[10] Gilda was founder Gilda Marx, a self-described former "chubette" and Pittsburgh native who had relocated to southern California, where she found exercise gave her the confidence to fit in and earn a livelihood. Marx had started out instructing homemakers who gathered in her San Fernando Valley living room, but her workouts became so popular that she expanded to multiple locations and in 1975 even launched a fashion line, featuring nylon-spandex body stockings branded as "Flexatards," which ultimately became a multi-million-dollar business.

But it wasn't fashion, or even Marx, that entranced Fonda and convinced her of the transformative potential of exercise. It was the classes taught by petite former ice skater—and current smoker—Leni Cazden that Fonda found nothing short of "a revelation." In the company of forty other women sweating and leg-lifting to pounding music over ninety minutes, Fonda felt "in her gut" how "exercise could affect a woman's body and mind."[11] Sure, she lost weight for *California Suite* as she initially intended, but she did so in the company of women strengthening rather than starving themselves. Marx was a contemporary of Orbach and Nidetch, and she also never challenged the conventional physical ideal of "sleek and flexible," despite proclaiming, "I am against dieting!" But even as her studios perpetuated the timeless pursuit of thinness, Marx insisted that the real transformation that exercise enabled came from the "first-rate feeling" and "self-assured attitude" borne of "mental and physical harmony."[12]

Fonda soon hired Cazden to teach her privately, and even led a version of the class herself when she was on a movie set.[13] If Fonda didn't yet explicitly associate her growing passion for fitness with her burgeoning feminism, she did understand it as a concrete way to energize progressive politics. Six years earlier, she had married activist Tom Hayden, a founder of Students for a Democratic Society, and his antipoverty nonprofit, California's Campaign for Economic Democracy, desperately needed cash. Cazden's workout, with Fonda's celebrity imprimatur, could be their ticket. Within a few months, they moved forward—that is, Fonda did, as Cazden remembers painfully: over lunch one day in 1978, under pressure from a lawyer, Fonda told Cazden, "This is going on, with or without you." The two made amends years later, but Cazden remembers that lunch as "literally taking everything from me." Cazden swallowed her pain, and took off for the next six years, sailing around the world with her third husband on a self-described "soul retrieval." She was not there in September of 1979, when Jane Fonda's Workout studio opened on Robertson Boulevard, in a space that Cazden had found, in Beverly Hills.

Fonda was far from first to the dance-fitness world, but her celebrity was crucial to making the format famous. Gilda Marx brushed off the idea that she was offended that Fonda's name had become more synonymous with working out than her own; the exposure benefited all of them. The choreography in Fonda's Workout was similar to that in Jazzercise, but liberal Hollywood was a markedly different environment than Missett's San Diego, and the Workout united women's fitness more closely with Fonda's overtly progressive politics. Clients who visited the three studios she opened over the next few years may not have known their class purchase supported a left-wing nonprofit, but they found a space Fonda described as designed explicitly to "create more realistic, less anxiety-ridden standards" for women, judges or janitors, who all struggled with body image and sexual exploitation.[14] Fonda was so famous that even before VHS tapes would make the Workout a global phenomenon, this ethos suffused the experience of exercise even for women who never set foot in one of her studios. Fonda made it acceptable "to sweat in public," countless women told me.

Gloria Steinem, no stranger to feminist consciousness-raising, marveled at the "Family of Woman" engendered by the intimacy of the locker room at her own women's gym. In a *Ms.* magazine essay, she remarked that Fonda-style exercise was unmaking the assumption that athleticism was unfeminine and frivolous. The camaraderie of the locker room was a powerful antidote to messages that women's bodies should look a certain way or existed primarily for male pleasure. Unashamedly changing together before or after a class was in itself a feminist experience, making "great beauties seem less distant and even mastectomies seem less terrifying."[15] Molly Fox, who had taught at Fonda's San Francisco studio, credited Fonda with inspiring a generation of women to be unabashed about their new exercise habits, proudly wearing the pantyhose they cut into crop tops, or the belted leotards and off-the-shoulder sweatshirts that advertised they were coming to or from a class.

Fonda had been inspired by Gilda Marx, and so was Kathy Smith, the midwesterner turned Hawaii marathoner. She had recently caught Marx's eye while running on the beach. Marx quickly hired her as a "hangtag model" to shoot in her Flexatards, which women were not only wearing to exercise, but increasingly pairing with jeans and skirts too. Smith was working at a small gym on Montana Boulevard, Sean Harrington's Nautilus, that under the banner "IT'S TORTURE, BUT IT WORKS" advertised a twenty-minute circuit on Nautilus weight machines that were then cutting edge, but rarely at clubs that welcomed women. Smith not only loved the workout herself but found herself lining up with the likes of stars like Linda Evans, Bo Derek, Cher, and Morgan Fairchild.

Smith sensed an opportunity, and asked Harrington if she could build out a small, unused space in the gym to sell workout wear: Flexatards, but also the tiny, clingy Dolfin shorts favored by the growing ranks of active men and women. "People wanted them in every color," Smith recalled. Decorated with a Superman logo and repainted in bright colors, the space was called "Kathy's Knockouts." Around 1977, Smith remembers, she asked Harrington if she could take over another space in his club as "an exercise room," to teach her own version of the class she loved at Body Design by Gilda—but with more choreography. He built it out, and before long, Smith built "a huge following." And because it was at a gym, not a "studio," Smith told me, it was unique in being "really male-female."[16]

Another Body Design by Gilda regular, Richard Simmons, went still further in launching a fitness phenomenon that redefined both exercise and who could participate in it. A frizzy-haired Louisianan working as a waiter in Los Angeles, Simmons had always struggled with his weight, and had "felt like a failure" at every workout he attempted. But a friend sent him to Marx, whose red lips, nails, and matching leotard reminded Simmons—before the music even began—of a warrior princess. Marx's luminous smile, the live piano, and the room full of music and movement were a game changer. Simmons broke into song several times and signed up for a multi-class membership on the spot, practically floating with joy at having found such a fun version of exercise that made him feel his "body was really alive." But that night, as Simmons worked the dinner shift, Marx and her husband showed up to deliver some bad news: Simmons was "too much of a cutup, too much of a disruption" to be welcomed back to class. She returned his money and walked away, leaving him heartbroken and furious.[17] This was Simmons's interpretation of the snub, but Marx clarified that the problem was really that "women were not comfortable with a man in the class."[18] He was skeptical, and doubly hurt because he dreaded returning to unwelcoming men's gyms, where the trainers were militaristic and his emerald-green tracksuits with white piping stood out uncomfortably amid the sea of stained, gray sweats.

Simmons took matters into his own hands and opened a studio called the Anatomy Asylum in 1974. His classes were performances as much as workouts, and he declared everyone was welcome. Gay men and fat women in particular would effuse that the studio was unique in that it "made them feel at home," since "you didn't have to look like you already go to the gym to belong there." Unlike muscled weight lifters or his slim, white, female contemporaries in dance-exercise, Simmons did not immediately present like a die-hard exerciser, and in favoring spangled, multicolored hot pants and clownish makeup, refused to suppress his flamboyance or joy.[19] The *Los Angeles Times* described him as "a kind of freaked-out Jack LaLanne" determined not to run "another phony hangout for the beautiful people," despite the Beverly Hills location. There *were* limits to his inclusiveness, as one hundred dollars would buy only ten introductory classes (four dollars apiece thereafter), rather than a year's membership at the Y. Despite these democratic pretensions, Simmons explained, "it's a matter of life-style," likening the experience to that of luxury department store Bonwit Teller: "Some people like to buy a dress at [bargain store] Lerner's. . . . In our field, we're the Bonwit's."[20] Anatomy Asylum also featured a salad bar, Ruffage, which at the time was an amenity found only in steak houses.

If dance-aerobics represented a convergence of the slenderizing spa, athletic field, yoga retreat, and ballet studio, Anatomy Asylum was equally influenced by the men's gyms that had long been vibrant social spaces. What had been underground meeting places for most of the twentieth century were by the height of gay liberation in the 1970s far more visible in urban landscapes; even famed conservative attorney Roy Cohn was an investor in a Greenwich Village men's gym. The nightclub and fitness scenes often overlapped in New York City and Los Angeles, sometimes explicitly: party promoter John Blair opened The Body Center in Los Angeles in the early 1970s and described it as "the first gay gym: Nautilus machines, tiny shorts, tube socks, and Abba all day long." Blair invited the best-looking members to parties to attract crowds, which in turn sold gym memberships to revelers who aspired to look like them. In 1978, Blair opened a New York gym and later told the *New York Times* he "would give one month's free gym membership to every cute boy I met at Studio 54." Gay culture—in what some considered its most superficial form—flourished in fitness clubs, but also began to become normalized in mixed spaces like the Anatomy Asylum.[21] As recently as 1971, *Good Housekeeping* had published the aesthetic exercise routine of a "remade man" who warned readers: "Before you get some idea that this is a little strange, let me tell you I'm not one bit ashamed of it, and I don't feel effeminate either." Within a decade, Simmons helped make obsolete such caveats from men who worried exercise would emasculate them.

A Culture of Narcissism?

"Jane Fonda's Exercise Salons Aiding Her Husband's Candidacy," reported the *New York Times* of the crucial role of The Workout in funding Tom Hayden's congressional aspirations.[22] He didn't much appreciate the idea that his wife and a bunch of sweaty women in legwarmers held so much power over his political career, and he needled her about this activity he perceived as incommensurate with their serious activism. Hayden echoed a chorus of intellectuals such as Christopher Lasch and Tom Wolfe who derided yoga, aerobics, jogging, and other aspects of New Age "encounter culture" as part of a lamentable "fadeout" of legitimate political and civic commitments that had been supplanted by a "culture of narcissism."[23] According to these critics, the popularization of fitness was enabled by this dubious, self-centered spirit of the seventies, which Lasch disdained as the "prevailing passion . . . to live for yourself, not for your predecessors or posterity." Interestingly, Joel Kramer, a former resident yogi at Esalen, agreed with Lasch that the culture was becoming terribly self-absorbed, but saw an authentic yoga culture "gobbled up by the Me-Generation" as a casualty rather than cause of this troubling trend.[24] Such laments resonated with a very different criticism from the Right, which argued yoga was part of "an evil tide sweeping America," worshipping the body but "scarring the soul."[25] So too were the groups of women sweating together in scanty body stockings discomfiting to religious conservatives; Missett, who sought to rent space in churches, had to convince clergymen that Jazzercise was no tool of the devil. Lasch argued that the "cult of expanded consciousness, health, and personal 'growth'" was actually similar to religious fundamentalism, and a similarly unfortunate response to despair about a changing society.[26] These blanket dismissals—mostly issued by men—overlooked or misunderstood the nature of the transformations afoot. Americans were channeling their spiritual, emotional, and—at times—explicitly political energies into a new sort of movement culture.

Redefining exercise beyond calisthenics, weight lifting, and organized sport—and as an activity appropriate for everyone—*was* revolutionary. And some who flocked to new spaces like yoga retreats, dance-fitness studios, and jogging trails saw participating in these activities as bound up with the fight for bodily liberation that powered activism for reproductive and civil rights, and a general search for authenticity in an era of disillusionment with so many social and political institutions. Others created and participated in these new arenas for physical expression as a path to a less explicitly political, but no less personally important, self-possession. Title IX, and the 1970s fitness boom more broadly, enabled women athletes to break into the mostly male realm of competition, but the broader democratization of physical activity also came to engage girls and women with little desire to participate in an athletic culture defined by men. Many of these enthusiasts specifically disavowed the revolutionary effect of their ambitions, emphasizing instead the uncontroversial benefits of fitness for beauty (for women) or athleticism (for men), or just their own personal achievement, untethered from any greater cause. Companies happily capitalized on this new market, sometimes explicitly packaging a tepid politics with exercise apparel, as with the Nike "Liberator." The Presidential Council on Youth Fitness, which had barely included girls in its early days, released advertisements in the mid-1970s that also reflected this measured transformation in ideas about girls and women. A "lovely revolution," the ad announced, revealed a new reality: "Physical fitness is beautiful."

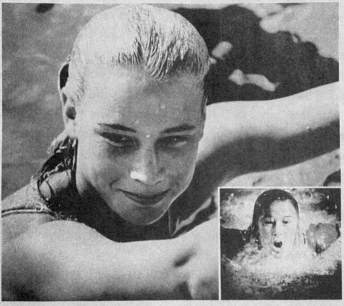

Physical fitness is beautiful, beautiful, beautiful.

There's a lovely revolution going on. It's girls! They are not just spectators anymore. They're into Physical Fitness—doing their own thing in Swimming, Diving, Tennis, Track, Skiing and Gymnastics. The results are beautiful.

Today, her beauty is more than skin deep. Her new healthy glow, well-coordinated charm and educated grace come from Physical Fitness.

When parents really support the Physical Education programs of their schools—something really beautiful happens to their children.

The President's Council on Physical Fitness & Sports
Washington, D.C., 20201

19

Figure 15. *Physical Fitness Is Beautiful, Beautiful, Beautiful!*, June 1974. By the mid-1970s, the Presidential Council on Physical Fitness and Sports had begun targeting girls and women as well as boys and men—in the process adding "beauty" to its list of the benefits that came along with the pursuit of physical fitness.

But what about those weight lifters and bodybuilders who had first brought national attention to the salutary, transformative possibilities of physical fitness? Muscle Beach had planted the seeds of the sensibility that made fitness as a form of work and leisure acceptable, and bodybuilding ironically both became more popular than ever *and* remained a relatively marginal form of the pastime it helped popularize. In *Stay Hungry*, a 1972 novel about an unambitious wealthy southerner who becomes captivated by a circle of Birmingham weight lifters, a Junior League debutante, Dorothy, stares at the massive shoulders of the "ruddy and foreign" protagonist, Joe Santo, in a mixture of awe and fear, mustering the courage to ask what on earth he does. When he replies he "lifts weights," she wonders "what the hell that meant."[27] By 1976, *Stay Hungry* was released as a feature film, starring a new actor as the eccentric, inscrutable Santo: Arnold Schwarzenegger. In the movie, a blushing Dorothy reacts to his unconventional appearance with a common misconception: she had "always heard that people of your profession were . . . homosexuals." He offers to prove her wrong.[28]

The next year, *Pumping Iron* made Schwarzenegger a national celebrity and gave bodybuilding—and the gym—cultural currency. He spoke about the mind-blowing thrill of lifting weights in a way that resonated with a culture in which exercise was increasingly intertwined with exhilaration that infused all aspects of life. "The greatest feeling you can get in a gym . . . is . . . blood is rushing into your muscles, and that's what we call the pump. . . . It feels fantastic." But his elaboration on the specifically heterosexual ecstasy of exercise was also evidence of the continuing pressure on bodybuilders to prove their sexual normalcy. "It's as satisfying to me as . . . having sex with a woman and coming," Schwarzenegger elaborated. "So can you believe how much I'm in heaven? I'm getting the feeling of coming in the gym. I'm getting the feeling of coming at home. I'm getting the feeling of coming backstage when I pump up. . . . I'm coming day and night. I mean it's terrific, right?"[29] He made the point even more clearly in a 1977 interview: "Men shouldn't feel like fags because they want to have nice-looking bodies."[30] If Schwarzenegger's breathless words resonated with Jeannine Medvin's celebration of yoga as a path to orgasmic self-possession, Jim Fixx's elegies to endorphins, or Jane Fonda's insistence on the "joy, excitement, vitality, and wellbeing" afforded by exercise, weight lifting felt oddly out of step with the moment it helped launch.[31] The macho brutality and bulging aesthetic were increasingly unpalatable for a main-stream culture more comfortable with the controlled family jog around the neighborhood first recommended by Bowerman, or the sorority of Jazzercise or a Lotte Berk studio, especially as women and gay men became more powerful presences at the gym and on the streets, if not in always in the marches and demonstrations that captured headlines and show up in history books—a different revo-lution brought about by these dynamic new movement cultures.

Part **Five**

FEEL THE BURN

Bigger than General Motors and twice as profitable!
ARTHUR JONES, FOUNDER OF NAUTILUS

There were still, of course, those who were unconvinced of the benefits of exercise, even as its popularity surged in the 1980s. Dr. Henry Solomon, a cardiology professor at Cornell University's medical school, was certain that the "women in stylish gear hurrying to exercise class; middle-aged men huffing to and from Central Park; people of every age and description panting and sweating their way to today's version of the healthy lifestyle" were making a potentially mortal mistake. In his 1984 book, *The Exercise Myth*, Solomon made a strenuous case against the idea that hitting the road in rubber-soled shoes was the path to a healthier heart and happier life. On the contrary, he walked just about a mile a day and warned of "stricken" exercisers who found themselves "lying under the sheets in the intensive-care unit with a coronary attack," feeling "guilty and ashamed" that they had been "stupid enough to buy the bill of goods" that rigorous exercise was good for you.[1] Aerobics evangelist Kenneth Cooper dismissed Solomon, noting that his alarmism was misplaced given there were no "streets full of dead joggers" or "hospitals overwhelmed by injuries because of exercise."[2]

While Solomon echoed a skepticism that was over a century old, he expressed fresh concerns about the risks to new exercisers who threw themselves too zealously into this craze for activities that were more intense, and more widely practiced, than those of past generations: only 24 percent of American adults had exercised regularly in 1961, but that that number jumped to 50 percent by 1968, and 59 percent in 1984.[3] The results of this "physical fitness epidemic," so styled by a dour 1980 *McCall's* article, spanned torn tendons to internal bleeding to delusions of athletic grandeur: "You can't reasonably expect to run a four-minute mile; nor is it likely that you will win the Open Tennis Championship at Wimbledon," it admonished.[4] Running could also wreak psychological damage, *Sports Illustrated* reported the same month, in a feature on the malaise of "marching to euphoria," afflicting wild-eyed "physical fitness devotees" whose passions rendered them a "bunch of Skid Row running addicts" as dependent on the "gossamer trance" of exercise as junkies and drunks. Ill-equipped to train as responsibly as athletes, "recreational runners" could be dangerously consumed by this new passion for feeling the burn.[5]

These perils had at least one famous face; on a crisp fall day the year before, President Jimmy Carter had been four miles into a 6.2-mile race when he collapsed, his skin pale and "rubbery of leg and gasping." Though Carter recovered quickly, the images of the president with his mouth hanging open and his heather-gray T-shirt soaked with sweat circulated widely, raising doubts about the connection between fitness and civic fortitude that boosters had long labored to establish.[6] Anti-exercise forces also found ammunition in the sudden death, five years later, of Jim Fixx, whose *New York Times* obituary dubbed him "the guru of running." Fixx, fifty-two, suffered a massive heart attack—while jogging. Fixx had taken up jogging in 1967 because he knew he was susceptible to hereditary heart disease, and his dramatic death—he was discovered by a motorcyclist on the side of a Vermont road—fanned the fears of exercise skeptics but left enthusiasts mostly unperturbed. New York City Marathon founder Fred Lebow figured that if Fixx had kept smoking two packs a day as he had before he had taken up running, "he'd have died five years ago."[7]

But a few tragic running incidents and pleas from contrarian physicians did nothing to dampen the enthusiasm for fitness flourishing in the open air of city streets, the protected enclaves of exer-

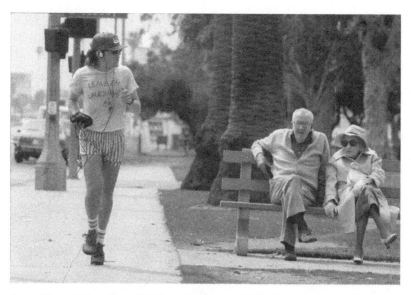

Figure 16. Jose Galvez, *Man with Walkman Jogging past Elderly Couple Seated on Park Bench in Santa Monica, Calif.,* 1981. A jogger, no longer a rare sight by the early 1980s, exercises on a Los Angeles sidewalk. He wears sneakers and a Walkman, both consumer products aimed at growing ranks of fitness enthusiasts, part of a generational phenomenon distinct from anything the elderly couple on the bench would have experienced.

BLACK-AND-WHITE NEGATIVE. *LOS ANGELES TIMES* PHOTOGRAPHIC ARCHIVES, SPECIAL COLLECTIONS, CHARLES E. YOUNG RESEARCH LIBRARY, UCLA. COLLECTION ID: UCLALAT_1429_B1260_29483. HTTPS:// CALISPHERE.ORG/ITEM/ARK./21198/ZZ0002RVHV/.

cise studios, and the immaculate health clubs that catered to young, attractive patrons who, some scoffed, perhaps with a touch of envy, hardly looked in need of hitting the gym. From 1977 to 1990, the number of commercial gyms grew exploded from just 2,700 to nearly fourteen thousand, and from 1972 to 1995, from 1.7 million to 24.1 million engaged clients, changing the shape of not only bodies, but more importantly, the landscape of daily life.[8] And these figures didn't even account for the community centers, workplace gyms, and small studios that multiplied in the 1980s, or the era's biggest innovation: exercise on home video.

By the end of the decade, anti-exercise naysayers would be lonelier voices, relics of an era when a society that did not include the pursuit of fitness as a defining feature—or maybe bug—was still imaginable. Over the course of the 1980s, the pursuit of exercise became encoded in everyday experience, in an expanding web of fitness facilities, products, media, and an increasingly organized profession. Yet the group best prepared to take advantage of this enthusiasm—physical educators—found itself marginalized by a popular culture and policy environment that hacked away at the public institutions in which they served, and by an industry that rewarded entertainment and individualism over expertise and collective endeavor, or at least one that channeled them toward civic ends.

16

Daytime Disco

Newly ubiquitous, and often glamorous, brick-and-mortar gyms were the most public signs of the evolving fascination with fitness. Jack LaLanne licensed his name to a chain of gyms that strove to differentiate itself in this crowded market. Surprisingly, given LaLanne's association with an earnest, on-screen wholesomeness that had transformed a generation of 1950s housewives from exercise skeptics to acolytes, Cher signed on as its spokeswoman. Known not only as a celebrated contralto but also for her public divorce from Sonny Bono and daring fashion choices such as head-to-toe chain mail, Cher's presence signaled an edgier aesthetic. Typical of the LaLanne campaign was a print ad in which Cher, clad in a crop top and leg warmers, stared suggestively, kitten heel poised atop a barbell.[1] "Getting blonde was easy," she intoned in a 1985 television spot, pumping a weight with her bicep. But, she confided, as a row of iron plates slams down and the camera zoomed out to show her sculpted body, "getting this body wasn't."[2] The ad evoked the nineteenth-century ideas that fashion signaled laziness while exercise was a sign of disciplined virtue, but its real message was that working out was not just salutary but sexy and celebrity-adjacent.

Cher's bare midriff got the print ad banned from *TV Guide*, but her presence signaled a more controversial association. America was in the midst of the HIV-AIDS epidemic, which the Reagan administration dismissed as a uniquely "gay plague" and only acknowledged after forty-seven thousand Americans had been infected.[3] Cher was not just an unapologetically sexy and edgy divorcée but a figure especially adored by the gay community.[4] When most straight public figures remained silent about the epidemic, she actively supported HIV-AIDS research funding—while the ubiquitous face of decidedly middlebrow LaLanne Health Spas.[5]

For decades, LaLanne, his fellow Muscle Beach alumni, and fitness enthusiasts in general had labored to distance themselves from associations with homosexuality. Many performed an exaggerated heterosexuality that often veered into homophobia. Yet even as gay liberation had made important inroads, fitness spaces often continued to provide solace from pervasive ostracism.[6] LaLanne acknowledged as much in 1984, when *Playboy* asked him whether "gays have ruined health clubs for heterosexuals." "This is bullshit!" he rejoined. He acknowledged that since opening his first club in 1936, men who sought sex with men had disproportionately gravitated to the gym, especially when he had offered massage; "guys who were pillars of society . . . bank presidents, lawyers, judges" would offer him money for sex. LaLanne stopped short of condemning them— "Whatever you want to do is your business. . . . This stuff has been going on forever"—but made sure to distance himself: "You could write me a check for $1,000,000 and I would never let a man touch me." LaLanne trafficked in various stereotypes: his acceptance didn't extend to "old queens" who "take 12, 13, 14-year-olds who give them money and force them to go around with his friends," but he appreciated that "homosexuals love to look good . . . clean, neat . . . fastidious, well-mannered, and well educated. They like aesthetic things. They like good, firm, tight bodies. Health."[7]

Thanks to the successes of gay liberation, the connection between queerness and the gym only intensified in the late 1970s and early 1980s, but it became significantly less controversial. At the Sports Connection in Los Angeles, openly gay Simon Doonan, dressed in patterned spandex, would take his place daily in the front row of aerobics classes after he worked designing window displays at the boutique Maxfield's, mixing with gay and straight men and women.[8] The first "real gym" that teenager Brian Moss experienced as a member was "a men's gym" on West 76th Street in New York City, which to him in the 1970s "meant a gay gym." He wondered,

"Could a straight guy work out there?" Yes, it turned out. Unlike the clientele at some of the downtown gyms known as "cruise spots," Moss found most, like him, "just wanted to get strong." As a brainy kid attending a public arts high school, he "barely had PE," much less contact with the kinds of sinewy human specimens he knew only from the television show *Kung Fu*, and now the gym floor. Moss was "mesmerized," and when a physical education teacher lent him a small weight set he kept in his office, he got hooked on developing his own strength, and on joining a growing world of enthusiasts.

Working as a museum educator after graduation, he kept hearing his father's advice: "If you start a business, you can own a forest, not just teach about them." Moss sold his car and took out a loan to open his own gym: a "really hardcore" coed strength-training facility. "But you're going to get all lesbians," his friends protested. Moss didn't care; the homosocial environment at West Side Body-building had inspired rather than revolted him, and sexuality was not the organizing principle of the gym he envisioned anyway. In 1982, Moss opened Better Bodies, filling four thousand square feet of warehouse space on West 21st Street with equipment he bought from the father of famed bodybuilder Lou Ferrigno. Openly gay men and lesbians were among the clientele, but Moss was more struck by the "outliers" and "underground people" who took advantage of his day passes, always offered for no more than the price of a movie ticket: adult film actress Vanessa del Rio, late night public-access television personality Robin Byrd, and writer Kathy Acker, whose 1993 essay about the liberatory potential of bodybuilding became a cult favorite among contemplative gymgoers.[9] Other clubs used initiation fees and membership contracts to cultivate exclusivity, but to Moss, accessibility and transience made Better Bodies more interesting.

Such mixing wasn't limited to liberal coastal cities. Minnesota native Michael Perron grew up playing ice hockey and skiing, but as a college student in Arizona resorted to cycling. When he returned home, snow and ice kept him off the road, so when a friend invited him to aerobics—an activity impervious to the elements—Perron

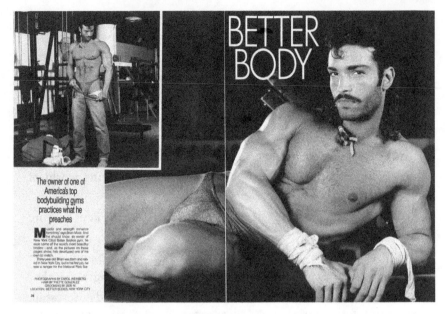

The owner of one of America's top bodybuilding gyms practices what he preaches

Muscle and strength enhance femininity, says Brian Moss. And he should know, as owner of New York City's Better Bodies gym, he sees some of the world's most beautiful bodies—and, as the pictures on these pages show, he's developed one of his own to match.

Thirty-year-old Brian was born and raised in New York City, but in his first job, he was a ranger for the National Park Service.

PHOTOGRAPHS BY CAROL WEINBERG
HAIR BY YVETTE GONZALEZ
GROOMING BY DEBI M.
LOCATION: BETTER BODIES, NEW YORK CITY

Figure 17. Brian Moss in *Playgirl*, July 1988. Brian Moss poses in *Playgirl* in a photo shoot at his gym, Better Bodies, in New York City. Better Bodies marketed strength training to women (as well as men), a unique offering in the 1980s that attracted a diverse group of downtown artists, actors, and others interested in physical cultivation.

PHOTOGRAPH BY CAROL WEINBERG. COURTESY OF BRIAN MOSS.

agreed, though he associated the word only with "slouchy socks and women." Before long, he was not only wearing fitted tights himself, but immersed in a "full-blown subculture" of fitness enthusiasts who did everything together: taking and teaching classes, sharing meals, and hitting the nightclubs. "Tight-knit" didn't mean exclusive: "There were no expectations on people; anyone could join us," Perron remembered: it was "probably the only time in my life I was in the minority as a straight guy." But it didn't matter; most exercisers in this new dance-fitness culture seemed to be more interested in learning the latest choreography or landing a gig at a new studio than in parsing each other's sexuality.[10]

Across the country, Monique Dash, a young Black woman who taught aerobics after finishing her shifts in the bookings office of Carnegie Hall, reflected similarly on how her race somehow felt less salient in the expanding fitness world than it had in other contexts.

At her mostly Black high school in the Bronx in the mid-1970s, she overheard her white friends discuss hikes and bike rides, activities not on her family's weekend agenda although they were middle class. In the halls of her dorm at SUNY Buffalo, which was predominantly white, her classmates explicitly discussed politics and race, played Frisbee and threw keg parties, and gossiped about who acted "appropriately" white or Black.[11] After switching majors from business to dance, she met her first "jock-y friend," a fellow New Yorker who owned a copy of Jane Fonda's recently published *Workout* book. Dash wanted to "work on her thick legs," so the two began exercising together, and she soon found this training complemented her rigorous dance program. She moved back to New York after graduating in 1982 and was accepted to two dance companies—but life as a performer in New York City was expensive. Teaching fitness provided a way to make money, stay fit, and enter a world that felt less racially fraught to her than Buffalo or the Bronx. "In the fitness world, it was just different," she remembered, "I felt like it was really about your talents. Could you fill a room or not?" In the early years of Reagan's America, racism and homophobia found quarter at the highest reaches of government, but this inchoate, emergent fitness culture could provide surprising pockets of solace.

But this climate of tolerance fostered by certain gyms could be tenuous. At Jim's Gym in the Montrose neighborhood of Houston, Texas, founder Jim Densmore proudly described the elaborate amenities of the gym he opened in 1980 on two refurbished floors of a former beauty school: tanning booths, a health bar, ample parking, and instructors freshly certified by Nautilus. In the local paper, he announced that "this is not necessarily a gay only gym."[12] Even in the more conservative south, the idea of straight and gay clients mixing at a fitness facility was plausible. Houston's "days of intolerance are over," the *New York Times* affirmed in a 1981 article about the city's growing gay community and the sophistication of its Gay Political Caucus, which approached that of Washington, DC, and San Francisco. The Texas city was gaining a reputation as "a place where homosexuals can find the freedom and mutual support that make life easier." Gay activists reassured the public of their collaborative nature, emphasizing "what's good for the city is as a whole good for the gay community"—like getting fit.[13]

Six years after Jim's Gym's auspicious launch, an electrical fire shut it down, and when it reopened, it had a fresh coat of paint, a new name—Parkway Athletic Club—and a new owner.[14] Mark Schmidt, a slim, mustachioed real estate developer from Indiana, undertook a massive renovation, and he cast a wide net advertising the thirty-thousand-square-foot facility's "INCREDIBLE" additional amenities, from a full basketball court, saunas, and solariums to Nautilus machines and nutrition classes. Members of other gyms were invited to join at discounted rates.[15] But the relatively accepting climate Densmore had embraced was fraying. Houston was home to an entrenched conservative contingent whose homophobia was emboldened by the AIDS epidemic and catalyzed in 1986 by a proposed antidiscrimination measure.[16] "Opponents Fear Another San Francisco," the *Los Angeles Times* wrote of the Houston situation, relaying the belief of the coalition of Baptist ministers, organized labor, and the Ku Klux Klan who rallied against the measure that it would invite a "rapid influx of homosexuals" to the South, turning the city into a hellscape of "sadomasochistic bars" and sickness. When the legislation failed to pass, conservative magazine *Human Events* relished this "devastating setback" for the "pro-homosexual" movement.[17]

Defining gay men as deviants, and the spaces where they gathered—like gyms—as dangerous, was a key strategy for homophobes. "Gays don't call normals 'straights' for no reason," opined one 1985 pamphlet on "criminality, social disruption, and homosexuality" that presented gyms as especially pernicious. Acknowledging "sometimes we must be nude or semi-nude in group-settings . . . 'time out' from sexuality is a requirement of good social order," the pamphlet explained. Citing dubious statistics to argue "gays" were overwhelmingly more likely to enjoy "being ogled by a homosexual in such a circumstance" than "normals," the pamphlet said such behavior paved the way for more "crimes against humanity" like child abuse and political insurrection.[18] Such stigmatization undercut the mixed environment Densmore had imagined and advertised just a couple of years earlier—in one magazine spread, he emphasized that despite nude locker rooms, sex was "absolutely not permitted" due to the negative effect of notoriety on the community—though he continued to resist such negative associations. "Building for your future" became the Parkway slogan, and ads now featured smiling, muscular men who looked nothing like the emaciated images of AIDS victims in the news or the swaggering bodybuilders of gay pornography.

Parkway was offering far more than fitness, providing a space for community, information-sharing, and activism. Reflecting the time before effective treatments for AIDS, when one doctor remembered feeling devastated by being unable to recommend remedies other than exercise and healthful eating to patients who were obviously gravely ill, not all the resources shared at the club were equally sound.[19] The month of its reopening, Parkway offered seminars about nutrition and the AIDS crisis, featuring alternative health practitioners such as meditation advocate Louise Hay and William Hitt, an amateur doctor whose three local clinics injected AIDS patients with their own urine—until they were shut down by the Food and Drug Administration.[20]

Schmidt, who had also hosted a "gay-sports radio show" and participated in bowling leagues and local business organizations, died of AIDS in early 1988, at thirty-four. But like many contemporary gyms in areas with sizable gay communities, Parkway became only more important as a haven, expanding its mission from gym to "community fitness and wellness center," organizing events like a Christmas card contest for HIV-positive artists, and hosting seminars on "self-healing" and AIDS.[21] A month after Schmidt died, one ad trumpeted the "Parkway Philosophy," in which working out was only one component—among positive self-image, safe sex, good nutrition, exercise, and relaxation—in the "ammunition that can make us all winners in the victory against AIDS. . . . Become a Parkway man today."[22]

For gay men, especially those affluent enough to join private gyms, the importance of these spaces for cultivating the self and community persisted, even as medical advances slowly began

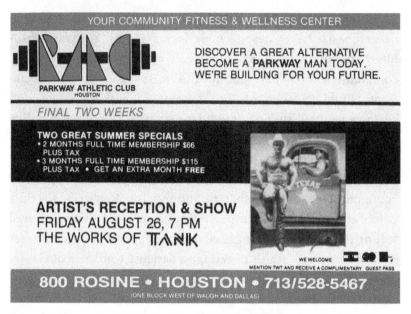

Figure 18. Parkway Athletic Club advertisement, *This Week in Texas*, August 12–18, 1988. Parkway Athletic Club began as a gym but throughout the 1980s became an important cultural hub for Houston's gay community. In 1988, PAC advertised gym membership rates and an art show of the work of Paul Tankersley, who was inspired in equal parts by male physique and cowboy culture.

ADVERTISEMENT. IMAGE COURTESY HOUSTONLGBTHISTORY.ORG. HTTP://WWW.HOUSTONLGBTHISTORY.ORG/MISC-JIMS.HTML.

to lessen the threat of AIDS. For Simon Doonan, the endorphin rush afforded by aerobics "offered an asylum, a refuge, an escape," from the reality that "all of [his] friends were getting sick," even the designer of his favorite spandex shorts.[23] "Bill" was one such Angeleno diagnosed in the 1980s; he relocated to Palm Springs, where a community of HIV-positive men made him feel "like less of a freak." His "very worked out, muscular body" served as "an armor, almost," visibly projecting robustness. (By the early years of the '00s, Bill's younger friends actually preferred HIV-positive men, he said, "because they're generally more healthy and muscular and look . . . more manly.") Doug, another HIV-positive Palm Springs resident, who had fallen sick while performing in *Cats* on Broadway and was then pushed out by the panicked management, agreed on the centrality of the gym when other social supports felt so tenuous:

"If anything is a church, it's the gym for me. . . . I go in there almost like I am entering a temple." The collective experience could also be refreshingly lighthearted; "Doug" describes an uplifting "fun and flirtiness" that makes him feel, "you know, sexy." Coincidentally, Doonan likened his favorite classes to a "disco version of *Cats*."[24]

Culture often migrates from edgy environments to the mainstream, but the case of Molly Fox Studios is less clear. As a twenty-three-year-old dancer in the Bay Area, Fox was aware of the most popular dance-aerobics workouts, specifically Jazzercise. In 1979, she learned that, due to the success of her Beverly Hills studio, Jane Fonda was opening a San Francisco location and would be there in person to teach a class. Fox phoned her friend, ballet dancer Peter Dudley, and told him that they absolutely must attend, confiding her fantasy: Fonda would spot Fox in the crowd and, on the spot, invite her to teach. Dudley, an established and employed dancer, grudgingly agreed to go along. Fonda approached them, all right—to hire Dudley, not Fox. "I had to scratch and crawl and sub for someone who drank all the time," Fox remembered, but she was ultimately hired, too. Armed with Fonda's choreography, a stack of cassette tapes, and the sense that the only other dance-fitness outfits in Manhattan were a Gilda Marx club and the famed Lotte Berk brownstone, Fox relocated to New York City the next year. She rented out "a dance room" for a three-hour slot in the West 19th Street building that housed the prestigious Actors' Institute and dubbed it "Molly Fox's Heavenly Bodies at the Actors Institute." By her own account, Fox knew "zippo about business," relying on informal advice, her own reading, and a prescient instinct that there was a market for creating transcendent experiences of exercise.

The "artsy types" who showed up had mostly never heard of the "Jane Fonda Workout," but they loved that Fox generated such an electric environment they would sometimes break into song during class. Every day at the Molly Fox Studios, she remembered, felt like a "daytime disco . . . sanctioned as healthy but really a sexy, sweaty, body-oriented" environment with "a disco edge." Before class, instructors would gather in a little dressing room, swathe themselves in Capezio dancewear they refashioned into "sexy tight

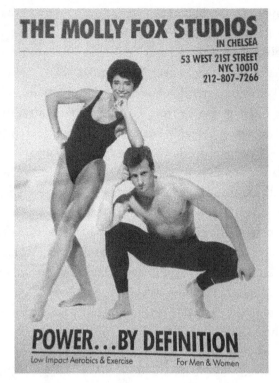

Figure 19. Magazine advertisement for Molly Fox Studios, ca. late 1980s. Molly Fox Studios, a dance-fitness studio in Manhattan's Chelsea neighborhood, became known for its "downtown disco" mood—a mood that made it a destination for fitness professionals from all over the country.

ADVERTISEMENT. FROM THE COLLECTION OF MOLLY FOX

things," stamp out their cigarettes, and stride into the main studio that was invariably packed well beyond its thirty-person capacity. A small boutique soon offered racks of lacy exercise togs, which one client preferred to bulky sweatpants or standard-issue black leotards because "you feel feminine even when you're sweating."[25] Unlike Jazzercise Centers, where mirrors were removed to make women less self-conscious, Fox installed wraparound mirrors "so people [will] look at themselves and feel good about what they see."[26] To the beat of twelve-inch records on the turntable—and then cassettes in a boom box—they would, to other tenants' chagrin, dance and revel until the floor shook, in an experience "just so much bigger than the sum of its parts."[27] Within a year, Fox moved two blocks away to a larger space, right by Better Bodies.

Even within the dance-fitness studio subculture, "Molly Fox's" felt like a refuge, and not only because Fox organized fundraisers for City of Hope, an HIV-AIDS advocacy group, or because she was out herself. For these extravaganzas, Fox invited the most popular instructors from all over town to teach in "workout-a-thons" that lasted many hours, her clientele enjoying impromptu cabaret performances from singers and dancers she counted as clients, while picking at sushi platters donated by local restaurants. Jeff Martin, an uptown instructor and studio owner whose outpost became equally popular, would take the subway to Molly Fox's to take the only dance-fitness classes in the city that he remembered attracted gay male clients, and where he felt he could be himself in a way he was not uptown—in part because it felt so much more like a nightclub than a gym.[28]

Franchising Fitness

By the middle of the decade, twenty-two million Americans did a version of the dance-aerobics workouts studio owners like Molly Fox and Jeff Martin popularized and helped associate with urban coolness. Like Fox, Martin described himself as an unlikely business owner, having imagined a career path as a cantor or a Broadway actor—not running two studios so busy that six phone lines couldn't accommodate the booking requests. But the majority of the growing ranks of American aerobicizers were not part of an avant-garde "gritty, funky downtown studio where a mix of lifestyles just came together," or even of Martin's uptown location, three and a half stories above street level—your warm-up, he would say—where *A Chorus Line* was filmed and "you could just feel the energy."[29]

It was Jazzercise, with its wholesome, suburban sensibility, that corresponded to more Americans' experience of this fitness boom—especially because it became a franchise business with locations all over the country, and the world. In and around San Diego, Missett had been running her vocal cords raw to meet the demand for her classes.[30] She always seemed to find a way to add more local classes, especially as tennis and racquet clubs were ripping out courts to build dance-aerobics studios to meet demand for the craze she helped create. But Missett couldn't clone herself, or create more hours in the day.

Unsure of how to proceed—"I was just a dancer!" she insisted, despite her Northwestern degree—Missett turned to her accountant, who made clear she couldn't hire tens, much less hundreds, of employees or independent contractors. She would have to adopt a structure more usually associated with fast food restaurants and gas stations: a franchise. And as historian Marcia Chatelain has written, the barrier to entry to a franchise business—"the most American idea in the world"—is intriguingly low. As the myth goes, "an owner's manual and free will" is all a franchisee needs to unlock entrepreneurial success.[31] In Missett's case, the decision proved propitious, and by 1984, Jazzercise was the second largest franchise business in the country, just after Domino's Pizza. Missett counted $40 million in revenue, 350,000 students and 2,700 instructor-franchisees worldwide, 99 percent of them women. Countless homemakers attested to experiences more transformative than exercise, recounting how Jazzercise let them earn a living and find community without disrupting their domestic lives.[32]

Franchising became common even among smaller fitness brands, as it remains today. In Yakima, Washington, Women at Large welcomed "large ladies" with "encouragement, friendship, and caring" rather than the disdain its founders had experienced at gyms. At first, the owners were unable to find instructors whose bodies looked like their own or their desired clientele, so they postponed their opening and got certified to teach fitness themselves. They carefully managed the environment in which they operated: instructors were required to wear a full face of makeup and leotards in a conventionally feminine color palette, and fat women were called "fluffy" and bestowed "incentive baskets" to improve their appearance. After an initial false start, business boomed after their 1984 reopening. By 1990, Women at Large had franchised across the United States and in Canada.[33] The inclusion they offered stopped short of self-acceptance or fat liberation, but their very presence was an important counterweight to the outright hostility toward fatness common in the fitness industry, such as the matter-of-fact pronouncement by the manager of the swank New York Vertical Club that "we have no fat people here."[34] When fitness felt more like a dance party than drudgery, it turned out, more people were inspired to exercise.

17

The New Gospel of Fitness

Exercise was undeniably becoming more apparent in the lives of all sorts of Americans. Even before Molly Fox officially taught "master classes" at newly organized conferences and trade shows convened to serve the emergent fitness profession, she noticed teachers and club owners from all over the country appearing in her classes, taking notes on the rhythmic "toning" and "low-impact" classes she had devised in part to placate her downstairs neighbors, who complained about the thudding feet and booming music.[1] Studio owners were rooted by their real estate, but the instructors they hired and the students they inspired spread this fitness gospel through growing networks.

Michael Perron felt the gravitational pull of Los Angeles's fitness scene, and relocated there from Minneapolis to teach at Voight Fitness Center, a five-studio facility where he found he could make a living—fifteen dollars a class, plus a dollar a head in classes that could reach a hundred people, three times daily—and industry connections. "People would fly out for the weekend to take classes at Voight Fitness . . . and we would go to Detroit and other regions and do master classes," Perron recounted. He was succeeding in this expanding universe, but pushed himself so hard to perform that he "escaped reality" by "tweaking out" on methamphetamines in the bathroom before teaching. But he loved the work. After moving again, this time to suburban Dallas to teach at a gym, Goodbodies, he was surprised to see buttoned-up straight men exercising with their girlfriends and wives, in a shared experience he could liken only to church.

Perron ultimately "hung up his sneakers" and became a pastor, creating experiences of spiritual fellowship that he related to me, choked up, reminded him of the intense community that had formed in his exercise classes. Perron is not a household name and did not go on to launch a fitness brand, but like other charismatic instructors, he attracted the attention of brands eager to capitalize on this new movement. Ryka, a brand-new aerobics shoe company, sponsored him to fly to Denmark, Mexico, and Sweden to teach huge classes to cavernous halls full of aspiring instructors fascinated by this American export. Monique Dash seized a similar opportunity to see the world beyond New York City through exercise. In 1983, an ad in *Backstage* caught her eye. It was a call for instructors—no training required—to teach at newly established "aerobics centers" in Italy. Drawing on her dance training, Dash easily booked the job, and her new bosses expedited her first passport. Proud of her elementary Italian, she announced her new place of employment as a chain of *centri di aerobica*. But her Italian managers and clientele insisted she call the studios "aerobics centers," for their American-ness was key to their appeal.[2] Dash spent a year abroad with a cadre of other expatriates, none with working papers, teaching "an exact copy of the Jane Fonda Workout" to Italians intrigued by aerobics, this American phenomenon they had seen mostly in movies and magazines.

The work of working out was even making its way into vacation. Tamilee Webb, a self-described "farm girl" and bodybuilder with a master's degree in kinesiology from Chico State University, got her big break teaching fitness at San Diego's Golden Door Resort and Spa. Webb hailed from Rio Del, a town of thirty-five hundred so sleepy it was known as "Real Dull," before arriving at the Golden Door in 1983, had taught at Chico's first aerobics studio, near campus. Founder Deborah Szekely "hired" Webb to work for free for a weeklong trial, helping guests "decompress." Webb was dazzled by the people and the place. Model Christie Brinkley was one of her first charges as "basically a personal trainer" before such a job title existed. Such posh amenities as individually dedicated exercise professionals established Golden Door, in Webb's words, as "the first elite fat farm." Webb excelled at the job—a role that existed at the intersection of taskmaster, coach, and therapist—and stayed for three years, teaching several daily classes sandwiched between 6:00 a.m. hikes and afternoon spa visits. She soon joined the Golden Door traveling staff, teaching fitness on cruise ships that introduced her—and her teaching style—to Japan, Alaska, and China.[3]

Golden Door, with its lush surroundings and extensive programming painstakingly designed to pamper and support the physical health of affluent clients, had opened in 1958, a luxury version of Rancho la Puerta, the spa Szekely had run since 1940 that Webb characterized as "hippies in tents." Golden Door retained some of this countercultural spirit—Szekely hired a Native American chief and a Japanese priest to bless the land—but as the clientele became more monied, Golden Door billed its vegetarian cuisine and "international patchwork of health ideas" as a counterweight to the soullessness of a life symbolized by Muzak and plastic flowers. In the late 1970s and eighties, Szekely began to emphasize the opportunity to "exercise constantly" in jazz dance, body-conditioning class, or walks among the deliberately far-flung buildings on Golden Door's six-hundred-acre property as an essential "antidote to soft western paunch" caused by a "languid-paced society."

Some clients checked in to complete a book manuscript or recover from trauma—one couple so loved the lifestyle they stayed ten years—but most guests came to "the reducing ranch" to lose weight, the emphasis on exercise being a major attraction.[4] Such "fitness vacations" were not only catching on among the wealthy; in 1982, both *Reader's Digest* and the African American *Chicago Metro News* recommended "week-to-month-long vacations" organized around exercise for "Americans of all ages" seeking to "take a breather from life's pressure-filled pace." Resort prices ranged from $450 to $2275 a week, but the point was that even a "simple do-it-yourself program" sufficed—and that while rigorous exercise might be interpreted as in itself stressful, it was essential to proper rest. The "basic principle" of "total activity" that governed such "vacations" was admittedly hard to envision as relaxing: "Work on everything at once—exercise, diet, attitudes, and habits. . . . Try to do something you'll do every day from now on (like running before breakfast)."[5]

If exercise enabled escape, whether through drugs, travel, or endorphins, it was also becoming a workplace staple, elastic enough to be framed both as a boon for personal health and productivity, and an antidote to corporate monotony. In 1980, Exxon—hardly a company with health at the core of its mission—launched an elaborate, eight-month executive fitness program, a sufficiently novel initiative that *US News and World Report* published its particulars, from examination by a company doctor to a cool-down (curiously) with a punching bag, and the universal recommendation that all employees exercise, eat right, and stop smoking.[6] The next year, a public service announcement by the President's Council on Physical Fitness and Sports queried "Can you pick out the greatest employee health hazard?" in a caption below obviously perilous images of a bubbling test tube, a meat slicer, and an electric drill. The correct answer, however, was the upholstered swivel chair, that "keeps us sitting on the job—with no exercise—no chance to keep physically fit." Consistent with its Kennedy-era messaging, the copy harped on the dangers of "our bodies growing soft." But the ad ran in *Cosmopolitan*, targeting working women rather than men facing military combat. Even more expansively, the council advised employers to "provide direction and opportunity for employee fitness" both for individual health and to avoid "losing billions" due to "lowered productivity, chronic fatigue, absenteeism, and early retirement."[7] Bank of America was one of many companies to follow suit, in 1986 touting its "Bankercize" program as increasing productivity and leading to a steep drop in stress-related worker's compensation claims.

Gyms were becoming fixtures in the office towers that were the habitat of upwardly mobile, predominantly white young urban professionals, or "yuppies," working ever longer days to fuel Wall Street's bull market. Timothy Pytell, a former college athlete who had relocated from Colorado to Manhattan in 1985 to pursue a degree in intellectual history, found work as a private coach at a slew of the opulent gyms that were centerpieces of office renovations. A far cry from the dank gymnasiums where early-twentieth-century clerks had warded off sloping shoulders and droopy paunches, these spaces were shiny and immaculately maintained, with uniformed attendants distributing towels to the clean-cut, overwhelmingly male, executives sweating on Nautilus machines and whirring treadmills. These gyms could establish new hierarchies even within these rarefied office buildings. Sweeping views of the Hudson River and the Statue of Liberty surrounded the exercisers on the top-floor gym where Pytell trained executives; other employees used a crowded, less luxuriously appointed space on the fourth floor. Such innovations could backfire when they reproduced corporate power structures too harshly. At one midwestern firm, only vice presidents and up were entitled to a gym discount, in part as "an incentive" to work toward promotion. Some junior employees interpreted this darkly: "They only want vice presidents and above to be healthy."[8]

These corporate gyms so reproduced the stark homogeneity of their firms that Pytell joked his Irish ethnicity made him a minority among the overwhelmingly WASP workforce.[9] The growing association between regular exercise and "yuppies" was just as powerfull on the streets outside these gyms, where jogging had mostly shed its countercultural cast to be known as a fancy affectation, like croissants or an expensive juicer.[10] The multi-city "Corporate Challenge," which by 1987 organized sixty-eight thousand runners—sporting T-shirts emblazoned with employer logos—from over four thousand companies in a three-and-a-half-mile contest, was celebrated by *American Banker* for promoting personal health and company morale. Along with a proliferation of urban marathons in these years, such road races were so prevalent because they were inexpensive and highly visible ways for city officials to market an image of fiscal and personal health that offset depictions of urban crime and decay.[11]

Yet the yuppification of fitness in general and running in particular increasingly served to define "legitimate" recreational runners as white, in contrast to poor people of color not only underrepresented in this fitness culture but antithetical, and even threatening,

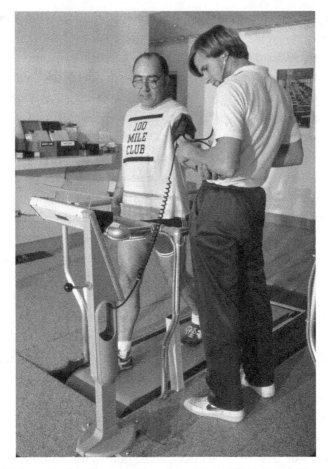

Figure 20. Bernard Gotfryd. *Corporate Fitness, General Foods*, 1984. A General Mills corporate employee exercises at an on-site facility. Corporate gyms, often offering personalized attention, became increasingly common in white-collar workplaces that framed fitness as both a health-enhancing perk and a technique to boost productivity.

PHOTOGRAPH, COLOR TRANSPARENCY, 35MM (SLIDE FORMAT). BERNARD GOTFRYD PHOTOGRAPH COLLECTION, LIBRARY OF CONGRESS PRINTS AND PHOTOGRAPHS DIVISION. CONTROL NUMBER 2020737225. HTTPS://WWW.LOC.GOV/ITEM/2020737225/.

to it. The *Los Angeles Times* wrote that the presence of joggers—and croissant shops—in gentrifying Black ghettos were the telltale symbols of how such neighborhoods were coming to resemble the sterile suburbs that white residents had ostensibly escaped.[12] As jogging became solidified as another accoutrement of 1980s affluence, the formerly male pursuit came to include white women. But in public spaces, people of color, and especially Black Americans, despite professional excellence in running, were increasingly seen in opposition to white joggers. Perhaps most tragically, when two young Black men went jogging in Salt Lake City with white, female teenage friends in 1980, they were murdered by a white supremacist who interpreted this behavior as a mortal provocation.[13] The juxtaposition was usually more subtle, such as an image of marathoners in Los Angeles in 1988, streaming down Sunset Boulevard—which had been closed for them—under a Spanish-language billboard advertising Camel cigarettes.[14] The implication that the predominantly white runners had a right to the streets, while Latino Angelenos might be smoking on the sidelines, was palpable. In 1985, the African American periodical the *Crisis* identified the dynamic explicitly: "The homeless and downtrodden are most times a 'disgusting' irritation to the jogging, orange-juice drinking yuppie who must step over or past them on his or her way to the office."[15] Nothing solidified this notion of the Black threat to white joggers as viscerally as the 1989 frenzy over the "Central Park jogger," when five men of color were wrongfully convicted of the rape and attempted murder of a white female investment banker who had been out running.[16]

But jogging culture was never as white as dominant media portrayed it. Ted Corbitt himself was an elite competitor, but had been a key member in the New York City distance-running community, and in establishing the city's marathon that brought so many casual exercisers out to compete. Far less famous Black Americans embraced and engaged in this pastime. On the South Side of Chicago, a Black mother of six who had fallen in love with running after participating in an Avon women's race mobilized her fellow postal workers to join the city's Corporate Challenge.[17] *Ebony* magazine recommended jogging as part of an active lifestyle, and a full-page color advertisement for Bell Telephone featured a middle-aged Black couple in powder blue tracksuits teasing each other about the pace of their five-mile jog.[18] When a sanitation worker jogging through Central Park en route to church intervened in a mugging to protect a woman who dubbed him a "Black superman," the press

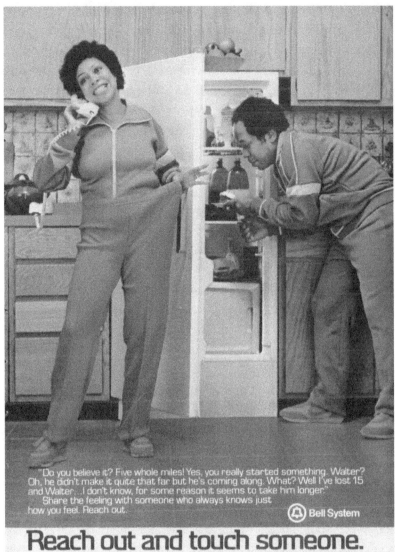

Figure 21. Bell System, "Reach Out and Touch Someone," June 1982. In an advertisement for the Bell phone company, a Black couple playfully competes about their five-mile jogging pace. By the 1980s, jogging—and dressing for it—was, like the full refrigerator in their kitchen, a sign of upward mobility.

minimized him as a "do-gooder" and omitted his race or the fact that he was jogging too. "It's ironic that when a Black person is the perpetrator of a crime, we are quick to learn of it," the *Amsterdam News* acidly observed.[19]

Exercise as Entertainment, on Demand

Screens became an even more powerful medium to spread these fitness activities and their attendant ideologies. Exercise television had been an established genre since LaLanne coaxed homemakers to intersperse loads of laundry with leg lifts. But in these years, exercise became much more enmeshed in broader television culture. On the one hand, fitness—its instructors and acolytes—retained some sense of strangeness. *Real People*, an NBC program that profiled people with unconventional jobs, visited Richard Simmons at the Anatomy Asylum in the late 1970s. Described as the "Billy Graham of muscle building," Simmons whooped and danced, playfully slapping the buttocks of his ebullient male and female students. The host, in a three-piece suit, awkwardly observed from a chair at the back of the room. The segment dwelled on the special class for women "larger than Simmons ever was," who, in leotards and aglow, gushed about the confidence and courage the classes inspired, and encircled Simmons as he tallied up their pounds shed. For the peculiarity of Simmons's theatrics—in between movement cues he sometimes waved around black-and-white photographs of internal organs damaged by high-fat diets—and the spectacle of fat people exercising and enjoying it, the number of people packed into the carpeted studio suggested those outside the asylum might be the crazy ones.

Simmons soon landed a repeating role on the soap opera *General Hospital*, leading to his own syndicated program, *The Richard Simmons Show*, which integrated a full-length workout with life advice, invariably concluding that exercise and diet modification were imperative to happiness, virtue, and fulfillment. In the opening sequence, Simmons, dressed as an angel, intercepts a woman at the grocery store to replace the junk food in her cart with vegetables.

LaLanne personally found Simmons's style "too fast," but accepted an invitation to appear on the show because his wife was a fan.[20] "You and I are exact opposites," LaLanne told Simmons, in that he had been so underweight and malnourished that he was "psychotic," while Simmons had overcome obesity. But really, they learned on set as they co-led a rhythmic workout combining calisthenics and aerobics, and then cooked stuffed peppers, they were both "born again" through exercise. Addressing the audience, they shared this epiphany with platitudes such as "the only thing that is constant is change," concluding that America's only salvation was "every single person realizing the value of fitness."

Talk shows such as *Donahue* and *Oprah* were becoming a fixture of daytime television, and exercise programming both reflected and was absorbed into this broader "therapeutic culture" that connected physical fitness to self-fulfillment.[21] On *Donahue*, fifty-two-year-old actress Debbie Reynolds swore to the silver-haired host that the secret to youth and vitality was exercise. Lack of experience, agility, or desire was no excuse for sedentariness, she insisted, as the program she had designed and endorsed was suitable for all ages and abilities. "So *this* is what you're supposed to look like in your fifties," Donahue remarked appreciatively of Reynolds, clad in wine-colored tights and leotard, before he and the studio audience gamely joined her in a Big Band dance warm-up. Exercise was imperative to a youthful, can-do attitude as much as appearance. Connecting bodily cultivation and individual virtue still more intensely, in 1988, Oprah Winfrey wheeled out a red wagon filled with sixty-seven pounds of fat to help viewers visualize the magnitude of her weight loss from fasting and exercising. She later regretted the stunt, but it articulated and amplified a powerful set of assumptions: prioritizing weight loss as "the most important thing in your life" demonstrated enviable self-possession that was more than skin deep.

Less lofty talk shows often featured an exercise segment, inviting viewers both to watch and participate in a fitness performance before settling in for more sedentary entertainment. Cable television became a powerful tool in the proliferation of such programming. *Alive and Well*, an ambitious two-hour program that first aired on the USA network and was then syndicated, broadcast aerobics—taught by Kathy Smith—and stretching, along with guests from sex therapists to scientists. Such shows were inexpensive to produce, in part because they could be shot outside, in a natural landscape that resonated with popular ideals of a healthy, "California lifestyle." The format's potential felt boundless.

Gilad Janklowicz, a track-and-field athlete, fitness instructor in the Israeli army, and erstwhile aspiring Olympic decathlete, had taught for Gilda Marx and at the Sports Connection while recovering from an injury. His Achilles' heel healed, but he realized new potential for his "militaristic" style that distinguished him from choreographed formats. Shooting on Hawaii beaches that evoked beefcake calendars, in 1982 he launched *Bodies in Motion*, the first fitness show on the sports network ESPN, blurring the boundaries between feminized fitness and masculine sport, and which ran for three decades.[22] This trend was international; on the BBC morning segment "Twice as Fit," Tony Britts, a Ghanaian-born instructor who favored mesh tank tops and tiny shorts, performed athletic feats before white hosts who awkwardly gaped at, and commented on, his body: "His hips must be on ball-bearings."[23]

Videocassettes, not television, became "the product of the decade" and contributed more than any other medium to the expansion of fitness culture.[24] Invented and produced in Japan, videocassette recorders debuted in the United States in 1977, costing over twelve hundred dollars apiece (nearly $5,000 today). Clunky and counterintuitive, VCRs were no guaranteed bestseller.[25] But by 1982, 4 percent of American households owned one; by 1989, an astonishing 65.5 percent did.[26] Empowering "consumer liberation" by allowing viewers to skip commercials, pause programming, and literally "time-shift," the ethos of VHS seemed to have a natural affinity with the individualism of the fitness industry.[27] Even Arthur Jones, the founder of Nautilus, the manufacturer of the painstakingly designed teal-blue exercise equipment that defined the facilities that invested in it, understood video was the industry's future. Out of a two-hundred-thousand-square-foot studio, he recorded instructional videos for his exercise equipment, and he planned to "cover every facet of education" far beyond fitness, from "math to how to cook a pot roast or how to perform an appendectomy." Vowing to "be bigger than General Motors and twice as profitable," Jones imagined "owning the video self-help market," a segment he correctly identified as ascendant.[28]

Jane Fonda, whose *Workout Book* had stayed on the *New York Times* bestseller list for two years, so long it reportedly inspired the establishment of a separate "how-to" category, was the biggest star of the exercise video market; she arguably created it. Initially, Fonda had been unsure about the future of home video at all, much less about making one herself. In 1980, when Stuart Karl, a former waterbed salesman turned aspiring video entrepreneur, suggested Fonda produce a workout videocassette, she offered "a firm no." Karl's wife had read Fonda's book and swore it would translate well to this new medium, but Fonda didn't even own a VCR, and as a prominent figure, she worried she would look silly or vulnerable exercising on-screen. But the chance to support the Campaign for Economic Democracy (CED) in a more scalable way than the in-person studios allowed piqued her interest, and she relented, on the condition of a relatively low-budget shoot. Fonda outlined the script in pencil and eliminated hair, makeup, and teleprompters from the budget. She discovered that she had to "mirror" her imagined audience, which meant calling out cues for kicks or arm reaches opposite to the way she was actually moving, all while "going full out" on an unforgiving concrete floor. The result was exhaustion, but also the video version of *Jane Fonda's Workout*, which ultimately sold seventeen million copies, reportedly reaching women in Guatemalan mud huts and Basotho villages.[29] Her tape boosted the popularity of dance-aerobics at large, and she became its biggest star.

Molly Fox would have her friend Peter Dudley, who appeared in Fonda's videos, send her videocassettes from which to draw inspiration for her New York City clients. "No one even knew what I was talking about at first," Fox recalled, but thanks to Fonda, they had heard of dance aerobics. Missett focused on building physical franchises but also released videos, a natural technological progression from her vinyl records in the 1970s and increasingly a requirement of any 1980s fitness outfit. Fonda took an opposite tack, closing her Encino and San Francisco studios, and using the Beverly Hills location as a laboratory for video concepts. By 1987, she offered a "Video Fitness Library" to viewers encompassing senior citizens, pregnant women, children, professionals, and homemakers who appreciated the convenience of video and the joyousness of aerobics.[30] Despite the fortune Fonda's fitness business raised for the CED, and the breathless testimonies of how many lives she had changed, Hayden constantly disdained it as a vanity project. Deciding she had had enough of his "disparaging remarks," Fonda separated the business from the CED, and eventually left Hayden altogether.[31]

Exercise *was* perfect for video, as Karl predicted, for Americans were more likely to watch a fitness tape repeatedly than a film, especially as the recommendation to incorporate exercise into daily life became commonplace.[32] The success of the *Workout* intensified demand for VCRs, as prospective buyers justified the purchase by envisioning themselves virtuously exercising rather than lounging on the couch. Established fitness personalities emulated Fonda's formula while differentiating themselves in a crowded marketplace; fifty fitness videos were released in the two years following Fonda's.[33] Simmons "didn't need to be convinced" to team up with Karl on his first videocassette in 1983, *Everyday with Richard Simmons*, though he had already had a television show and a best-selling cassette of original music. (Ironically, Simmons's show was canceled the same year because, he said, so many shows by then offered people an outlet to "talk endlessly about their problems," an offering that had always been his calling card.)[34] Karl's association with Fonda intrigued Simmons, but despite feeding the same demand for exercise, inspiration, and entertainment, "Dick and Jane" did so differently. While "bunches of men lined up in the video stores at night, just staring at [Jane's] tape" and enviable figure, Simmons recalled, he endeavored to show people as they were, rather than as unrealizable versions of celebrities.[35]

Everyday opens with a close-up shot of greasy fries and viscous ketchup. Diner patrons gorge on fattening food in a scene that links overeating to other excessive appetites—a heavily made-up woman stuffs her face with a heaping corn dog, a couple barely pauses to chew their pizza before locking lips, and a Black patron douses his fried chicken in salt. A miniaturized Simmons leaps from a banana split and beams everyone into yellow jogging suits and then into his studio, just as class begins.[36] As the exercise video market exploded, Simmons's videos became more elaborate. The most famous title, *Sweatin' to the Oldies*, was a real "lavish affair."[37] The multiday shoot took place in the Santa Monica Women's Gym, included a live "aerobic concert," a new look for Simmons of tiny Dolfin shorts and logo tank top, and expensive licensed songs such as "Peggy Sue" and "Great Balls of Fire," a world apart from the "boring old elevator music" common in lower budget productions. Simmons soon drove a shiny black Mercedes-Benz with the license plate "YRU FATT." Along with his cookbook and "Deal-a-Meal," a diet tracking system, *Sweatin' to the Oldies* was available exclusively by mail order from a telephone hotline featured in Simmons's "infomercials," extended advertisements that became a television staple in the 1980s after federal deregulation lifted time limits on commercials—a particular boon to the diet and fitness industry.[38]

These videos created a new sort of intimacy. Fonda was a Hollywood star, so she was accustomed to being recognized in public. But she noticed a difference in how those who "did Jane" for exercise approached her. One woman started demonstrating her pelvic tilts in a store, while her husband commented that the first voice he heard each morning was Fonda's, emanating from the living room where his wife religiously exercised. Such familiarity conjured the "instant sisterhood" Gloria Steinem described experiencing in health-spa locker rooms, the same sense of supportive sorority that had drawn Fonda to establish the studio. Apparently, the distance of video did not diminish the intensity of the personal connection, even if it only went one way. Simmons had similar stories, including a request in a men's room to autograph toilet paper for the adoring wife of a man who also happened to be using the facilities. Simmons had originally thrilled at the "personal contact" and performative aspect of his shopping mall classes, where crowds like that which packed a South Bend parking lot felt like a "mini-Beatles experience" and created a kind of energetic feedback loop of "acceptance and respect." But it was the response of viewers he would likely never meet—some homebound, others too intimidated or deconditioned to feel they could exercise publicly—that convinced him of the power of video to spread the message that even a "former fattie" could be a "living example" of health and fitness. When he visited one suburban New York woman who had been inspired to lose over two hundred pounds through his video workouts, she awaited him on a custom-made bench, displaying a sign reading, "WELCOME ST. RICHARD, I LOVE YOU."[39]

Some found such on-demand access invasive. Cal Pozo, who became a video producer, recalled hearing concerns from white men about their wives watching a video featuring a "hunky" Black male instructor, whose presence "in" their homes they considered improper.[40] Some feminist-sports advocates bemoaned the absence of athletic community in this solitary pursuit. Film scholar Margaret Morse argued that aerobics videos all but eliminated the aspects of women's physical culture that challenged the cult of thinness, instead enticing viewers with an elusive, on-screen mirror image of a "superstar" tantalizingly "supernear, sharing intimate secrets" of how to *become* her. Due to the "time-shifting" of VHS, pursuit of this "passive femininity" could colonize an infinite amount of women's energy; the "me time" of LaLanne's thirty-minute program was now potentially all-consuming, thanks to the rewind button. Moreover, the success of the *Workout*, with Fonda as its slim white star, encoded as "fit" a physical ideal scarcely different from those on runways or in fashion magazines.[41] A Fonda spokesman called Morse's findings "absurd," while Raquel Welch opined, "I resent the research." Kathy Smith—whose videos sold almost as well as Fonda's, and who was also blonde, white, and slim—conceded Morse "definitely has a point." The videos featuring "girls puckering, or arching their backs and throwing up their fannies in contorted positions," she acknowledged, were "offensive." Simmons conceded

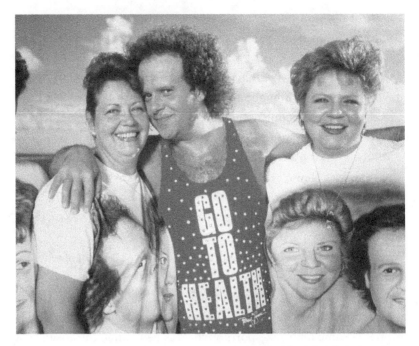

Figure 22. Evan Hurd, *Women Go on Richard Simmons 'Cruise to Lose" Which Sails through the Caribbean,* January 14,1996. Richard Simmons poses with women on his "Cruise to Lose" fitness vacation in 1996. Simmons began his career with the Anatomy Asylum, a standalone fitness studio in the 1970s; twenty years later he was a global fitness personality known for his television appearances, home videos, vacation cruises, and merchandise.

PHOTOGRAPH. ALAMY STOCK PHOTOS. IMAGE ID: EDWHCF.

the study had "some validity." However reluctantly, critics participated in the fitness culture they questioned; Morse's research was inspired by her own "slavish devotion to aerobics videos."[42]

The market dominance of mainstream videos that featured thin, able-bodied white women obscured smaller, but significant, demand for videos that featured people with different bodies, abilities, and sensibilities. In Debbie Reynolds's 1983 tape, she banters with fellow students of varying size and age about their past lovers, their bodies and bawdiness challenging images of demure, disciplined femininity.[43] Some fat women who criticized the industry for only acknowledging them as marks for weight-loss products established alternative fitness media. One such video, the Canadian *Grand Form,* sold two thousand copies in 1986, reflecting a "more down-to-earth approach."[44] Four years later, Women at Large bolstered its North American studio franchise with an award-winning video they "couldn't keep in stock."[45] It opens with the two founders, clad in black-and-white chevron-striped leotards, breaking out of a jail cell signifying "the self-imposed prison" of fat discrimination—notably, not fatness. The video was an opportunity to prove "larger ladies" could be fit and beautiful, if they chose to reject the sentence of "unsexy, unattractive, uninsurable, and even unemployable" that society foisted upon them.[46] Exercise videos for the elderly proliferated, some by personalities like Fonda, Simmons, and Reynolds, who marketed modified "prime time" or "silver fox" programs, and others by specialized therapists such as Maura Casey, who self-financed *Wheelercise* and *Walkaerobics* videos for nursing homes and rehabilitation centers. The benefit, Casey described, was emotional, physical, *and* cultural: "being able to identify with programs available to the general public."[47]

There were limits to even these relatively gentle challenges to the industry's normative assumptions about thinness, youth, and physical ability. Participants were overwhelmingly white, though by the end of the decade videos began to reflect a kind of "Benetton multiculturalism" that showcased occasional Asian, Black, or Brown faces. Simmons's *Reach for Fitness: A Special Book of Exercises for the Physically Challenged*, a book and video developed from his work with the Spina Bifida Association, went further, featuring children in leg braces and wheelchairs happily exercising.[48] Simmons knew from personal experience that people with disabilities were often more enthusiastic participants in exercise than the general population, though they were rarely portrayed as physically energetic or robust. Yet retailers would stock only a few copies of *Reach for Fitness*, and they refused to publicize events Simmons scheduled with the children involved in the project, despite demand for the titles that he knew existed, or that could exist if sufficient promotional resources were expended on them. "This doesn't look good," one critic insensitively told him in the presence of a girl whose leg had been amputated, highlighting the obstacles to full inclusion and visibility, even as fitness culture continued to expand.[49]

18

Turning Up the Intensity

Ironically, video made fitness "placeless" in that exercisers no longer had to go to a facility—even as they multiplied—or even appear before the television on a fixed schedule. But exercise was not the only industry transformed by video. So was pornography, and the two were intertwined in their natural appeal for repeated viewing in the privacy of one's home, and to a certain extent, in their cultural associations. Fitness, with its unapologetic physicality, revealing apparel, and often sexually subversive associations, had long been the topic of pulp novels with titles like *Lesbian Gym* and *Midtown Queen*, and VHS took this convergence between exercise and eroticism to new levels. The linkage was both conceptual and practical.

When the owner of the male exotic dance revue Chippendales released an exercise video in 1983, he drove from his west Los Angeles office to a pornographer's warehouse in the San Fernando Valley (a.k.a. "Porn Valley") to evaluate a better deal on production and distribution. Chippendales already catered to grandmothers and suburbanites more likely to see the muscled men on daytime television or coffee mugs at the mall than at their Culver City nightclub, but the video, *Muscle Motion*, was undeniably racier than most exercise titles. The Chippendales dancers lifted weights to achieve their signature muscles, but the video showed them doing an aerobics routine, an exercise aimed at women. Invited in with an opening nightclub scene, the viewer was coached in a breathy voice to work up a sweat with double entendres about keeping the men's "hands busy," visuals of "wasted" champagne being splashed across the men's waists, bare above tight, unbuttoned, acid-washed jeans, and intermittent moans. After a "cool down" winkingly intended to achieve the opposite, the narrator sighs that it *"had* to be a good workout."[1]

Pornography star Traci Lords's 1990 foray into the genre, *Warm Up to Traci Lords*, made this connection even more explicit. In 1986, an FBI investigation revealed Lords had starred in adult films while a minor, rendering them child pornography and her a tabloid fixture. Her workout video served both to sanitize her image and sexualize the genre. Clad in a demure yellow bikini and matching ballet slippers, Lords leads stretching and core exercises in an unremarkable, even dingy, living room, the camera emphasizing cleavage, crotch, and slow-motion neck rolls that exuded ecstasy as much as good form. The voiceover took the tone in *Muscle Motion* up a few notches; evocative lines were "Don't jerk it hard / Twist it out / To be thin is your route," and "Bend on down / Your legs do spread / Stretch your thighs / Fat you'll shed" as Lords straddled and pulsed with her rear in the air. Unlike many other videos, there was no storyline in Lords's production, perhaps because the plots of her films—such as they were—were implied.[2] Chippendales and Traci Lords laid it on thick, but many exercise video producers deliberately used sexy lighting and suggestive camera angles, even on tapes that purported to offer exercise without innuendo. The effect was such that—producer Pozo recalled—incarcerated men, permitted to order exercise videos but not pornography, often found the former a satisfying substitute.

In 1984, at the height of the exercise-video craze, a controversy suggested the reach of the medium and the declining power of the figure that had for decades embodied fitness instruction: the physical-education instructor. Alice Zook had been teaching physical education in the Bartonville, Illinois, public schools for twenty years when a student suggested she engage her apathetic class with *Muscle Motion*, the Chippendales exercise tape. Known for her quirkiness—like sporting bright green hair—Zook obliged, and most of the high school girls, giggling, followed the breathy cues without complaint. Three refused to participate on religious grounds, however, and registered a grievance. Zook was suspended and became a national cause célèbre. On *Donahue*, she insisted the Chippendales men "are experts in aerobic dance" and that she just "wanted to show students how the professionals did it." On the *Today Show*, she argued that the workout held "a lot of educational value," and wasn't even "mildly erotic," especially compared to "provocative" exercise media featuring women. To the delight of Chippendales's media-genic management—the producer and choreographer-narrator flew in from Los Angeles for Zook's hearing—and talk-show audiences, Zook declared herself the victim of a sexist double standard: "[The school district] isn't used to women being liberated and being able to say and do what they want to say. . . . If I had shown women doing aerobics, there probably wouldn't have been any objection."[3]

Framing *Muscle Motion* as feminist pedagogy was debatable, but the controversy illuminated the rapid spread of fitness videos, and the new authorities to which Americans appealed for exercise expertise. Zook, who was reinstated, defended her decision to show not only *Muscle Motion*, but also tapes featuring Simmons and other fitness luminaries, arguing she was exposing students to cutting-edge exercise science.[4] Characterizing the genre this way was equally questionable. The Chippendales men were primarily self-taught bodybuilders, and while their choreographer swore to the safety and effectiveness of the workout, she had no exercise-science training. Such improvisation was common in commercial fitness, an industry arguably growing faster than the expert knowledge of its biggest stars. In one dramatic example, when Simmons opened Anatomy Asylum, he noticed that one regular at the Ruffage salad bar, who regularly brought him gifts of plush, handmade teddy bears, ordered only vegetable juice. With each visit, she—and the teddy bears she presented—noticeably shrank. Simmons was unbothered until she stopped showing up, and a neighbor shared she had died of anorexia, an affliction Simmons had never heard of. Disturbed that he saw her daily but hadn't detected the severity of her struggle, Simmons began reading health books and convening thirty-minute meetings with students to "discuss anything that came to mind regarding exercise and weight loss."

The health challenges he witnessed his clientele faced were formidable—women collapsing with bloody noses due to snorting cocaine before class, a client wiring her mouth shut to prevent herself from eating—but Simmons's goal remained emotional connection more than imparting expertise: "We weren't professionals—just people of all different shapes and sizes who were sharing information and our feelings with each other," he explained.[5] Molly Fox also remembered the early 1980s as a "wild West" in terms of the lack of an established body of scientific knowledge and best practices; she and other instructors would roam the Strand bookstore in Greenwich Village in search of teaching inspiration from dance and anatomy titles. But few consumers seemed to care about credentials: charisma, beauty, and passionate communication could suffice.

Defining Experts, Not Educators

Of course the most organized cadre of fitness experts, beyond the military, were physical education teachers like Zook. Heirs to a profession over a century old, some physical educators saw the 1980s fitness craze as the moment they, long underappreciated by fellow educators and the culture at large, could be vanguards, and not just by popping in a videotape. Exercise for both women and men was widely celebrated; overweight, newly medicalized as "obesity," was making headlines again; and the commercial demand for fitness was unprecedented in its intensity. In 1985, physical-education stronghold Springfield College enthusiastically announced expanded programs and facilities to meet this "ever-increasing popularity and interest in sports and fitness activities."[6]

Curiously, the most expansive response of universities to the "new opportunities" this "fitness craze" presented were emerging programs in exercise science and kinesiology—the study of human movement—that largely defined themselves in *contrast* to school-based physical education. Kinesiology had for a time been known as a marginal field often lumped in with "holistic techniques" such as foot leveling and vitamin cures; in 1963, the American Medical Association's Committee on Quackery dismissed it, along with chiropractics, as "a cult." By 1981, however, the field had attained greater, if grudging, respectability: a skeptical Michigan public-health official conceded that perhaps kinesiology was "a legitimate study for physical education . . . [but] not a form of health treatment."[7] Kinesiology's most vocal champion, physician George Goodheart, made the opposite argument, but expressed a similarly dim view of education. He touted his participation on the Olympic medical team and the incorporation of kinesiology into the health, medical, and business fields—but *not* schools—as indicative of its success.[8]

Such legitimization of exercise expertise—apart from teaching physical education in schools—was happening everywhere. At Chico State, Webb's alma mater, the physical-education department added exercise-science classes in 1984, specifically highlighting career opportunities in commercial fitness and medicine, rather than in schools.[9] The kinesiology division at the University of Michigan was established the same year, and in operating distinctly from physical education, invested a sense of professional legitimacy and dynamism on the new program. Nearly forty years later, only one of the nearly fifty careers on its website alludes to education.[10] Similarly, in South Carolina, Lander College recruited longtime physical educator Jerry Hawkins to establish the state's only degree program in exercise studies, intended to provide "exciting opportunities for careers other than coaching or teaching," including "hospital-based adult fitness, cardiac rehabilitation, [and] corporate fitness." The point was to disassociate a slew of new, private-industry fitness-related careers from the unglamorous image of the physical educator, rather than to invest the field with new status and resources. Indeed, a journalist covering the Lander program revamp began by mockingly noting a Somerset Maugham quote in the promotional materials: "Such a lofty figure, you might think, to promote 'P.E.?'" Such pretense only made sense given the department's reimagination as something *other* than physical-education preparation.[11]

Programs that failed to effectively rebrand could be casualties in an age of austerity: the University of Washington kinesiology program, so renamed in 1979, had been established in 1897 to teach "physical culture and hygiene" and served 250 students, but was cut in 1982 despite its chair's despair that "never in the history of mankind has interest in exercise, health, and sports been greater than now."[12] This burst of interest was no match for decades of disrespect. As a freshman physical education and recreation major at San Jose State in the 1960s, Lynda Huey strove to distinguish herself from both the sorority girls more concerned with their pancake makeup than sports and the "overweight and mannish . . . Hercs . . . the worst male chauvinist pig's description of a woman athlete." The discrimination was institutionalized, as only women students in her department were required to wear skirts. While Huey's running excellence had led her to the field, she found as a student and a faculty member that its ethos was uninspired: "respect athletic mediocrity" and don't "make it about winning."[13] Ultimately, she sought athletic esteem and challenge by training with the men's track team and deliberately trying to set a different example as a professor of the discipline, but a decade and a half later, physical education and organized athletics would be only one of several options for students of her interests and talents.

Many on the physical-education track who witnessed this dynamic industry emerging wanted in, and immediately. The stakes were especially high for women, for while athleticism was long seen as evidence of male suitability for many professions, for women it usually meant the PE track. "Girls become teachers, and you should teach gym because you like sports," Carol Scott, who grew up excelling at softball and basketball in 1970s Queens, was told. As a physical-education major at the State University of New York at Cortland, she was especially disappointed by her student-teaching experience. "No girl wanted to play gym, and the guys who loved sports played, and those who didn't got beaten up or never picked, and sat out." Her chosen career didn't seem like it would do much to improve the lives of the next generation of tomboys like her, or to change any kids' attitudes toward exercise. Plus, the curriculum had apparently remained unchanged since Scott was a schoolgirl. "The stagnation of 'roll out the balls' and stand on the sidelines was not going to light my fire," she said.

What am I going to do? she thought as graduation neared. On a walk in her Long Island town, she came upon a scene she could describe only as "fabulous": an aerobics studio, full mostly of women sweating, laughing, and moving together. The instructor was hardly passively chaperoning from the sidelines but was right in the action with her students. The athletic, dramatic performance Scott saw before her eyes seemed to perfectly merge her passions, from the acting and piano she had taken up in school to her natural extroversion. *This*—whatever it was—and not the school gym—was clearly her calling. By 1983, Scott taught four to six classes a day, worked the front desk, and sold memberships to the small club, which also included a childcare center. Part of the electric energy, Scott described, was because it was "absolutely more inclusive" than any physical-education class in her experience. "If you came into the room and tried,"—and paid—"we were happy to see you."[14]

Fred DeVito was teaching physical education and coaching sports in suburban New Jersey when he had a similar revelation. A musician, DeVito would travel into Manhattan on weekends to play and hear music, staying with his girlfriend, Elisabeth "Lis" Halfpapp. She was a professionally trained ballerina teaching barre fitness at the Lotte Berk brownstone. To DeVito, Lis's new job first seemed "very cultlike and exclusive, almost like a speakeasy." The facade was nondescript, and clients would ring a buzzer and slip upstairs to the chintz-carpeted studio, often balancing a cigarette and a coffee. "I never really probed very much or knew about the potential," he remembers, because as a man, "I wasn't invited."[15] But the owner, Lydia Bach, saw Halfpapp's talent—and asked her to open a West Hollywood studio in 1983. Fred and Lis headed west, and he got a job teaching PE in Catholic schools while trying to make it as a musician. Within a year, Bach, panicked because her manager and several instructors had quit, summoned Halfpapp back to Manhattan. At first, the newlyweds balked at this transcontinental ricochet, in part because DeVito had left a tenured teaching position to make the move. But Bach offered DeVito a job too, doing essentially everything but teaching, despite his degree. He cleaned toilets, ran payroll, and checked in clients at the front desk: the closest any man had gotten to the inner sanctum of the studio.

Bach was reportedly a difficult boss, and instructor turnover became a problem. DeVito struggled to fill a hole in the schedule until he and Halfpapp had an idea: *he* would teach. First, he took one of Halfpapp's classes himself, and even as a fit twenty-four-year-old, was "shaking and sweating" like the regulars, women in their fifties and sixties. Positively "blown away with the effectiveness of the exercise," DeVito, possibly the first male barre student in the country, was an interloper in the deliberately women's-only environment, but as "Lis's husband," the clients welcomed him, letting him "get away with" proximity to women pulsing and tucking in leotards. His classes filled, and Halfpapp and DeVito were soon teaching six classes a day, five or six days a week, and living on the fifth floor of the brownstone. DeVito added a men's class, offering intense upper body work and "using words like 'glutes' instead of 'tushie'" to strike a more acceptably macho tone.

DeVito chuckled remembering telling his father, who was "blue-collar" and into "things that were grounded and stable," that he was abandoning a union job for work that barely had a name in the mid-1980s, much less one legible as a career for a college-educated, tenured teacher-coach. But as different as the studio was from the gymnasiums and athletic fields where DeVito had envisioned spending his career, he found in this cosseted environment a surprising inclusiveness that had eluded him in his physical education career. The "type of environment that caters to the athlete, while the kids who need [exercise] sit mostly on the sidelines," dreading a class that "always eliminated them," had dispirited DeVito while he worked in schools. He could feel those kids' intimidation upon entering the gym, and the sad fact was that physical education, hamstrung by "bureaucracy" and budget cuts, he told me, was unlikely to alter their experience. The brownstone was undeniably exclusive by dint of its cost and the relative homogeneity of the clientele, but there at least he saw exercise changing bodies and lives—mostly of women whom decades of presidential councils had barely thought worth targeting.

DeVito and Halfpapp became the most renowned barre-fitness teachers in the country. When they opened their own Santa Monica studio two decades later, DeVito stopped by a blacktop court where he had taught physical education, and he marveled at the different path his life had taken. Tamilee Webb, a few years younger than DeVito and Scott, likewise relayed with palpable relief the luck of her moment of birth, given her gender and passion for athletics. "Can you imagine?" she told me. "I could have been a PE teacher."[16]

Eschewing careers in physical education, this new generation of professional fitness enthusiasts strove to deepen their knowledge of the disciplines and pedagogies that would distinguish them in a growing industry. Competition was so fierce that Bach reportedly forbade other instructors from entering the brownstone, for fear they would copy the method. Yet at other studios, instructors would show up, show off, and distribute business cards to impressed clients.[17] In southern California, a young married couple saw an opportunity to meet this need for professional development and collaboration in an atomized, emergent field. Peter and Kathie Davis had met as undergraduates at San Diego State University in the late 1970s, she a physical education major and he in the business program. Both played tennis, and Kathie moonlighted teaching for California Aerobic Dance, "a knockoff" of Sorenson's and Missett's programs. The couple always wanted to work together and had imagined doing so in the tennis world. But they noticed that the health clubs around them were ripping out tennis and racquetball courts and building out fitness studios—a new leisure pursuit with a far lower barrier to entry in terms of skill and equipment. What began as "mostly women looking for a fun income and way to stay fit, more of a hobby," they realized, was becoming a profession.[18] For all this enthusiasm and investment, no organization existed to systematize, and legitimize, this fragmented field. Bureaucracy was a common frustration in the education system, but the fitness industry suffered from the opposite problem: insufficient structure to disseminate knowledge about teaching, pay equity, injury prevention, or insurance.

The Davises saw an opportunity in this obstacle. With Kenneth Cooper's *Aerobics* as their "bible," the Davises founded an organization that supported fitness in order to "get healthier, not just build muscle." To establish credibility, they worked their local connections to establish a board of "the top people in San Diego," including a cardiologist, exercise physiologist, and a sports-medicine physician." Notably, they did not gravitate toward Kathy's training in physical education or emulate or collaborate with the multiplying programs in exercise science and kinesiology, but looked to the United States Tennis Association as a less "cumbersome" organizational model. In 1982, they established the International Dance Exercise Association (IDEA), and issued a newsletter to a membership of three hundred—mostly women ages twenty-five to forty—just months later. The following year, membership grew tenfold, even as the competing Aerobics and Fitness Association of America also incorporated. IDEA held its first convention at a San Diego Holiday Inn in 1984 and expanded the newsletter into a magazine more loftily titled *Dance Exercise Today*. Over the next few years, the magazine published widely, on topics ranging from remedies for vocal strain to an instructor code of ethics. In 1985, the IDEA Foundation—which became the American Council on Exercise—established a certification exam covering anatomy, physiology, exercise programming, and health screening, administered over three and a half hours by the Educational Testing Service, which also administered the SAT. "Hiring ETS was huge," Kathie said, "because it showed we were serious ... it was standardized and legally defensible. Someone couldn't sue us if they didn't pass." Four thousand instructors took the first exam.

Injuries in the industry were high—over 75 percent of instructors and nearly half of participants suffered lower-leg ailments—but the specter of regulation presented an equally serious threat.[19] "Wary of government control," one article characterized IDEA's outlook, adding that "the industry is moving ahead to regulate itself by training and certifying instructors through rigorous testing procedures." The issue was urgent, as mounting legal and insurance costs indicated that these credentials were not sufficiently widely adopted, or rigorous, to keep pace with the appetite for exercise, often satisfied by untrained instructors. "The onus is on the consumer to ask questions and observe instructors carefully for signs of unsafe or unprofessional practices," IDEA's executive director advised in an eight-point checklist whose line items ranged from asking about CPR certification to assessing how smoothly instructors integrated warm-ups and cool-downs.[20] Even the certifications "can't make a person a good teacher," said Ken Alan, an IDEA educator who helped design the standards. Alan trained celebrities like Raquel Welch and Sylvester Stallone, held a bachelor's degree in kinesiology from UCLA, and warned that "for someone with no formal training, certification programs are a good place to start" but hardly a guarantee of a safe or effective program. Ultimately, he advised clients, the market would dictate fitness instruction: "Make it your business to talk to the instructors and tell them what you want. . . . If you get nothing but a hard sell, go somewhere else."[21]

Carol Scott was one of the first instructors certified by IDEA—before a manual even existed—and in 1986, she flew to California to attend a convention. She discovered "a whole population" doing what she did: stacking eight-counts of grapevines and step-touches, integrating them with sports drills, and getting painful shin splints along with paychecks. Most taught fitness "on the side," but in New York City as in Los Angeles, the rates of the most popular instructors could sustain a livelihood: fifty dollars an hour flat fee, plus a dollar a head. As Scott watched the IDEA events spawn regional gatherings, she was inspired to organize. "There's just so much talent in the East," she thought. "What if we make our own convention in New York City?" she asked Jeff Martin and Molly Fox—by then known as the "king and queen of aerobics," reigning over uptown and downtown realms, respectively—and several other instructors, who seemed interested but who ultimately left much of the fundraising and logistics to her. Scott used fifty thousand dollars she and her ex-husband had saved, and with a Reebok sponsorship, in 1991 launched ECA World Fitness, which despite its global sobriquet began by holding conferences in New York and Florida.

Instructors like Alan, Fox, and Webb were becoming nationally known thanks to the master classes and workshops they offered on this expanding conference circuit, which included bustling trade shows featuring tanning sprays, remixed workout cassettes, protein powders, and aerobics apparel from brands like Carushka and Capezio. The convention highlights, however, were the aerobics exhibitions that served as finales. While daily sessions often focused on accessible, "low-impact" formats for casual exercisers, the competitions were dazzling performances that combined dance and sport and shiny costumes—like "ice skating without the blades." Since 1982, Jazzercise had hosted freestanding conferences, which Pozo remembered felt like rock concerts when Missett took center stage, "practically levitating," Pozo remembered of one Florida convention, accompanied by the "Jazzercise Band," to teach to thousands of participants and their families—events covered by far-flung newspapers in towns that sent Jazzercisers to attend.[22] Many instructors saw themselves as serving a growing professional class that shelled out for health-club memberships and VCRs, but the idea that *they* constituted a coherent profession was still incipient. Yet even for those pursuing performance careers or raising families, these conferences and the networking, education, and peacocking they offered helped coalesce this inchoate profession. Careers were made in the corridors of convention hotels: Tamilee Webb, who became the most visible face of Buns of Steel, landed the gig thanks to a chance encounter at IDEA. Most experiences were quotidian but no less life-changing: Judith Berlin, a New Jersey homemaker who had first found Jazzercise at the YMCA, traveled to the 1989 Chicago convention, her first time alone on a plane and in a hotel.

The widening chasm between these erstwhile physical educators and private-industry fitness instructors was subtle, for as cultural esteem for exercise grew, many popular fitness instructors and entrepreneurs continued at least some involvement in public programming, although not always in a sustained way. Jacki Sorensen was named to the Presidential Council on Fitness, and developed curricula based in Aerobic Dancing format. During California's newly declared Wellness Week, Missett taught large, free classes at the University of California's San Diego campus. This national enthusiasm—and the apparent partnership between industry innovators and policymakers—appeared to infuse energy into the public provision of fitness and recreation. President Ronald Reagan posed grinning astride a Nautilus adductor machine, celebrating his gym-going as equally crucial to his health as the more conventionally presidential activity of chopping wood outdoors—an activity he jokingly described as "chopping iron," presuming his listeners' familiarity with both working out and the bodybuilding movie *Pumping Iron*. In 1981, more undergraduate degrees in physical education than ever—nearly 18 percent of education degrees—were granted than in the preceding decades. But this elevation of exercise culture was, at least in policy terms, mostly symbolic. Federal and state legislatures emboldened by Reagan's rhetoric of "trickle-down" prosperity and freeloading "welfare queens" slashed budgets for social programs that served poor and working-class Americans, including those affording access to healthy food and safe recreational spaces.

Public education, especially in any form deemed frivolous by policymakers committed to a "back to basics" curriculum emphasizing only core academics, was usually first on the budgetary chopping block. *A Nation at Risk*, the influential 1983 federal education report that decried a "rising tide of mediocrity" afflicting American children who were unprepared to safeguard the country's geopolitical supremacy, omitted physical education entirely. While an earlier generation of Cold Warriors had imagined physical education as key to global preeminence, *A Nation at Risk* implicitly lumped it in with other supposedly intellectually unserious subjects perpetuating national decline, perhaps because it had become so linked to popular culture rather than civic duty. The number of teaching degrees climbed slightly in the ensuing decade, but the proportion of physical-education degrees dropped by a third and has since continued an uninterrupted descent.[23] Cosmetic efforts such as the Presidential Council on Fitness's "Academic Athletes" initiative did little to counter the reality that while fitness was a desirable consumer good, it was no longer a policy priority. Notably, in 1986, President Reagan anointed Missett a "top woman entrepreneur," emphasizing her success at business rather than at democratizing access to fitness. (Fonda, who was best remembered, and reviled, among conservatives for her progressive activism, would never have been so honored.) By the middle of the decade, it was clear not only to potential physical educators who embarked on different paths, but to parents, that public institutions could not be counted on to support their children's physical fitness. Cutbacks to physical education and the lure of television, the *Chicago Metro News* told its African American readership, meant parents must support their children in leading a "disease-free life" by instilling exercise habits early, while businesses promising as much to those who could afford it only became more of a fixture in the city's more affluent neighborhoods.[24]

19

Not Quite Sports

The strongest indication that fitness had attained an enduring place in American culture, if not in the school gym, was its new proximity to the world of sport. In the opening ceremony of the 1984 Olympic Games in Los Angeles, Missett led three hundred Jazzercisers from fifty states, decked out in tight red tops and flippy white skirts, in a performance orchestrated by a Broadway choreographer and set to Big Band music. Seen by 180 million television viewers in the United States alone, the spectacle brought the traditionally masculine realm of competitive sport together with the predominantly female world of group fitness in a public, celebratory way unimaginable even a few years earlier.[1] Across the country, at the Vertical Club in New York City—known for the celebrity clientele that pedaled on computerized stationary bikes, pumped up on Nautilus machines, and sweated through aerobics class—tennis champion Billie Jean King started offering lessons. Such adjacency to athletics conferred new legitimacy on fitness, but it was not always an enthusiastic embrace. Crystal Light, the powdered diet drink that sponsored national aerobics competitions, was sarcastically likened to the "Virginia Slims of women's tennis," as fitness events occurred in small venues or niche conventions that paled in visibility compared even to the relatively low billing of professional women's sports.

King felt this awkwardness acutely. *WomenSports*, the magazine she had founded on a shoestring budget in 1974 amid excitement about her own celebrity and the inspiration of Title IX on a generation of sportswomen, was rebranded a decade later as *Women's Sports*

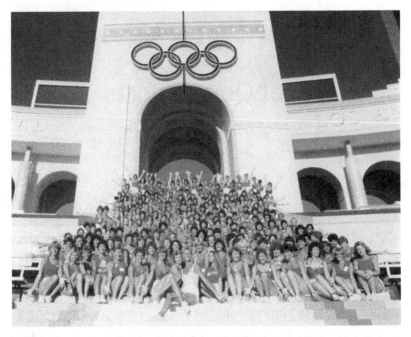

Figure 23. *Jazzercisers Perform in the Opening Ceremonies of the Los Angeles Olympics,* 1984. Hundreds of Jazzercisers came together from all fifty states to participate in the opening ceremony of the Olympic Games in Los Angeles. This moment was pivotal in terms of women's fitness earning legitimacy in relation to the realm of sport.

PHOTOGRAPH. FROM THE COLLECTION OF JUDI SHEPPARD MISSETT. REPRINTED WITH PERMISSION. HTTPS://WWW.BUILDINGABUSINESSWITHABEAT.COM/?PGID=JUHDIDN5-B259BEC3-5EF2-11E9-A9FF -063F49E9A7E4.

and Fitness. From the start, King had endeavored to stay true to the publication's feminist principles while delicately courting advertisers such as Clairol that were equally as interested in aesthetics as in athletics. Editorial content that prioritized recreational exercise and fitness enjoyed a somewhat larger audience, but such articles could promote precisely the disempowering dynamics King had founded the publication to disrupt. Editors struggled to cover athletic achievements while also portraying the women as conventionally feminine, as in one cover image of a runner that was discarded because her grimace might have put off advertisers. Ultimately, the magazine changed hands and titles several times, and was folded into fitness publication *SELF*, upon which one editor lamented: "if *womenSports* was a magazine for women who were either interested in women who competed in sports or for women who competed in sports . . . *SELF* magazine was how you can do sports to keep your man."[2] Given that by the early 1980s, King was not only a champion of women's sport, but the first professional athlete to come out as a lesbian, the irony of this turn was especially poignant.

Clearly, the popularity of fitness could uphold old hierarchies as much as challenge them—as was evident at Nike. The athletic-apparel giant long dominant in running was at a crossroads in 1984. Just a month after Nike's president warned shareholders of the company's precarity, it cut a deal with a rising basketball star initially reluctant to even meet them: Michael Jordan. Jordan met with Nike executives when he was in Los Angeles to play at the same Olympics Jazzercise had kicked off. Turning to basketball courts in predominantly Black neighborhoods for design inspiration and new customers was a sharp pivot from the lily-white Oregon track and field world where Nike originated, and the deal is remembered as unprecedented in orchestrating product and marketing around the image of a single athlete. But it was just as bold in elevating active-wear popularized by Black youth as aspirational fashion.[3]

The shoe behemoth was less bold in chasing a market its mostly male executives deemed to be beneath them. Female sales representatives had been pushing Nike designers to develop a shoe for the women they saw lining up for aerobics classes all over the country, but were reportedly rebuffed by one vice president that a serious sports company had no business designing apparel for "a bunch of fat ladies dancing to music."[4] The company's own internal history acknowledges that "he was not the only Nike executive with that opinion," and few were surprised that a *fitness* practice that was largely the realm of women did not impress co-founder Phil Knight, who didn't want to risk Nike looking like a "sissy fashion" label or "diluting a brand founded on testosterone."[5] Reebok, however, exhibited little such ambivalence, and released its Freestyle aerobics sneaker in 1982, announcing it had "put its heart into the athletic shoe business so you can put your sole into aerobic exercise,"

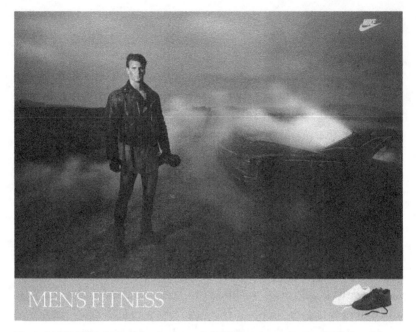

Figure 24. Nike "Rake" shoe advertisement, ca. 1986. In an attempt to capture the aerobics market—and to appeal to men—Nike released the "Rake" aerobics shoe and marketed it with over-the-top macho imagery, including in *Sports Illustrated*.

ADVERTISEMENT. COURTESY OF NIKE, INC., BEAVERTON, OR.

quickly dominating a shoe category that was undeniably exploding, though not among those conventionally understood as athletes.[6]

Nike had little choice but to rush an aerobics line to market, despite "incredible resistance" internally that this was a fad, and would only "legitimize what Reebok was doing." But the models Nike released—the Aerobi-Tech, the Fame, and L'Aérobique—were hastily designed and plagued with production and quality issues, confirming the executives' skepticism. The company's attempt to market aerobics to men ages twenty-eight to forty-five was just as muddled. In the internal *Nike Times*, a marketing manager announced somewhat optimistically that while "at first, men considered aerobics as strictly a women's activity, now men are getting involved." The response to the new line they released, however, was just "lukewarm" due to the incongruous pairing of a "soft, very feminine shoe"—Nike had recently started using the supple leather and

more flexible construction that made Reebok shoes so popular—
with an advertising aesthetic based on the violent, gritty action film
Mad Max. This was going to be "an incredibly masculine product,"
said a member of the advertising department, reflecting on the
hulking, chained male figure breaking stone pillars in the ads, but
the "Rake" shoe and the line of which it was a part did not prove
successful.[7]

Strongly signaling this distinction between sport and fitness,
Nike did advocate for women's running at the same time that it
held aerobics at arm's length, successfully lobbying the International Olympic Committee to include longer women's events in the
1984 Games. Yet the failure to take aerobic fitness seriously suggested a deeper distaste at Nike for women who were not conventional athletes. A 1988 advertising montage featured triathlete Joanne
Ernst jumping rope, lifting weights, and doing aerobics, and then
looking at the camera to sneer: "It wouldn't hurt to stop eating
like a pig, either." On the all-male advertising team, "all the guys
thought it was very cool." One woman at the shoot remembered
arguing against this line, and being told to relax: "We're doing it
just for fun, we would never use it." But then, she remembered,
somehow "it ends up on TV." Women viewers were uninspired by
"the macho sensibility" of a workout series more akin to the programs marketed by Bo Jackson and Michael Jordan, but they were
downright enraged that Nike appeared to be making light of dis-
ordered eating.[8]

Soon after, advertising firm Wieden + Kennedy proposed a new
spot, to run in the 1989 Super Bowl, for a women's line of sports
bras and bike shorts. It opened with slow-motion shot of a jock-
strap bursting into flames, set against a soundtrack of a joyous
gospel choir. At first no one spoke, until one member of the executive team asked, "Do you want to lose the men's part of our business?" The nearly all-male room of executives chuckled nervously
and immediately scrapped the idea. It was a turning point, remembered executive Nancy Monserrat, one of the few women present.
"After 'Burning Jock Strap,' they all said, we need to go out and do
some research, because it is pretty clear we have no idea how to talk

to women." The result were two brands—teen-focused Side One and i.e., which marketed "cheap and cheerful" vanity-sized shoes with fashion photography—that felt so out of step with Nike's performance-driven culture that their existence caused internal rancor and lost the company nearly thirty million dollars; both were shuttered by the early nineties. Nike was clearly increasingly convinced of the profitability of women's fitness, but not yet of its athletic legitimacy. Significantly, nor was the larger culture: Madonna had tentatively signed on as a Side One spokesperson, but balked when she realized it wasn't for Nike proper. "I liked the product . . . but it wasn't sports product," one employee said. "We weren't at a point where we needed to grow beyond sport. . . . It was important to stay on track."[9]

Staying Hard as a Lifestyle

Exercise became encoded as essential in the 1980s, but it was not the introspective, enlightened, self-actualization of the previous two decades that fitness now helped its acolytes achieve. Rather, the work-hard-play-hard ethos and conspicuous consumption that defined the era shaped the expansive fitness culture bequeathed by back-to-the-land joggers, aerobic dancers, and yogis. The name of Puma's running shoe, the Predator, for example, intimated how the countercultural activity of jogging had been recast as a pursuit of mercenary individualism. Fitness culture was tightly bound up with the appearance of affluence, if not always its presence. Predictably, this enthusiasm inspired an avalanche of material stuff.[10] Videocassettes and contraptions hawked on infomercials overflowed the closets of American homes, while fitness vacations, corporate gyms, and the omnipresence of exercise on television, from soap-opera subplots to prime-time prescriptive programming, made fitness hypervisible.

Many such examples involved no actual exercise. "Physical," the 1981 pop anthem by Olivia Newton-John, presents fitness as foreplay. In the music video, piercing blue eyes matching her leotard, Newton-John breathily serenades muscled, tanned men positioned on workout equipment primarily to flaunt their physiques (as much to each other as to her). *Perfect*, a feature film starring John Travolta and Jamie Lee Curtis and set in the carpet-and-chrome Los Angeles Sports Connection, elevated the health club to a believable backdrop for big-screen drama. Adapted from a 1983 *Rolling Stone* cover story that portrayed gyms as "the new singles' bars," the film both glamorized and disdained fitness. Travolta's cerebral Manhattan journalist character falls for Jessie, Curtis's California aerobics instructor, who impresses him with her sexy athleticism and devoted following. But even as he appreciates her talent, he inquires ever more incredulously, "You don't want to be an aerobics instructor forever, do you?" Jessie's celebrity in this superficial, louche environment both makes her intriguing and intimates her misguided priorities.[11] Meaningfully, Jessie, who is white, is ultimately portrayed as respectable, in contrast to a Black exotic dancer who performs almost identical moves in similarly revealing attire—in the strip club rather than the aerobics studio—and is portrayed as secondary and irredeemable.

"The gym" had not completely rehabilitated its seedy midcentury image, but was sufficiently sanitized to be ever more ubiquitous in a surprisingly wide range of products, from the 1987 slasher flick *Aerobicide*, in which semi-nude women with feathered hair and fake tans are murdered in between aerobics classes, to the children's mystery novel *The Haunted Health Club*, premised on a brother-and-sister detective team who "stop into The Fit and Trim Health Club to find out about the grand opening specials" only to find the inviting facade hides a dingy interior and a corpse.[12] At shopping malls, one might not only find a Richard Simmons exercise event, but a cartoon book of the character Cathy complaining about her lack of willpower to exercise, a Workout Barbie doll, a shirtless Chippendales dancer promoting his beefcake calendar, and racks of Dolphin shorts, Lycra, and legwarmers that telegraphed one's affluence to seek leisure, discipline, and entertainment in ritual exercise.

This commercial success and cultural acceptance also meant the dulling of whatever edginess was still associated with working out. In 1980, Charles Gaines, who had become famous for chronicling the lives of bodybuilders in *Pumping Iron*, released *Staying Hard*, an exercise book for "housewives, children, old people . . . anyone" who "didn't want to look like [his] muscle-men buddies" but who merely worried about "going soft."[13] The offshore expansion of apparel man-ufacturing—in 1970, 75 percent of apparel purchased by Americans was manufactured domestically, while in 1990 only half was—meant many suburban aerobic dancers could afford to swathe themselves in leotards and headbands, reliably stocked in hosiery and sports-wear departments and Jazzercise Centers. The fashion mostly shed its glamorous association with the sylphlike young women in night-clubs who once inspired it, or even the chic Beverly Hills ladies who outdid each other with the stripes and prints of the leggings they paired with oversized, off-the-shoulder tops.[14] The Vertical Club recruited its notoriously attractive staff and clientele from nightclubs like Studio 54 and Chippendales, but its proximity to the highway meant that as it became more famous, and fitness more aspirational, it began to draw a "bridge-and-tunnel" crowd that dulled the luster of exclusivity.

The bodies that powered this boom paid the price too. Rachel Sibony, who began her career teaching fitness at a gym while work-ing at a beauty salon, remembers both worlds ravaged by AIDS. "We started to see people turning gray. . . . It felt like AIDS just killed them all off."[15] Monique Dash agreed, "AIDS was atrocious. . . . We just lost so many." The seamlessness between a drug-fueled night-life and the "daytime disco" of the exercise studio became unsus-tainable for some of its stars, who snorted lines of cocaine to teach consecutive classes straight from the clubs. In 1984, even Jack LaL-anne—at age seventy—told *Playboy* he saw punishing workouts and equally intense weekend debauchery as mutually reinforcing. "Who are the greatest dissipaters in the world? Professional ath-letes. They're in such good shape they can drink, they can screw they can smoke. . . . We're living in a promiscuous society now. People want sex; they want drugs; they want lots of things."[16]

But it took a toll, and more quotidian forms of physical depletion played out as well. Doctors regularly recommended skipping meals and popping diet pills for weight control, while the concrete floors common to many gyms "destroyed" the knees and joints of the most avid exercisers. Variable standards of knowledge and expertise could also cause injury; DeVito and Halfpapp later realized that the constant tucking of the lower back that they had once recommended caused postural problems.

A generation earlier, physical-fitness boosters and policymakers had warned of the civic and social health risks posed by the "soft American," a flabby figure best whipped into shape in the school gymnasium. By the eighties, a privatized fitness culture not only continued to overtly celebrate the virtue of "staying hard" through physical exercise, but defined it explicitly and as universally desirable. In *Staying Hard*, Gaines promises his program will stave off a sagging chest and buttocks, but that "*being* hard is something more than the tactile result of physical conditioning." It is not just a life philosophy, but "outsmarting life" itself: " 'Hard,' " he wrote, is "durability, discipline, energy, potency."[17] As committed exercisers shared how difficult it was to commit to this new requirement of regular exercise—"I have to go when I'm unconscious," one woman confessed, while others confided it was only the fear of early death or of "feeling myself jiggle"—that motivated them, the question became pressing: how long could Americans really afford to play, work, and work out *this* hard?[18]

Part **Six**

HARD BODIES AND SOULFUL SELVES

A knock-down, drag-out yoga bootcamp for . . . endurance-test-style serenity.
YOGA WORKS ADVERTISEMENT, 1997

"I used to do aerobics until I dropped," confessed a smiling Suzanne Somers in a 1991 infomercial. Best known for playing the ditzy but well-intentioned Chrissy Snow on the sitcom *Three's Company*, Somers was almost equally familiar as the spokeswoman for the Thighmaster, a wishbone-shaped contraption covered in royal-blue foam, joined by a red plastic hinge, that promised "toning and strengthening" to women and men who dialed the toll-free number splashed across the screen in gold letters. The inexpensive and easily stored Thighmaster became a bestseller, but Jack LaLanne was disgusted. "Have you seen some of the crap they're selling as exercise equipment now?" groused the octogenarian credited with inventing the jumping jack, in 1995. "How about that Suzanne Somers? She should have been thrown in jail for selling the piece-of-crap Thighmaster. It just develops a little muscle on the inner thigh. What good is that?"[1] Even at his advanced age, LaLanne rose before dawn for self-directed two-hour "systematic, vigorous, and violent" workouts, and bemoaned the something-for-nothing premise of a sprawling industry that enticed exercisers with the false promise that they could perfect "problem areas" with little exertion.

But *The Jack LaLanne Show* had been off the air for nearly a decade, and his Trimnastics program, with its quaint entreaties to homemakers to tone "the front porch" or the "hippy parts" with gentle movements like standing leg lifts, had always been more similar to quick-fix, spot-training contraptions like the Thighmaster and other such programs and devices than to his own punishing personal regime.[2] Both were becoming relics, however, as was the instant, intense—and sometimes painful—thrill of high-impact aerobics that dominated the 1980s.

Yet, even more than the accessible exercises LaLanne popularized on television, the grand language of exercise as absolution that he had trumpeted since the 1930s, and that coursed through the counterculture in the intervening years, came to powerfully animate the fitness industry in the 1990s. In these years, fitness—now entrenched everywhere from shopping malls to network television to children's literature—came to represent a path to actualizing an athletic, affluent, and physically and spiritually flexible self. As men sweated through Step aerobics, women trained for triathlons, and they increasingly met each other on the yoga mat, this fit ideal became ever more ambitious and expansive. But it was only nominally more accessible, since such pursuits were pay-to-play—or work—depending on how a growing number of participants defined the sweat they sought in pursuit of physical *and* spiritual transformation.

20

Beyond Aerobics with Chanting

As ever, how Americans exercised evolved with their engagement with the world at large. When the Berlin Wall fell in in 1989, the global conflict that had served as a key unifying aspect of domestic culture also collapsed, and the results were both geopolitical and existential. "Without the Cold War, what's the point of being an American?," Harry, the middle-aged protagonist of John Updike's 1990 Pulitzer Prize–winning *Rabbit at Rest* wondered. Absent a Soviet enemy, Americans turned inward with new focus on diversity—that afforded by both inborn identity and voluntary affiliation.[1] "Multiculturalism" became a buzzword as ubiquitous in education as in advertising, elevating "tolerating difference" over values once thought to be universal. Such unmooring was disorienting.

Introspection could be a way to make sense of it all, as "building self-esteem" and "personal responsibility" became core learning objectives in some schools. A bipartisan California commission, for example, recommended that the solution to social ills from teen pregnancy to obesity to academic failure to suicide was to devote as much attention to students' "inner space" as Cold Warriors had dedicated to the space race.[2] "Beating stress" among overworked adults became their equivalent public-health preoccupation. Road rage, high blood pressure, weight gain, insomnia, cancer, and premature aging were just a few of the ailments caused by "stress," not to mention the general malaise of feeling one's "natural reservoir of energy" depleted by daily life.[3] Tellingly, Updike personified Harry's loss of political purpose in personal, embodied terms: it was depression, overeating, and a lack of physical vitality that led the former high-school basketball star to a nearly fatal heart attack.[4]

This new questing sensibility carried a whiff of the counter-cultural politics of the sixties and seventies, which at times was expressed as a rejection of the commercialism and cutthroat individualism of the 1980s, and at others as a repackaging of it. Cultural critic David Brooks eviscerated the superficiality of the era's "bobo" (bohemian-bourgeois) affluence most expansively, identifying a pervasive ethos that only nominally "renounced accumulation and embraced cultivation." Cloaking consumerism in a patina of virtue, this ethos invested even leisure pursuits with rigor and discipline and often found expression through bodily cultivation.[5] "Bobos" disdained the rank flashiness of collecting power boats or designer purses, but spent just as lavishly on technical hiking gear, ethically sourced granola, and yoga classes. A spirit of Woodstock prevailed only aesthetically, and barely, over that of Wall Street, as they converged in this worship of a "serious"—and seriously expensive—commitment to health. If some of these same individuals had once understood the aerobics studio as an extension of the nightclub, and sensed little contradiction in snorting cocaine to fuel them in both spaces, a competing conception of exercise as part of an almost religious, often ascetic, pursuit of health now prevailed in some workout cultures. Smiling health and fitness experts were as present as sermonizing preachers on morning television, Brooks wrote, but their entreaties to exercise were simply other means "to encourage moral behavior through the back door." For Brooks, the unsmiling and achievement-oriented, if nearly naked, "bra joggers" in local parks embodied this austere, joyless version of exercise.[6] (Joyless in his regard, it is worth mentioning, as the perspectives of the nameless bra joggers were not included).

"Jogging," now upgraded in common parlance to "running," grew in popularity such that "the loneliness of the long-distance runner" of the early 1960s felt like a distant memory. Oprah Winfrey completed the Marine Corps Marathon in 1994, and Disney launched its own contest the same year. Overall, "frequent exercisers," defined as those working out more than one hundred days per year, grew to

51.3 million in 1998, up by nearly ten million since 1987, with their interests gravitating to include resistance training and cardio equipment, in gyms and at home.[7]

It was in newly popular, athletic forms of yoga that the impulses to exercise intensely and to enlighten and improve oneself intersected most powerfully. By the 1980s, yoga participation had fallen from a 1975 peak of about five million, and the twenty-two million aerobics enthusiasts absolutely dwarfed this always relatively niche pastime. But by 1994, the number of yoga practitioners had climbed to six million, with seventeen million more interested in trying it. Data vary, but by 1999, it seemed that about eighteen million Americans considered themselves regular practitioners.[8] This growth was in part because yoga's quieter, meditative forms were increasingly "fused" with competitive, unapologetically individualistic physical fitness in programs such as "yoga bootcamp" and "power yoga." At a conference on "The New American Yoga" held at the Kripalu Center for Yoga and Health, a retreat the *New York Times* described as a "yoga power spot" full of "yoga personalities" recognizable from ESPN and the exercise aisle at Blockbuster Video, John Friend, founder of the athletic "Anusara Yoga" style, defended yoga's move from the "confines of the counterculture to the mainstream of American fitness."[9] Significantly stewarded by white Americans like himself, some of whom were derided for offering mere "aerobics with chanting," these eclectic new forms were bringing yoga to fresh audiences, and "any spiritual influence is better than none at all," Friend pointed out. Later that year, *Yoga Journal* cosponsored the World Fitness Convention, targeting gym owners and instructors, and the magazine's new corporate owner, John Abbott, explained his pursuit of the partnership: "Our culture likes the physical stuff. . . . We're all ingrained from the earliest age that it's good to do exercise. And then you find this, wow, this is more than exercise."

This evolution was not sudden. *Yoga Journal* had launched in San Francisco as a pen-and-ink newsletter in 1975, advertising Eastern bazaars and primarily featuring bearded, male Indian gurus on its covers. Ambivalence about the undeniably growing popularity of yoga-for-fitness soon permeated its pages. "Yoga is not simply exercise," one 1980 editorial proclaimed, affirming the centrality of "spiritual community" rather than physical technique. The same issue, however, included leading yogis excitedly announcing a new frontier for yoga, including its use as "static stretches" for sports programs, now that its "peculiar connotation" with "an imprisoning cloud of religious affiliation" was dissipating.[10] By the 1990s, this secularization continued apace. "Namaste, Jane," read the caption on a photo of Jane Fonda in lotus pose in 1994. Thirteen years after the release of her best-selling *Workout*, Fonda had integrated "user-friendly, non-mystical, nonfat yoga" into her personal fitness routine and expanding video library.[11] "When in doubt, breathe," replaced Fonda's famous injunction to "feel the burn." She was ecstatic to popularize "the most exciting new exercise trend," which had been introduced to her by basketball star Kareem Abdul-Jabbar, and which emphasized "fitness and stress reduction" over spirituality.[12]

Yoga Journal editor Rick Fields proudly declared Fonda's evolution as evidence that "the mainstream has discovered the benefits of yoga . . . and we are glad to be here."[13] That mainstream was white, metropolitan, and upper-middle class. A plaintive letter from a reader who had found yoga helped her recover from three miscarriages took no issue with this focus on fitness, but did criticize the emphasis on Fonda to the exclusion of Raquel Welch, another movie star who headlined aerobics and yoga videos. At the same time, other readers were frustrated by favorable coverage of a "Yogalympics" competition and of an expensive Tantric couples retreat in Hawaii—writing that such events are "the antithesis of what yoga is about." That retreat, focused on romance, gourmet meals, and luxurious vacationing for "rich yuppies," was—they complained—"a bunch of crap" disconnected from the true, and unglamorous, Tantric aim of realizing that even while "fucking and shitting, in the most gross of physical settings, whether a cremation ground or a stripper bar, nothing can escape Spirit."[14]

But this mainstreaming of yoga, due in large part to its increasing interconnectedness with exercise, felt almost inexorable. In

Los Angeles, one self-described "fitness junkie" who had long dismissed yoga as "a passive pastime performed by religious fanatics" who misguidedly believed that "'it is better to feel good than to look good,'" realized in 1988 that a new genre of yoga was "attracting hundreds of jocks" such as himself seeking "healing and balance, as well as the body beautiful." One such program was "Urban Yoga," whose founder, Billy Porter, dismissed aerobics as "repulsive to my soul." But so too was yoga, conventionally understood, excessively "airy fairy" for Porter's tastes. Urban Yoga, the practice he developed and offered twenty-seven times a week, plus special classes for people with AIDS, was exercise for "the whole person. It strengthens and tones. It releases stress. It releases blocked emotion through sound and breathing." Yoga Works, which had opened the doors in the fall of 1987 to its "beautifully designed studio with an ocean view," also catered to those seeking "secular yoga" from the established Ashtanga and Iyengar traditions. The Yoga Works "house blend," a seventy-five-minute "hybrid 'yogaerobic' workout for the very fit" was especially popular.[15]

Yoga Works already had a location in the "high-rent district" of east midtown Manhattan, and it launched a national teacher-training program in 1990 that spread this more athletic version of yoga. While Yoga Works studios continued to host events such as a sitar and butterfly harp concert, offered with a dinner of Indian curry rice, by 1997 it was also advertising "a knock-down, drag-out yoga bootcamp for . . . endurance-test-style serenity." That sort of programming fueled its expansion.[16] Such standardization led detractors to diminish the format as "McYoga," a criticism only amplified when in 2001 two technology executives, with backing from a venture capital firm and an investor in a big-box gym chain, began buying up studios to emulate a model more familiar in the fitness industry: Yoga Works became "America's first major non-franchised yoga studio chain."[17] *Yoga Journal* underwent a similarly corporate shift. After its 1998 acquisition by John Abbott, it became a glossy magazine increasingly available in supermarkets beside equally shiny fitness publications such as *SELF* and *Shape*, featuring content by contributors such as "power yoga" proselytizer Baron

Baptiste, whose writing about accessing one's "awakened athlete" melded with stories on stress reduction and sculpted arms.

Many lamented how a shallow American fitness culture was corrupting yoga's transcendent, often ascetic, spirituality to sell yet another technique for thinner thighs. When *Yoga Journal* featured two new "power yoga" programs established by students of Ashtanga yoga luminary K. Pattabhi Jois, he wrote from Mysore, India to distance himself from such "ignorant bodybuilding" borne of bastardizing his teachings into "a circus for their own fame and profit."[18] A Los Angeles teacher watching "power yoga" classes swell to fifty or sixty students warned that "it's getting harder and faster, and you're going to see a backlash."[19] But the influence worked both ways, and yoga just as powerfully shaped, and helped legitimize, fitness culture. To many Americans, yoga's heady vocabulary of "transcendence," "holism," and "practice" elevated the cultural esteem of exercise among those who had dismissed gyms as little more than "body shops" for dim-witted narcissists; "The Body Shop," of course, had been the name of Lucille Roberts's first gym.

Certain evocations of this newly metaphysical approach to exercise were over the top, such as "astroyoga," whose creator customized "yoga tutorials" based on her daily reading of her clients' astrological signs and "the astronomical position of the sun, moon, and planets to determine what kinds of asanas, meditations, and pranayamas ought to be practiced." Popular among a Beverly Hills set "blown out from aerobics" in whose milieu "personal fitness trainers are as plentiful as bottled water," astroyoga was just one beneficiary of a new, voracious appetite for niche exercise programs with ever loftier goals.[20] Yoga elevated exercise to "something more," even something cosmic, legitimating the pursuits of millions of exercisers and intensifying pressure for others to follow suit.

While fitness certifications from the profession's growing number of alphabet agencies evaluated aspiring instructors on CPR, basic anatomy, and facilitation skills, the instructor application used in the 1990s at New York City's Jivamukti Yoga reveals a search for a different standard of leadership that also upped the ante on exercise instruction. The single-spaced document contained eighty-four questions, some including up to twenty-six subsidiary parts. While a few were typical—"Do you currently teach yoga?"—others required Sanskrit translations, essays about specific yoga traditions and comparisons of various schools of yoga and their leading gurus' philosophies, or metaphysical personal reflection: "Many of the Yoga scriptures label human birth as the highest birth and that human consciousness is the most evolved consciousness. What are your thoughts on this proposition?"[21] The Jivamukti application communicated a far more exalted place for the instructor than was typical in the fitness industry. The studio's newsletter reaffirmed this vaunted role, featuring on its cover co-founder David Life, clad only in briefs, his braid falling over his muscled shoulder, perched in *pincha mayurasana*, a modified elbow stand. Inside, co-founder Sharon Gannon, known as a spiritual teacher and animal-rights activist, reflected on the "magic of the yoga center" that "infected and inspired" her and all who came together in the "spiritual practice" she and Life had enabled.[22] Before establishing Jivamukti in 1984, Gannon was sucessfully teaching aerobics, an earthly past that explains her innovation of using music in class and her regular comments in the press about the strength-building qualities of the "new yoga," as opposed to the older "watered-down version, easily managed by mostly older, female patrons."[23] In some ways, Jivamukti was part of an older tradition that sought to "remystify yoga" by insisting on the centrality of spirituality, philosophy, and lineage, according to Leslie Kaminoff, who taught there after closing his own studio, Yoga Tone, in 1992. But its prominence in a world where fitness and yoga were becoming ever more enmeshed spoke to a new conception of an authoritative, knowledgeable, athletic, and inspired teacher—even guru—at the head of the room.

Such esteem could be easily abused. To Kaminoff, the uniquely extensive Jivamukti application was meant to signal to aspirants that "humiliation is part of the process" of joining the community.[24] Kripalu's founding guru, Amrit Desai, stepped down as spiritual director when it was revealed he had had "inappropriate sexual contact" with three female disciples, breaking his vow of celibacy, his bond of marriage, and the trust of a community that regularly dismissed members for such behavior, and to whom he had lied.[25] This public dismissal in some ways served to underscore and unearth—but not resolve—severe abuses of power perpetrated in yoga communities led by revered teachers. "We are really experiencing the fire at Kripalu," one resident teacher and lawyer, Daniel Bowling, confided in a letter to Kaminoff. "Amrit continues to be in serious denial about the true nature of his abuses of power, sex, and money." Many members of the community were angry at the "strong stand" taken against Desai, while others were disgusted at his hypocrisy. Either way, guest enrollments were "way down" and "many senior residents were leaving." Perhaps most disturbingly, in one "group process" led on-site, "lots of suffering [was] spoken," including other accounts of sexual abuse that had not yet come to the fore. "It is a mess," Bowling confided.[26] Notably, Desai was only the first prominent male leader of American yoga to embody how fluidly esteem could enable abuse. In the coming years, John Friend; prominent Jivamukti teachers including Gannon and Life; Ashtanga Yoga founder K. Pattabhi Jois; and Bikram Choudhury, who pioneered his own heated, eponymous program, were all accused of serious misconduct born of the power afforded to them as stewards of this "new American yoga."

Choudhury, an Indian immigrant who favored loincloths, Rolex watches, luxury cars, and a topknot, most famously and lucratively blended intense physical fitness and yoga. After he was accused of rape, intimidation, and displays of general misanthropy in 2013—such as publicly yelling at a student to "suck in his fat fucking stomach"—his name became inextricable from such abuse. But a certain grandiosity had always been core to his rigorous, heated yoga program, likened to "a steambath with an obstacle course" that propelled him to celebrity in the 1980s and 1990s.[27] Choudhury fancied himself a "human blacksmith" who fashioned flesh instead of metal, and favorably compared himself to physicians, boasting that his cures lasted a lifetime whereas doctors' waiting rooms were damningly always filled with patients battling the same unresolved afflictions. Typical coverage mentioned his blissed-out followers who resolved physical ills and "traded their shrink for yoga class."[28] One journalist admiringly relayed Choudhury's belief that no one in top physical shape needs more than four hours' sleep and described him, in between sips of Coca-Cola, yelling at a student who missed one day of class that "24 hours without me, it's no wonder you can't sleep and are having a bad day."[29] At his studios in Beverly Hills and Hawaii, with the temperature turned up over one hundred degrees Fahrenheit, Choudhury sat atop a red plush barstool he styled his "throne," instructing students through his signature combination of twenty-six postures and breathing exercises over ninety minutes. Celebrities such as Shirley MacLaine, Raquel Welch, and Kareem Abdul-Jabbar sang his praises.[30]

As Choudhury recounted his life story, he had emigrated to California, by way of Japan, in the early 1970s after a successful career as a bodybuilder and competitive yoga champion, a discipline he discovered when an accident with a barbell shattered his femur and threatened permanent incapacitation. Believing only "false yogis" charged for their wisdom, he began teaching yoga for free at Los Angeles's Ambassador Hotel and at weight loss spas. But by 1974, he realized how much wealth signified status in his adopted country, and he opened studios in Hawaii and Beverly Hills, the latter reportedly bringing in one thousand dollars a day by the 1980s. He penned a 1978 mass-market book, *Bikram's Beginning Yoga Class*, and appeared on the *Tonight Show*. According to Choudhury, this ascent to fame and fortune was a function of his most prominent pupil, President Richard Nixon, who granted him a green card after his yoga therapies saved the president from a leg amputation due to thrombosis. This narrative is unsubstantiated—from the yoga championships, which did not commence in India until the mid-1970s, to the Nixon anecdote—but its uncritical repetition contributed to Choudhury's material success, which was undeniable.

By the early 1990s, "Bikram's Yoga College of India" was up and running, and in 1994 it began offering teacher trainings. Thirty-five enthusiasts showed up initially, paying five thousand dollars each for twelve weeks of instruction and a certificate granting them "all rights and privileges to teach Bikram's Yoga System." These programs soon swelled to over three hundred registrants, consolidating Choudhury's wealth and firmly establishing the connection between spiritual refinement, physical exertion, and unsparing instruction. His officially affiliated network of schools exploded from ten in 1996 to nearly seven hundred worldwide by 2003, but hotels, recreation centers, and health clubs from Brattleboro, Vermont, to Miami to the Jersey Shore advertised "Bikram-style yoga" even if they possessed no formal credentials or license to do so. He had sued former student Raquel Welch for ripping off his series (they settled), but the scale of pretenders was becoming unmanageable. Since his first training in 1994, Choudhury had wanted to establish a trademark and franchise his schools, but advisers had dissuaded him with warnings of red tape. In 2002, cognizant of the value of his brand and angry about impostors cutting into the profits to which he now felt his due, he took action. Choudhury trademarked his name and "the sequence," the series of postures that he had adapted from his own teacher, Bishnu Ghosh. He then aggressively went after imitators.[31] But in a move many thought befitted a consumer goods manufacturer—or gym owner—more than an enlightened yogi, he also franchised his business, and relentlessly protected and expanded it with an "anger and capriciousness" which alienated many and often went unchallenged due to his extensive resources and authoritarian personality.[32] Inspired by the fitness industry, Bikram set the standard for the "ultimate commodification" of transnational yoga by establishing its most recognizable brand, making it inextricable from commercial fitness culture, and defining yoga as a consumer product.[33]

Exoticizing Exercise

Choudhury attributed his "yoga mogul" status—a phrase that became a fixture of his frequent media coverage—to his unapologetic embrace of aggressive American capitalism and his astute understanding of a certain sort of consumer's willingness to hand over large sums to self-styled experts and showmen, who promised, as Choudhury did, to both enlighten and eliminate "cottage cheese thighs."[34] But unlike P. T. Barnum or Norman Vincent Peale,

Choudhury's popularity stemmed in part from the tendency to invest "exotic" figures with authority and even otherworldly power. This subtle sort of racism has deep American roots, especially as directed toward Asia, but it took on new forms in the 1990s, when a broad if often superficial celebration of ethnic and cultural diversity germinated in education and politics, but also informed popular culture and the fitness worlds it encompassed.[35]

Bikram Yoga was hardly the only exercise business that benefited from this shift. In fact, the *New York Times* commented that Americans put off by yoga as "weird and painful and elitist" or even boring—if not "writhing around with all your pierced buddies down at Jivamukti"—were embracing a more accessible and cathartic program, one also inspired by an Eastern movement practice: "Tae Bo."[36] Developed by African American martial-arts champion Billy Blanks in the basement of his suburban Boston home, this program combined cardiovascular training with martial arts. In the early 1980s, Blanks found little interest in the program, which he first styled "karobics"—before learning the name had been patented—at the karate dojo he ran. But two decades later, having relocated to southern California, Blanks found an enthusiastic audience for the program he repackaged as "Tae Bo," a portmanteau fusing Tae Kwon Do and boxing. Effusive endorsements from celebrities as diverse as pop star Paula Abdul and welterweight boxer Carlos Palomino soon followed.

The premise of Tae Bo—"one fantastic body shaping fitness system" offered in a suite of video tapes "without bulky, expensive equipment"—was familiar, but its appeal was distinct. One print ad featured "Tae Bo" in spray-painted, graffiti-style letters separated by a yin-and-yang symbol, centered below a banner of two eyes staring out from a black background, ambiguously symbolizing either a ninja mask or Blanks's own skin.[37] Scholars debate whether martial arts originated in Asia or Africa, but in the United States, these forms were often "polycultural." Boxer Muhammad Ali and karate master Bruce Lee inspired one another in the 1970s, and they understood the fights against racism and colonialism as intertwined, especially in the Vietnam War era. African American boxer

Sugar Ray Leonard—who became friends with Blanks—commented in 1982 that he "patterned himself" after Lee.[38] In the Black Panther Party and beyond, dojos were spaces where Black men, women, and children practiced martial arts as a part of a program of racial self-determination. Some practitioners imagined these "movement arts" as a rejection of capitalism and racism.[39]

Blanks professed no such politics. Indeed, though he had initially struggled to find a video production partner because a Black star was perceived as a risky proposition, especially in a workout targeting a white, female audience, he downplayed race and racism, saying he didn't "really let that bother him," that his "goal was to touch the hearts of people, not just touch white or black people."[40] Like many Black celebrities whose mainstream success was predicated on political discretion, such statements might have been a prerequisite for Tae Bo's runaway success: by 1999, its infomercials played two thousand times daily on cable television, moving $80 million of videos.[41] But its popularity reflected new attitudes about racial diversity even in the politically restrained fitness industry. Both appealing to and challenging stereotypes of Black men, Blanks was the first Black trainer to headline a mass-market home video whose sweat glistened visibly on his muscles rather than being quickly toweled off, fitness video producer Cal Pozo remembered.[42] Pushing the genre's boundaries while perpetuating the image of superhuman Black physicality was a profitable proposition.

Blanks was appointed to the President's Council on Physical Fitness and Sports, appeared on *Oprah*, and prompted so many imitators that his lawyer estimated she issued sixty cease-and-desist letters a week to businesses marketing classes such as "Y Bo" (at the YMCA) or "Tae Combo."[43] Television direct sales had become an important avenue for selling fitness videos, while those in stores often sat "rotting on the shelf." Blanks, however, had "single-handedly reignited the fitness category at retail," *Billboard* magazine gushed, and was the rare exercise personality whose videos sold successfully via both channels. Praising Blanks as "the guy who can bring [retail fitness videos] back from the dead," *Billboard* chronicled the similar success of a video distributor that had for decades struggled to find an

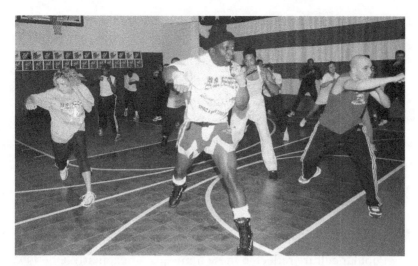

Figure 25. Todd Reeves, *Signalman Seaman Jeremy Cavaretta of New York (right) Works Out with Billy Blanks (center), the Creator of "Tae Bo," during His Visit aboard the Sixth Fleet Flagship USS "La Salle,"* 2002. Billy Blanks, who popularized the fusion workout Tae-Bo, teaches a group fitness class for men and women.

PHOTOGRAPH. COURTESY OF BILLY BLANKS.

audience for its "gay-and-lesbian-oriented videos," but in the late 1990s had prospered because "it's not just gay and lesbian people who buy and rent them: the potential for the genre has changed dramatically."[44] Tae Bo is "the Macarena of exercise," effused the *New York Times* with a hint of mockery, likening its irresistibility among both men and women to another cultural crossover phenomenon, the catchy Spanish dance song ubiquitous at the time.

The social and cultural progress that Blanks's individual success story suggested was incomplete, however. Notably, former Massachusetts studio manager Patricia Pierce told the *Boston Globe* she had financed Blanks in the 1980s and designed the workout with him, though her work had never been acknowledged.[45] Another woman, Patricia Moreno, who had developed a martial arts/cardio fitness program called Powerstrike with her partner Ilaria Montagnani, remembered their disbelief as Blanks became a global celebrity teaching a program nearly identical to the one they had developed in New York City gyms almost simultaneously. "I think it's because they were women," one devoted student reflected as to why Powerstrike did not achieve such recognition. "As amazing as they were, many women are drawn to the thrill of working out with a tough Black guy." Blanks's celebrity absolutely challenged the color line, but it should also be understood against the backdrop of the rise of mass incarceration of men of color during the 1990s. As Blanks inspired many to take up exercise, a series of weight-lifting bans in prisons explicitly curtailed the rights of others to do so. Such restrictions were rooted in long-standing fears of overdeveloped Black men, which were reignited by talk among policymakers of a generation of "super-predators."[46] But they also reflected a new attitude about exercise as a positive, even enjoyable form of self-improvement, and thus an activity with no place in a penal institution.[47]

Popular culture reflected these limits just as explicitly. One 1992 episode of the popular soap opera *All My Children* takes place at a health club, where adults of all ages toil away on Nautilus machines and weight racks. The presence of Livia Frye, a slender Black woman in a leotard pedaling on a stationary bicycle is notable, for white-owned gyms in affluent areas like fictional Pine Valley had for decades courted a "classy"—read "white"—clientele. A successful attorney who ultimately marries the white gym owner, Livia is clearly socially at ease in this exercise space. Her son Terrence, a college student who moonlights at the front desk, is less easily integrated. While folding towels, he is accosted by two white members, who address him as "boy" and demand he serve them grapefruit juice. The two men assure a white attendant he need not rush to get them a locker, but snarl that Terrence better drop the "bad attitude" and get his "step 'n' fetch it in gear." Appalled, Terrence's white friend Haley gasped, "Oh, not here! . . . Racist pigs make me sick!" The white owner was similarly aghast that such "hatred still exists," and assured Terrence such bigotry had no place in his club. But the two members, who were later revealed to be part of an underground white supremacy network, returned to beat Terrence unconscious. Pine Valley was "never the same again," the episode teaser describes. But Terrence had long been familiar with white people whose "frozen polite smile" revealed their racism; he was surprised only at their stridency in expressing it so openly at the gym.[48]

21

Strong Is the New Skinny?

Multiculturalism made the audience for, and experience of, exercise more variegated, but it was the increasing interconnection between fitness and sports that further entrenched recreational exercise in the mainstream. Fitness enthusiasts and athletic authorities had kept each other at arm's length since the 1950s: recreational fitness was supposed to be more inclusive than sports; to some athletic elitists who prized competition over access, that made it effeminate and unserious. But by the end of the twentieth century, this stark distinction was blurring. The male corporate athlete who had played sports in college and turned to running, swimming, or even aerobics to "stay hard" as he spent much of his time behind a desk was a familiar figure. But the first generation of girls who did not know a world without Title IX was also coming of age. In 1972, fewer than three hundred thousand teenage girls participated in athletics, but by 1995, the number had grown almost tenfold, to nearly 2.25 million.[1] "Daughters of Title IX, they've never been told what they can't do," quipped a *Time* editorial remarking on the uniqueness of a generation of girls who not only enjoyed unprecedented athletic opportunity but approached their male peers in educational attainment, achieved a greater degree of pay parity, and gained protection from campus sexual violence thanks to the 1990 Clery Act.[2]

This watershed was largely incomplete, however, as most women did not spend four years in college (where the Clery Act applied), and of those who did, only about 30 percent participated in sports, a proportion unchanged since the mid-1980s, and they received just 23 percent of athletic funding.[3] Especially after Democratic president Bill Clinton, with his wife Hillary by his side, vowed to affirm gender equity across educational and other public institutions, the conservative backlash to these advances was disproportionately intense. Opponents of affirmative action used claims of "reverse discrimination" to condemn how Title IX might adversely affect football programs, a tactic Donna Lopiano, the director of the Women's Sports Foundation, compared to IBM asking for protection under an antitrust law.[4] Sure enough, three years later, the right-leaning *New York Daily News* warned that the "evolution of Title IX into a quota program has been remarkable and perverse. . . . College sports programs have been scrambling to subtract males." It predicted that all sorts of institutions that received federal funding would "presumably be forced into gender balance."[5]

The popularization of this mutually reinforcing athleticism and femininity, however, destigmatized both fitness culture as frivolous and athletics as inappropriately mannish. A raft of new products announced that "strong is the new skinny," selling fitness and beauty with the language of athletic girl power rather than of the pursuit of thinness. "This is the first group of women that's had twenty years in the weight room. . . . You can see real definition on their bodies," Lopiano marveled in 1996.[6] That strength was often positioned as metaphysical. In 1990, chastened by having missed out on the women's aerobics market, Nike tasked advertising executives Janet Champ and Nancy Monsarrat with "dialing down the testosterone and starting a real conversation with women." Champ remembers her boss Dan Wieden poking his head in their office and saying, "Well, you guys are girls, so why don't you work on this?" Market research directed them to run ads in women's magazines, publications Champ and Monsarrat "despised" for their singular focus on "makeup or who you're dating." So they developed their first campaign, "The List," to subtly subvert all that "women are subjected to when they look in these magazines." Using a bold, sans serif font to make a statement "without feminizing the brand," an enduring priority for Phil Knight, The List was an inventory of the countless ways women were pressured to perceive themselves as problems to be fixed through fad diets, fanciful therapies, landing a man, and so on. "It was very tough, very anti-*Cosmopolitan*," Champ proudly recalled. The next campaign, "If You Were Born a Daughter" went still further in linking athletic endeavor—and the clothes to engage in it—with a broad sort of women's empowerment. The campaign took them to a new level, Champ felt, in that it "hit upon the universal and intimate things that make an athlete of any kind tick, or that make a woman of any kind want to be empowered." One of the partners at the advertising firm remembered visiting other clients and seeing the Nike ads pinned up on secretaries' walls; teenage girls did the same in their lockers.[7]

Buoyed by this success in print, Nike ventured into the pricier realm of television advertising. At one meeting, a male executive commented he would be upset if his son disliked sports but would be unbothered by his daughter's disinterest. What sort of ad could help erode such attitudes? "If You Let Me Play," a thirty-second spot released in the summer of 1995, drew on statistics gathered by the Women's Sports Foundation to link girls' sports not just to physical strength and skill, but to social outcomes such as improved mental health and decreased rates of domestic violence, breast cancer, and teen pregnancy. Tackling these intense topics in a spot to sell apparel was challenging. But permitting girls entry into sports, an area usually gatekept by men—by appealing to the broad uplift and empowerment associated with active womanhood that the fitness movement had helped mainstream—was a more natural sweet spot for Nike than, say, launching an aerobics line. (Notably, their early attempts at yoga apparel were also awkward.) Still, early versions of "If You Let Me Play," Champ remembers, had a "downtrodden, Dickensian feel." The "rag-tag" girls looked "like they were from Appalachia or something," an aesthetic unlikely to move merchandise that was supposed to make the wearer feel good. The final cut was cheerier, depicting girls of various ethnicities—if not sizes or abilities—happily playing, jumping, and repeating "If you let me play..." with all the ways sport would better their lives. To Champ's shock, the line "I'll be more likely to leave a man who beats me" was allowed to remain in the final cut, which was recognized by the White House, feminist nonprofits, and industry lists that still rank it among historic campaigns three decades later. Such ads unquestionably helped combat disempowering assumptions that girls and women didn't belong on the court or the gym, but also created new expectations of participation, and to associate an active lifestyle with affluence and an absence of disability.[8]

Such dynamics persisted as female athleticism was more widely embraced, and permeated the industry and broader culture. A sponsor of the US national women's soccer team, Nike "shocked" star Mia Hamm and her teammates by asking them for design feedback and customizing a "women's cut" uniform, a basic courtesy they had not been previously extended. Commercials on network television introduced these athletes to the public, but spots like "Soccer Vows," in which the teammates make promises to each other reminiscent of nuptials, persisted in centering the traditionally feminine virtues of collaboration and other-directedness. Champ said she wished she and her team had "been allowed to push it and be surprising and show that women can be just as bloodthirsty as men."[9] When the women's team won the World Cup in 1999, Brandi Chastain ripped off her shirt and fell to the grass in joy, unapologetically showing her muscular torso clad in only a black Nike sports bra. The historic image, captured on the cover of *Sports Illustrated*, fanned enthusiasm for women's athleticism more than any executive could have dreamed; media dubbed the nineties "the decade of the woman athlete."

Yet even journalists who celebrated this empowering shift could perpetuate the very dynamic they critiqued. *Time* praised the end of "heroin chic," but smirkingly pointed out that inspiring posters of Hamm or other "booters with hooters" that little girls pinned up in their bedrooms also titillated their brothers and fathers. Diminishing "the poster girl for jockette sex," tennis player Anna Kournikova, the article purported to celebrate the "healthy, full-bodied femininity" of this new athleticism, but concluded by listing the heights and weights of the "Babe City" athletes, arguably advancing objectification rather than undermining it.[10]

Still, specific fitness pastimes reflected this new sensibility, which could feel excitingly expansive. "Cross-training," the combination of diverse fitness programs, became an activity for gymgoers seeking variety as much as for professional athletes calibrating their exertions for better outcomes. Retailers from Nike to Tyr (swimming) to Danskin (dance) designed apparel for consumers as likely to hike, in-line skate, lift weights, or rock climb, and to sport their clothing for fashion as much as function.[11] New studies attested to the importance of strength training; back in 1990, the American Council on Sports Medicine had revised its prescriptions for regular aerobic exercise to include it.[12] Spinning, licensed in 1987 by South African cyclist Johnny Goldberg, who went by Johnny G, transposed the experience of competitive cycling into group fitness, a realm that had been mostly associated with the choreographed formats favored by women. In Atlanta, a former bodybuilder and gymnast named Gin Miller developed "step aerobics" after an injury in a high-impact class, integrating hand weights with a stair-stepping routine in a program she piloted at a Gold's Gym, and marketed to men and women—and later the military and athletic teams—as providing a short, intense, muscle-building workout.[13] Such "sportification" gave gravitas to recreational fitness, in part by bringing more men into the fold. Ruth Zukerman, who would go on to cofound boutique fitness studios SoulCycle and Flywheel, got hooked on Spinning classes taught by a Johnny G disciple whose smoothly mixed playlists recalled the dance studios of her youth, but who wore army boots and cultivated a competitive indoor cycling environment as inviting to men as women.[14] At the 2000 ECA conference, a full-day, two-hundred-dollar instructor-certification course for Powerstrike, the popular kickboxing workout founded by Moreno and Montagnani—two women—invited participants to experience the "thrill of hitting something" and specifically advertised the presence of punching bags as exciting to "a lot of men who otherwise would not be caught dead in a fitness studio."[15]

Even Pilates, whose American identity had been closely knit to the dance community, reflected this new focus on physical and mental fortitude and surged in popularity, despite an acrimonious trademark lawsuit that had many teachers awkwardly describing their method as "inspired by Joseph Pilates" or cryptically as "The Method." The San Francisco 49ers integrated Pilates into their training, and the number of studios exploded from seven in 1976 to 350 in 1996.[16] Joan Breibart, who had discovered Pilates in the early 1970s as an alternative to sports or recreational jogging, established a Santa Fe institute that certified over two hundred instructors and designed an at-home version of the Reformer sold via infomercial. Pilates still attracted women "getting bored with aerobics" as the path to weight loss, but it was now equally marketed as a way to build strength.[17] *Men's Health* touted Pilates as one of "the best exercises of all time," *Prevention* celebrated its "gentle moves for firm muscles," and *Essence* proclaimed its power to "strengthen body and soul."[18] "Pilates is not of the 'no pain, no gain' school of thinking or research . . . and for many others that thinking is also changing," declared a profile of Hawaii studio owner and dancer Anita Jackson, who contrasted the pursuit with that of "fitness seekers" seeking mere "body improvement." A Pilates class was not a lone painful hour to endure and then go about one's day, but a therapeutic, even transcendent, experience of "continual discovery" with a "master teacher" akin to "disciplines, whether spiritual, artistic, musical or athletic," that can yield "rich rewards and new feelings about all aspects of their lives."[19] Still, its broad popularity gave pause to some of Pilates's original disciples; one commented that "if Joe's watching what's going on down here today, the notion that anybody can learn it on their own or teach it, he is probably stomping his feet and shaking his fist, screaming, 'Stop it or I kill you!'"

"Abs of steel" are what many newcomers to Pilates really wanted, the *New York Times* reported, gesturing to the rock-hard abdominal muscles that were the corporeal core of a new ideal marketed to both men and women. The flip reference was to Buns of Steel, the fitness brand that became famous for the sculpted posterior it first promised and popularized before launching programs encompassing targeted workouts for every part of the body. Launched in 1988 by Alaskan ex–pole vaulter Greg Smithey, who awkwardly promised "a bun rebirth" to follow "squeezing the cheeseburgers out of your hips," Buns of Steel took off in the early 1990s, with a more polished production aesthetic and Tamilee Webb, the would-be physical-education-teacher-cum-bodybuilder-cum-fitness-professional, as frontwoman.[20] "'Buns of Steel' is grabbing fitness enthusiasts by the gluteus," trumpeted one 1993 article that credited the success of the program with its low-priced videocassette ($9.99, while Fonda's latest sold for $14.99), and targeting of specific body parts, which translated into a proliferation of offerings: in 1992, five different *Steel* videos—from the beginner and original *Buns* titles to Abs, Arms, and Legs—occupied the Billboard Health and Fitness Top 20. Webb had begun to feel that women bodybuilders looked "far less feminine" in the early 1990s, as competitions rewarded ever more bulging muscles and apparent vascularity out of step with most women's aesthetic aspirations. This appetite for muscular defini-tion, however, was shaping mainstream commercial fitness in a way that created a perfect niche for her skills and look, which attracted viewers "about 60/40 women to men," a far more equitable split than any other program she had taught.[21]

Exercise physiologists warned that spot training was futile, a gimmick to exploit insecurities and move new merchandise. But commonsense entreaties to a consistent, preventative commitment to exercise and diet did little to stem a wave of copycat products that specifically promised perfect posteriors: Kathy Smith, Cher, and Suzanne Somers all released targeted programs.[22] Its dubious scientific basis notwithstanding, this new obsession with a round, sculpted butt surely represented an expansion of bodily ideals to prize visible female muscularity rather than waifishness. But the specific obsession with a round behind, a body part long associated with, and celebrated in, Black and Latin cultures, also represented a dubious form of cultural inclusion. As Sabrina Strings has writ-ten, white Europeans had for centuries gawked at Black women's bodies, and their buttocks specifically, as "grotesquely oversized"; the sudden convergence, in the 1990s, of an aesthetic racial inclu-siveness and celebration of female muscularity meant a prominent posterior was newly perceived as desirable by the largely white, relatively affluent consumer audience for exercise products.[23] This appropriation could be self-conscious; at the top of the 1992 chart-topping song, "Baby Got Back," rapper Sir Mix-A-Lot's paean to round, sculpted backsides, a judgmental, white female voice opines, "Oh my God, Becky, look at her butt! It is so big. She's just so . . . Black!" Such a "healthy butt" had nothing to do with the "beanpole dames in the magazines" like *Cosmopolitan* and *Vogue*, or "workout tapes by Fonda" who had "no motor in the back of her Honda," the song explains in its celebration of Black women's bodies and critique of the narrow, white beauty standards.

But the song wasn't exactly about self-acceptance, either. A "healthy butt" was desirable primarily as a way to draw male attention, and most attractive in a small-waisted configuration that was mostly an accident of birth, not hours in the gym: "little in the middle, but she got much back." Ironically, Selena, the Tejana pop star whose backside became as much a part of her signature look as the sequined bustiers she favored, insisted she never exercised and preferred Coca-Cola to water. The slightly broader range of physical ideals did now include some visibly muscular or curvy women, but fell far short of full bodily diversity. Moreover, despite the flattering gloss, this focus on a single aspect of Black and Brown physicality could be dehumanizing, especially as a still predominantly-white industry proffered advice on attaining this ideal new ass, and profited from its pursuit. Black women suffered doubly, as the reductive notion that African American culture uniformly prized larger bodies meant Black experiences of eating disorders were almost entirely ignored, even as a great deal of media and scientific attention centered on the phenomenon of white "fasting girls."[24]

Girls and women who now went to bootcamp or Bikram were subjected to continued expectations that they look a certain way: still slender, but now with sinewy muscles and a "bubble butt." The limits of this new "celebration" of strong and curvy bodies were crystal clear in how freakish women who exercised too much—or looked to others like they did—were still considered. On a 1990 episode of his talk show, Geraldo Rivera begins by celebrating the evolution of "feminine beauty" over decades to ask—as a parade of five women bodybuilders pose to Madonna's *Vogue*—whether their muscled frames are becoming the "ideal body of the 1990s." The mood quickly turns. To audience laughter, Rivera inquires how the women feel about being seen as "female heads on male bodies," contrasting their bodybuilding with their previous lives as "feminine" cheerleaders and ballet dancers, and even their "civilian" skirts and blouses, and asking whether their strong bodies made men feel insecure.[25] The group of Black and white women gamely discuss their lives and training regimes, and how applicable they are for women who just want to "tone," create "the illusion of a bigger chest," or always "look great in a thong bikini." One woman, a rape survivor, deftly rejects Rivera's assumption that bodybuilders are unfeminine, and, ever smiling, explains that she and her fellow bodybuilders are actually redefining femininity, and modeling how women can reclaim their strength in the gym and on the street. But the moment is brief, as Geraldo asks the audience to weigh in on whether the move of bodybuilding from "the dark alleyway" to the mainstream is an affront to the intrinsic "softness" of femininity.

This messaging could be confusing, as women who were not conventionally slender were described as masculine for being too muscular or undisciplined in carrying more weight on their curves. On *The Richard Bey Show*, viewers watched a competition between mostly Black, more-muscular "voluptuous vixens" and thinner, mostly white "fragile waifs," all wearing heels, jewelry, and miniskirts or dress trousers, who competed in a mock "marathon" around the studio building. Meant to test if the more muscular "vixens" were actually more physically fit than the "waifs," the experiment "proved" that the thinner women were.[26] The spectacle of women exerting themselves was of course the point, and the event concluded with Bey draping his arm over the woman with large breasts who came in last, because "it's hard to run when you're amply endowed, isn't it," he drawled. She giggled, amid catcalls and a camera that focused on her visible nipples, that she could run fine, she just wasn't wearing a bra. Exhaustion was one effect of these confusing expectations of a generation of girls and women to exercise, and to look like it—but not *too* much. As historian Joan Jacobs Brumberg wrote in 1997, the "pressure to control the body . . . [had] ratcheted upward" and "a lean, taut, female body with visible musculature . . . requires even more attention, work, and control than the thin body" fetishized by earlier generations. And revealing fashions like crop tops and miniskirts made the "internalization of body controls" via the gym—not girdles or corsets—the only way to achieve the sort of body considered sufficiently desirable for display.[27]

The narrowness of these beauty ideals was proven time and again in media that simultaneously proclaimed their expansiveness. When *Seventeen* magazine featured a size-six bikini model on a 1993 cover, some readers cheered the presence of a woman who looked like she "forgets to do her Step aerobics once in a while" rather than usual "superskinny" figures. Another reader, however, chastised the editors for not choosing a cover model with a "better figure," *especially* if she was going to wear a bikini.[28] The struggles faced by publications that endeavored to address a female public primarily interested in performance were revealing. In the mid-1990s, Condé Nast acquired *womenSports*, and editor Lucy Danziger strove to keep the feminist editorial vision of founder Billie Jean King alive, but she found a public more likely to spend on general fitness than sports content, especially if it pertained to beauty. "We're all women as well as athletes," Danziger had thought optimistically of her ability to merge the two realms; "everybody wants their hair to look good after you get out of the pool." The strategy foundered, however, and the publication was soon subsumed into *SELF. Sports Illustrated Women* launched at almost the same time with similar goals that women hailed for their stark contrast with the sexualized portrayal of women in the publication's swimsuit issue and athletic coverage; it soon folded as well.[29]

The beauty imperative proved more durable than enthusiasm for athletics and health, or at least inseparable from it, in terms of transformations in mainstream fitness culture. The problem was bigger than women's ability to achieve appropriately sculpted abdominals or a big-in-precisely-the-right-way butt. A thoroughgoing "body fascism," according to philosopher Brian Pronger, that equated a visibly fit, deliberately cultivated body with social worth was permeating an expanding fitness culture in which men and women were both pressured to participate—a dubious form of equality.[30]

22

It's Not Fitness, It's Life

As the stakes of exercising—or not—ratcheted up, so did the opportunities to profit from this pressure expand. And as fitness culture became both omnipresent and apparently more inclusive, so too did it become more upscale and corporatized. Molly Fox might have had Madonna as a client, but her studio was small and the walls shook; a significant portion of her advertising consisted of paying underemployed actors to slip fliers under apartment doors, "like Chinese food menus." Uptown, Jeff Martin could count on James Taylor to come to class—and at a time, even hired aspiring young singer Mariah Carey to work at the front desk—but he collected payment in cash, which he packed into shoeboxes under his bed. "I had no business skills whatsoever," he told me.

When a trio of siblings from New Jersey, the Erricos, witnessed these successes in the gym world that they knew well as avid exercisers, they had an idea to scale it. Using their corporate experience—Lavinia sold fragrances up and down the East Coast, and her brothers worked in real-estate development and construction—they set about opening their own gym that would offer a different experience than those offered by small studios or impersonal chain gyms. Lavinia, in particular, who as a teenager had worked out on Ladies Days at a European Health Spa, then looked up to bodybuilder Rachel McLish and "lived at Jeff Martin's and the Vertical Club," had sensed opportunity in this space for several years. In the mid-1980s, when she moved back to the East Coast after graduating from the University of Southern California—where, armed with a boom box, she had taught impromptu aerobics to sorority girls in a campus atrium—she and her brothers had come close to opening a gym in New Jersey. But at the last moment, the landlord pulled out. "No one wanted gyms as tenants back then," she explained; "it was just not prestigious."[1] The stereotype was that gym owners sold deeply discounted memberships before opening, and then often never opened, leaving angry customers and landlords in a lurch. The Erricos' interest in opening a gym had been reignited by a "coming soon" flier for a grand opening of a New York Health and Racquet Club in their neighborhood that they had walked by for so many months that it became an inside joke—because it never arrived.

The Erricos could do better, they thought. Thanks to their connections in construction and health-club circles, they learned of a lease coming available on a large fitness facility going out of business in the Westchester suburbs. They decided it was a worthwhile investment. The siblings renovated the facility, installing sprung floors, a swimming pool, and that gym unicorn, a structurally sound aerobics studio with no columns that made teachers "just want to do their thing in there." Lavinia, whose corporate salary and expense account were too substantial to abandon, was still selling perfume from the club's back office, but she set to work recruiting the best New York City instructors, such as Jeff Martin, for guest-teaching appearances. The privilege of membership at Westchester Health and Fitness cost double that of area clubs, but this sense of elite belonging helped make it a destination, drawing suburbanites from four towns, including tony Bronxville, who drove over twenty minutes to make fitness a centerpiece of their social life and their spending.

The model might just work in the city, the Erricos thought, and in the fall of 1991 they opened a health club they named "Equinox Fitness Club," on West 76th Street, in plainsight of Jeff Martin's studio. The next location, on Broadway and East 19th Street, practically steps from Molly Fox's, soon followed. Designed by an architect who specialized in luxury hotels, each gym was structurally arresting and outfitted with a large group fitness studio and locker rooms and amenities such as juice bars to attract members to spend more time there. Meaningfully, they decided not to stock as many weights as gyms such as Gold's or World Gym, since new members found the sight intimidating. "Our goal was not to put anyone out of business," Lavinia Errico told me. It was to expand the clientele for fitness "far beyond" the crowd packing the smaller studios, to the "woman in navy and pearls to a guy who is all tatted up" and might never have thought about joining a gym. "You have no idea how new this all was to people," she explained. Prospective clients and new members would walk in, curious but unsure of how to use the equipment and even what to wear; one celebrity showed up to her first group exercise class wearing water shoes. "She'd never worn sneakers other than Keds," Errico told me. "Our competition was happy hour, not other gyms," she described as the essence of the obstacle and opportunity they faced. Unlike their Los Angeles counterparts, many New Yorkers still found spending time and money on fitness unfamiliar—so many, in fact, that there seemed to be an almost endless supply of souls to be converted, without any provider poaching another's publics.[2]

But one cold, snowy day a few months after Equinox opened, Jeff Martin remembers looking out the window and seeing a group of his regular clients who had just left his studio heading into the shiny new club. Perplexed, he realized that they were still taking classes at his studio but using the luxurious new showers and fluffy towels next door, amenities with which he could never compete. "I saw the writing on the wall," Fox remembers feeling just as acutely. Monique Dash, who was working for a husband-and-wife-owned small studio a few blocks north of Molly Fox's, remembered the tension that coursed through the place when they heard of Equinox's imminent arrival. Inevitably, the Erricos began hiring away the very teachers who packed the smaller, less luxuriously appointed studios that had energized the national dance-fitness trend. "No way I was leaving," said Patricia Moreno, who was a stalwart on Martin's schedule, represented his studio in competitions, and also taught for Fox. She stayed longer than many others, but ultimately, around 1993, she remembered that the classes were thinning at Martin's, and the Erricos came "begging me, courting me," offering health insurance and a rental apartment near Lincoln Center, perks unimaginable anywhere else. Moreno took the offer. "It was like, 'Holy shit, I cannot believe the power we have as teachers.'"[3]

Equinox wasn't the only player capitalizing on this intense appetite. Competition to capture the membership dollars of these affluent exercise enthusiasts was fierce and could play out almost comically. In Irvine, California, two similarly named chains, the Sports Club and the Sporting Club, each invested over twenty million dollars to open super-fitness centers that aspired to be the "Acropolis of physical fitness centers," directly across the San Diego Freeway from one another.[4] As each club broke ground on the hundred-thousand-plus-square-foot sites, they kept promising lavish amenities—tanning beds and massage rooms, but also rock walls, soccer fields, salons, valet parking, and marble lobbies—to differentiate themselves as the superior choice.[5] Some of them, like a kayak run, were never brought to fruition. Along similar lines, Bally's Corporation, after purchasing Jack LaLanne's low-priced chain and rebranding it as "Bally's Total Fitness," invested in the Vertical Club, and in the early 1990s opened several "executive locations" that offered a more "upscale and exclusive" experience than that provided in the majority of their clubs—which didn't merit the "Bally Sports Club" label.[6] After a 1994 IPO buoyed by its West Coast success, The Sports Club opened a 140,000-square-foot location on the Upper West Side of Manhattan, featuring a fake-granite rock climbing wall, gourmet restaurant, and pool with music pumped underwater.[7] Almost directly across the street, a World Gym franchise, once known for bodybuilding, remade itself more modestly to compete in this new environment, moving the heavy weights out of sight from the main entrance and featuring a large, glass-walled studio that showcased the step aerobics and yoga classes.[8] Classes became so full at these clubs that management would schedule popular instructors at inconvenient hours—to little avail, as diehard students confessed to fibbing to their bosses and spouses in order to make classes—and hire "aerobo-cops" for crowd control.[9]

Spacious locker rooms and a full class schedule steps from a stunning gym floor outfitted with the latest elliptical machines,

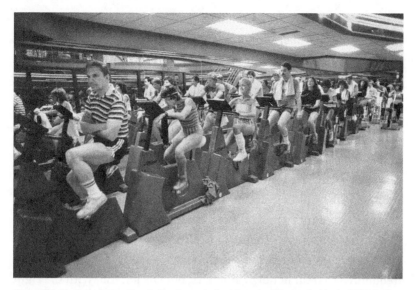

Figure 26. Marilynn K. Yee. *People Use Computerized Exercise Bikes at the Vertical Club in New York in 1984*, 1984. Fitness enthusiasts exercise at the Vertical Club, a large health club that offered many fitness and sports offerings under one roof, and that unapologetically marketed exercise as so glamorous that some members felt they had to get in shape *before* making an appearance at the facility.

PHOTOGRAPH. *NEW YORK TIMES*. REDUX PICTURES, IMAGE NO. 15486666. HTTPS://ARCHIVE .REDUXPICTURES.COM/?13460328111681950240&MEDIANUMBER=15486666.

StairMasters, and chrome weights wasn't all these new clubs sold. Jack LaLanne, Vic Tanny, Lucille Roberts had decades earlier understood the value of linking luxurious amenities to gym membership. Equinox and its peers went a step further, selling what they, and a growing raft of brands like Polo, Absolut, and even J. C. Penney called a "lifestyle."[10] While such a label made intuitive sense for apparel or alcohol that was ostensibly worn for, or inspired by, social activities from after-work drinks to a weekend in the country, working out was just beginning to attain this social meaning. These ever more consolidated upscale fitness brands not only marketed products and experiences that projected individual wealth and power, but linked discipline, health, and a vaguely defined "balance" to the aspirational state of existence attainable within the ever-expanding, and more handsomely appointed, four walls of the gym.

Not every idea worked seamlessly. The glamorous atmosphere that Equinox deliberately cultivated (with efforts such as granting models free or discounted memberships) could be so imposing that anxious prospective members would often demur, telling Errico that first they would "join Jack LaLanne to lose some weight" and would sign up once they felt more confident. "You have that backwards," she would protest, insisting that Equinox hired the best people to achieve weight loss. Errico launched a "wellness center" that offered alternative therapies such as aromatherapy, acupuncture, and craniosacral manipulation, practices they marketed as exceeding physical exercise in their ability to bring about "a luminescent glow of natural health."[11] At the time, these treatments were mostly offered "in Chinatown basements" that Errico frequented to treat her own ailments, but she felt that with the right luxury packaging, Equinox's clientele would love such offerings. In the late 1990s, Errico remembered, the idea of "wellness" barely registered with her skeptical brothers and their investors—"Is that even a real word?," they asked—and some members unprepared for a side of spirituality left angry comment cards about the "quackery" that had infiltrated the club.[12] Despite serving an enthusiastic subset of members enthralled by the new offerings, in 2000, after a management buyout, the wellness center folded.

Your Own Private Trainer

One innovation endured as a staple of high-end clubs and then the industry at large: personal training. Before the 1990s, the idea of a private coach for anyone but celebrities or professional athletes "barely existed," according to IDEA founders Kathie and Peter Davis. Yet the practice "trickled down" to become a lifestyle accoutrement for "Yupscale America—the population that lives by the buzzword 'busy,'" one of thousands of articles on the phenomenon declared in 1990. Rates averaged from fifteen to seventy-five dollars a session, an outlay that could quickly add up to more than a monthly membership at many facilities.[13] Still, as personal training promised individualized attention and interaction impossible in the large classes, videocassettes, or unsupervised exploration of equipment that had been the gateway experiences for so many now-aging exercisers, the phenomenon quickly expanded beyond affluent communities. In Eastern Iowa, where rates topped out about fifty dollars an hour, a typical feature on the popularity of personal training included a photo spread of a stern-looking trainer in a YMCA sweatshirt, taking notes on a clipboard while overseeing leg-curl technique in a manner that conveyed seriousness.[14] By 2002, 94 percent of commercial health clubs offered personal training, making it an industry standard and important revenue stream.[15]

The Davises perceived this growing demand and in 1990 presciently rolled out a personal-training certification that required deeper knowledge of anatomy and exercise physiology than the group-fitness credential. In keeping with the expanding reach of fitness beyond aerobics, IDEA had already distanced itself from the "dance exercise" aspect of its founding acronym in 1988, when it officially changed its name to IDEA: The Association for Fitness Professionals. By 1994, its personal training newsletter had become a full-on magazine, including practical tips for trainers and synthesizing a growing body of scientific research.[16]

"That's when the men started coming in," Kathie Davis remembered of IDEA membership. While the popular perception of an aerobics instructor was of a woman who was working part time or "looking for a fun income, more like a hobby," Davis recalled, the personal-trainer path offered a professional legitimacy inseparable from its decoupling from the realm of women's work. First, there was no choreography, shedding the association with dance. Then, the evolution of the fitness professional from a teacher-like figure at the head of a classroom—evoking the feminine world of education—to a one-on-one relationship that more closely approximated the role of professional adviser or medical clinician abetted the integration of men to the fitness world overall. Perhaps most importantly, so too did the compensation structure: private trainers are paid hourly, in direct proportion to their number of clients, and often to their level of certification.

While a group-fitness instructor was incentivized to collect certifications for individual formats, she was rarely able to command a higher rate from a gym where she taught Tae Bo, say, simply because she had also completed Jazzercise training. The fitness field remained three-quarters female; the figure of the personal trainer cohered more with that of the self-made, economically independent man. Yet that archetype was mostly an ideal. Despite a smattering of "celebrity trainers," most fitness professionals lacked bedrock workplace protections such as sick leave and health insurance. Likewise, they struggled to achieve financial stability in a career that required them to be "supersonic all the time," as one trainer described it, and not only to impart expertise but to embody it. "I knew I was getting to the end of working only as a personal trainer," she said, "when I was no longer willing to maintain my own looks in order to maintain my business." The credibility of credentials was conditioned by the most visible one: one's own body.[17]

The social function of the personal trainer was complex. Most visibly, hiring a trainer was a status symbol for clients who could afford it. At the same time, trainers also had a whiff of the muscled physical laborer—like a pool boy or gardener—tending to a wealthy white-collar client. Yet some clients specifically sought out an authoritarian instructional style. Sociologist Jennifer Smith Maguire interviewed trainers, male and female, who recounted how their clients gleefully likened them to Hitler, slave drivers, and drill sergeants.[18] The thrill of proximity to an individual who not only held expertise in health and beauty, but often physically embodied their clients' aspirations, could be a powerful and even titillating draw. Several dancers at Chippendales, the male exotic-dance revue, trained clients during the day, finding that their skill at charming women while scantily dressed translated well to the gym. For others—especially women—such eroticization was often less welcome. Terri Walsh, the first female trainer at the Vertical Club, described a pushy client who propositioned her over lunch with an offer of a free apartment and tuition if she would "see" him twice a week. "I almost burst into tears. I just wanted to work."[19]

The rapport could be exhaustingly intense, even if not overtly sexual: one client commented that stopping sessions with her personal trainer felt as momentous as "breaking up." In 2000, the *IDEA Personal Trainer Manual* published a code of ethics for personal trainers that revealed the challenges of navigating this new professional identity in a largely unregulated industry. Trainers should not come off like "meathead[s] or . . . bimbo[s]" and should strive to meaningfully connect with their clients, the manual advised, while carefully "maintaining boundaries" around touch, sexual banter, and discussion of personal life.[20] The pace of commercial health-club growth tapered off in the early 1990s, but the numbers of personal trainers grew tenfold. Interest in—and willingness to spend on—fitness intensified, and its arena expanded, as exercise increasingly appeared as a laudable, legitimate pursuit.[21]

This ever more expansive yet individualized approach to fitness endured. Though the wellness center at Equinox was short lived, Errico remembered how magazine editors thrilled to write about it and to experience firsthand the peculiar health pastimes of the affluent. Bodily fitness was required, but it was no longer the ultimate goal. "Our basic question was, 'Now that you're fit, what are you gonna do with it?'" And in 2004, Equinox introduced its long-standing tagline, "It's not fitness. It's life," a slogan revealing how all-encompassing the gym had become. Yet the loftiness of such claims overlooked how the amplification, through corporatization, of one sort of fit lifestyle could erase others—not only of the bodybuilders whose clattering iron plates were often literally sidelined in such luxe spaces. In West Hollywood, the all-men's Athletic Club, down the street from the coed Sports Connection, opened to women members in the early 1990s, reflecting the growing interest in fitness and destigmatization of a world that had once been a gay male subculture. Women did not exactly take over the club—the subpar changing rooms reportedly deterred many—but their presence meant shutting down the nude suntanning that had made the club's rooftop pool deck a destination for gay men. Without this draw to distinguish the club in an ever-more-crowded landscape of gyms making grander promises to their members, the membership of the small club dwindled and ultimately shuttered a few years later, after a brief stint as a Gold's Gym franchise.[22] Fitness might be marketed as "life" to a growing swath of exercisers, but that expansive framing could easily be experienced as exclusive.

The appetite for fitness grew apace, but it was not always satisfied in shared spaces, even luxuriously appointed ones that charged membership fees. As commercial gym membership plateaued, many of the small studios big clubs had displaced had either shuttered or still struggled. The movement toward private training helped keep some of the sprawling fitness palaces afloat, but liberated from the need for a large studio, affluent clients could now choose to bring their workouts home. In some markets, a new trend in home gym construction could cannibalize the clientele of the most cosseted studios and clubs. While most home-exercise devices had long marketed the fact that they were inexpensive and could be inconspicuously stashed away, both to save space and because owning a Thighmaster or an Exercycle might be a source of embarrassment, in the 1990s elaborate home-fitness setups became a showpiece of luxury real-estate listings.[23] A home gym staffed by a private trainer was a testament to one's ability to maximize efficiency in the gym and at life, said Kathie Davis. Many customers disliked lines for equipment or long commutes to a gym: personal training was the "wave of the future" because "people today are so busy they want to get the best possible workout in the shortest amount of time."[24] Fred DeVito recalled that his clients at one West Coast barre studio especially welcomed at-home private sessions, since the small, precise movements and minimal equipment their format required proved portable. Further blurring the boundaries between exercise and life, and discipline and leisure, in the 1990s committed exercisers could invite their personal trainer to their homes, while their teen daughter read glossy magazine articles on achieving "prom arms" and younger children played with a Get in Shape Girl toy set, Barbie Home Gym, or Nintendo Power Pad, a video game accessory that required players to exercise by moving their feet on a wired mat, all accoutrements to teach the next generation to practice the inescapable work of working out.

Who Needs PE When Exercise Is Everywhere?

Alongside this flourishing private industry, physical education might reasonably have been thought to also thrive. Its programs, however, graduated fewer teachers with each passing year. In 1987, a Congressional resolution had encouraged state and local educational agencies to "provide high quality daily physical education programs" to all grade levels. Three years later, the Department of Health and Human Services stepped up this commitment by articulating two goals that revealed how scant physical education actually was: increasing "to at least 50 percent" both the number of K–12 students who participate in daily physical education, and the proportion of physical-education class time meaningfully dedicated to physical activity.

These goals set a low bar, but by 1993 the federal *Shape of the Nation* report lamented that there was still "no federal law mandating [any] physical education," much less the recommended thirty minutes per day for elementary school students, and forty-five to fifty-five minutes for middle and high schoolers. The resolution remained advisory, with power left to the states to figure things out at a more local level. Four more states had implemented some physical-education requirements since the 1987 resolution (up to forty-six), but the more palpable trend was that "physical educators are under intense pressure to defend their programs in these cost-cutting times." Only Illinois required daily physical education of all students.[25] Budget pressures became so intense that local districts sought waivers from state physical-education requirements in order to fund core academic subjects. Even as the holistic benefits of exercise were so loudly proclaimed in the larger culture and growing fitness industry, the 1997 report lamented that "the wave of new technology combined with higher academic standards and cutbacks in school and municipal budgets" was marginalizing the physical fitness sorely needed by a generation that "sits more and moves less."[26]

Educators and policymakers were hardly unmoved by the value of exercise. By the early 1990s, new pedagogies focused on "building

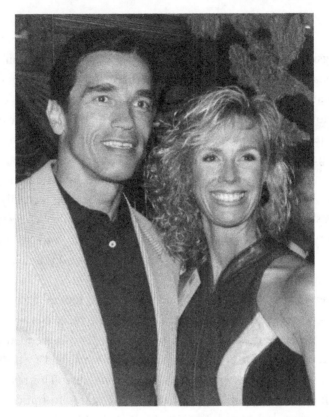

Figure 27. *Jazzercise Kids Get Fit Program Reaches 402,000 Children Worldwide and Is Presented to the President's Council on Physical Fitness and Sports with Arnold Schwarzenegger,* 1992. In 1992, President George Bush invites bodybuilding champion Arnold Schwarzenegger and Jazzercise founder Judi Sheppard Missett—by the close of the twentieth century, both architects of a wide-ranging but coherent fitness culture—to the White House to promote exercise.

PHOTOGRAPH. FROM THE COLLECTION OF JUDI SHEPPARD MISSETT. REPRINTED WITH PERMISSION. HTTPS://WWW.BUILDINGABUSINESSWITHABEAT.COM/?PGID=JUHDIDN5 -B25BDCAE-5EF2-11E9-A9FF-063F49E9A7E4.

self-esteem" often positioned physical fitness as important to achieving this goal. California's Task Force to Promote Self-Esteem and Personal Responsibility in schools suggested that adhering to a healthy diet and doing regular exercise were prime examples of the principle of "being accountable to myself."[27] But the school gym, presided over by a physical education teacher with a whistle, was not where proponents of these holistic pedagogies envisioned such self-fulfillment to transpire. Such externally motivated achievements—even if they got kids to do push-ups or climb the ropes—were insignificant when compared to the internal inspiration that derived from "a deeply felt sense of our own worth" that the report argued should be a learning objective.[28] John Vasconcellos, the California legislator who spearheaded the report, was mocked by pundits and comedians for its touchy-feely tone, but in stressing the importance of mind-body well-being and personal responsibility, he effectively articulated the underlying ethos of popular fitness culture, codified it as a public priority, and applied it to children. Untethering children's exercise from athletic performance not only departed from conventional understandings of physical education, but could also be controversial when schools attempted to implement it: when some districts offered yoga—usually provided by third-party instructors, not credentialed physical educators—Christian conservatives concerned about the transgressive power of this spiritual practice successfully lobbied the Alabama legislature in 1993 to ban yoga instruction in the state's public schools.

At the same time that some children were learning about the importance of bodily cultivation to self-esteem, another set of experts emphasized exercise from a more punitive perspective: as a way to avoid, or cure, the scourge of obesity. A generation of children weaned on fast food, television, and video games was fatter than ever, countless news programs screamed. Their girth, and that of their parents whose sedentary work and unhealthful eating habits wrought a similar effect, not only negatively affected their health and inhibited their individual abilities to thrive, but posed significant social "burdens" in the form of increased insurance premiums and military unreadiness. Reflecting on the bodily impact of the previous decades that had paradoxically also seen the elaboration of a booming commercial fitness culture, the Surgeon General issued no celebration, but rather a somber "call to action to prevent overweight and obesity," with individual commitment to exercise as integral to this path forward.

In 1997, fewer than a third of adults completed even thirty minutes of moderate physical activity several times a week, and 40 percent engaged in no leisure exercise at all. Over 60 percent of adolescents reported participating in twenty minutes of exercise at least three days a week, but data were far sketchier as to how many completed the accumulated sixty minutes daily recommended by the federal government. More conclusive data showed, however, that in 1999, over 40 percent of high schoolers watched at least two hours of television each day. Since the 1960s, the incidence of overweight among children had more than doubled; among adolescents, it had nearly tripled. Echoing Kennedy-era condemnations of the "soft American," these new calls to slim down a nation were civic and social as much as corporeal: the price of a deconditioned body was "premature death and disability," but also "lost productivity" and "social stigmatization."[29] Yet these calls to improve oneself and society through exercise were increasingly directed at poor communities of color, where obesity and associated illnesses were overrepresented, rather than at the leisured white suburbanites targeted four decades earlier. Yet such reports, issued by the government and the media, almost never commented on *why* that inversion had taken place or how to remedy it.

This mix of urgency and enthusiasm brought no commensurate investment in public recreation or physical education. Paradoxically, establishing physical fitness as fundamental to human thriving seemed to further diminish the status of physical educators. The intensity of concerns over obesity made it just as easy to vilify these champions of fitness and health as ineffective as it was to envision them as potential saviors. For the most part, pundits and public-health authorities took the former course or ignored the potential role of physical educators in improving health outcomes altogether. Moreover, a thoroughgoing logic of individualism coursed through fitness culture and the broader moment in which it was embedded, enshrining the idea that *not* exercising was primarily a personal failure, and that greater investment in public facilities or institutions was no viable solution to what was better understood as a crisis of willpower. Even as the *Afro-American Gazette* despaired in 1991 that "despite increased medical advancement and overall health/fitness awareness in this country, African Americans continue to get sicker and die younger than white citizens," it tempered its structural explanation of the "root causes" of such disparity with solutions that centered individual behaviors, from cutting down on "soul food" to managing the stress worsened by "destructive life-styles" pursued by choice.[30]

"Healthism," the false belief that physical health is an outward expression of inner virtue, served to prop up troubling new arche-types conditioned by identity: the "headless fatties" in ubiquitous B-roll on news segments about the "obesity epidemic" among the slothful poor, as much as the "Perfect Girl" on display in glossy magazines and activewear catalogs that pressured upwardly mobile (mostly white) girls to be attractive, assured, and athletic.[31] As each set of federal guidelines for fitness became more stringent—but were honored mostly in the breach—and as physical activity became elevated to a virtuous form of conspicuous consumption, what had been a "fitness craze" had evolved into a newly all-encompassing "lifestyle," one embraced by the relatively affluent few and imposed on many others. Fitness consumerism had escalated accordingly, from a closet full of colorful Flexatards and mail-order contraptions to expensive health-club memberships, home gyms, and fealty to a growing number of exercise "gurus," each signaling more serious commitments to self-improvement through sweat.

As enrollments in physical-education programs dropped to unprec-edented levels, the fitness industry kept expanding and infiltrating new environments, and encompassing new products and promises. No longer merely about the body but about the fully optimized *self*, fitness at the close of the twentieth century was invested with new moral valence, and more openly embraced as core to many more Americans' lives than ever before, whether they rejected or rejoiced at the competing ideas and sensibilities it evoked. Yoga could be Bikram Choudhury's empire built on banishing cottage-cheese thighs through buckets of sweat and boundary crossing, but it could also be a gentle, meditative practice for aging Americans wrung out from aerobics. Strength training could be an avenue to a perfectly sculpted ass, blithely decontextualized from the ideal's racialized origins, and it could signify a feminist rejection of frailty. Home gyms could represent humility, a refusal to participate in the peacocking taking place at ever-more-palatial health clubs, or the ultimate, snobby sequestration from the growing ranks of sweaty hoi polloi. However people embraced, eschewed, or were excluded from exercise at the turn of the twenty-first century, they increasingly had to acknowledge and engage with a set of practices that still define, and starkly divide, the contemporary fit nation.

Part **Seven**

IT'S NOT WORKING OUT

By the turn of the twenty-first century, exercise was certainly no longer just "working out" in the narrow physical sense, but neither was it "working out" as the collective, civic public health project imagined seventy years earlier. On *The Larry King Show* in 2000, an octogenarian Jack LaLanne was still evangelizing exercise, but pointedly decried the disinvestment in public education that had ceded health education to advertising firms who taught children that emulating their favorite athletes meant consuming sugary drinks and candy bars.[1] Participating meaningfully in America's expansive fitness culture was no right of citizenship, but a sign of aesthetic and economic status, or at least reflected a socially sanctioned striving on both fronts. Meanwhile, failure to exercise—whether due to access, ability, or absence of desire—signaled insufficient "hustle." The seeds of this divide were planted over a century earlier, but the first two decades of our millennium have been punctuated by three national crises, each of which bolstered defining aspects of twenty-first-century fitness. First, the September 11 terrorist attacks supercharged exercise as a form of self-determination, whether it meant the rise of "wellness" and its gauzy promises of empowerment and healing, or the militaristic self-sufficiency of CrossFit and its many imitators. Then, the financial crisis of 2008 ironically hastened the rise of the highest-end "boutique fitness" category and served to sacralize exercise as a legitimate expense and meaningful pursuit, for both professionals who imparted it and participants whom they served—an ethos that energized a "new economy of mind and body," as business journalist Jason Kelly styled it, embraced by a surprisingly wide socioeconomic swath of the population.[2] Finally, the coronavirus pandemic threatened to bring this evolution and expansion to a screeching halt. Going to the gym had, until March 2020, been an opportunity for self-congratulation and selfies, an act that proved one's commendable commitment to personal health and salutary forms of socializing. But even in the regions where gyms remained open, entering them—or even heading out for a jog unmasked—could feel transgressive, understood by many as self-ishly prioritizing individual pleasure over public health. Ultimately, the pursuit of fitness as a bedrock social and individual ritual was far too embedded in our experiences and ideals to be vanquished even by a pandemic, but the pause in its public consumption forced a reflection on the role of exercise in American life—if not, as yet, new and more equitable ways to provide it.

23

Exercising in an Age
of Uncertainty

Annbeth Eschbach was sure her investor meetings were canceled, and that the business plan she had so ambitiously envisioned as an MBA student was now destined for failure. It had seemed so promising: a "mind-body" space inspired in equal parts by the Lotte Berk barre classes that had caught her attention one summer in the Hamptons, the tranquility of a high-end hotel spa, the results-driven fitness industry where she had built her career, and the mix of lofty self-actualization and clinical expertise that had suffused her youth growing up with a father who was a medical doctor and a mother who regularly meditated. But just days before her slate of meetings in Los Angeles, on September 11, 2001, the terrorist attack on the World Trade Center threw the economy, politics, and culture into disarray. The Twin Towers crumbling against a perfect blue sky emerged as the emblematic image of the day that claimed nearly three thousand lives, and New York City convulsed with particularly intense panic. Eschbach doubted her meetings would be rescheduled: who would want to invest in a New York City–based wellness business now anyway?

But Eschbach, and the first crop of fitness entrepreneurs of the new millennium, found anything but failure in the world wrought by 9/11. Not only were her meetings rescheduled, but her pitch was well received. Investors bet that the mix of inner-directed healing and body work offered by her brand, Exhale, was precisely the salve a certain sort of consumer would crave in such a bewildering, disturbing moment. Sure enough, brands similarly embracing the mantle of "wellness"—not fitness—multiplied in the coming years, marketing "mind-body" variations on exercise at increasingly higher price points, and often in smaller, more intimate environments. IntenSati, a class that combined positive vocal affirmations and moves inspired by yoga, dance, and martial arts (founded by Patricia Moreno, and which I taught) launched in 2002. SoulCycle, an indoor cycling class that used bikes stable enough that riders could close their eyes and meditate while moving, opened its first, candlelit, studio in 2006. Today it is owned by the same real estate investment company that owns Equinox. What they were doing, in Eschbach's words, was taking a concept of mind-body wellness that had been associated with a "groovy, granola, hairy armpits" aesthetic and repackaged it as a luxurious—and efficient—experience. When the streets, subways, and schools felt unsafe, inner peace was a form of security many deemed worth the expense—especially if it was thought to simultaneously cultivate outer beauty. Such programs uniting enlightenment with exercise were becoming so common that the International Alliance of Yoga Therapists noted that while yoga participation grew by 95 percent from 1998 to 2002, so many new "mind-body" programs had arisen that yoga was no longer the only option for those seeking reprieve from stress and rehabilitation from injury.[1]

This new crop of workouts was undeniably challenging—complementing or even co-opting the intensity of the "traditional 'hard-body pursuits'"—but the aesthetic was soft. Pastel accents and signature fragrances complemented workouts that supplanted the old movement cues with positive affirmations—ranging from the solipsistic "find your truth, follow your bliss" to the self-assured "I am the master of my fate" to the earnest inspiration of "Impossible spells 'I'M POSSIBLE!'" Women were overrepresented in this realm that would come to be known as "boutique fitness," for its high prices and small storefronts, but the same complicated cultural moment and psychological impulse to find security through bodily cultivation gave rise to a different phenomenon with a distinctly masculine aesthetic: CrossFit. Conceived in 2000 in a Santa Cruz garage by then-married Lauren Jenai and Greg Glassman—the latter a former gymnast turned off by high-tech big-box gyms that fetishized low-intensity, steady-state cardio and prioritized appearance over performance—CrossFit represented the "anti-gym." Boxes, as CrossFit gyms were called, evoked garages, equipped with wooden boxes, pull-up bars, barbell racks—and no mirrors. "Functional fitness," accomplished through short, intense intervals, was inspired by military and police bootcamps that trained for survival rather than spiritual enlightenment or skinny jeans. The idea of the "body as a bunker," in the words of Lenore Bell, suffused the program, with daily workouts named for heroes who lost their lives in combat. Not until 2011 did the name of a female soldier ascend to this pantheon, but the first benchmark workouts—nicknamed "The Girls"—all bore women's names, though not for exactly feminist reasons. While some honored actual women who earned naming rights after being "wrecked" or "humiliated" by the workouts, Glassman maintained that "anything that left you flat on your back, looking up at the sky asking 'what the fuck happened to me?' deserved a female's name."[2]

As antithetical as a bare-bones CrossFit box and a cosseted Exhale studio might appear, these brands and the many that emerged out of the same ethos represent two sides of the same coin: tight-knit communities built around the optimization of bodily health in an era of intense uncertainty. Studio fitness die-hards wore studiously distressed crop tops announcing membership in a "posse" or "tribe" that gathered in darkened rooms to chant, move, and manifest at the behest of a charismatic instructor, often perched on a stage. CrossFit acolytes sported muscle tanks bearing series of digits inscrutable to the uninitiated, but legible to those in the know as the number of sets in specific "workouts of the day" engineered to steel them against enemies from old age to Big Soda to a mugger. The aesthetics of these spaces are easily contrasted as female/male and affluent/working class, but in the early 2000s, these highly specialized fitness communities *all* represented more significant spending on exercise than ever before, and across demographic categories, especially gender, age, and—increasingly—class.

Especially at CrossFit, women fed up with the diet-industrial complex thrilled at the opportunity to exercise in an environment devoid of mirrors and devoted to pure performance. Not just cops and cadets, but retirees and single moms joined local boxes. Conversely, men might still be a curiosity in the more choreographed group-fitness classes, but their presence was growing fast and perceived as a "mostly untapped potential constituency" in yoga and even Pilates.[3] The popularity of CrossFit-style high-intensity interval training workouts launched a raft of studio-centered boot-camp variants that served to diminish the association between group exercise and effeminacy. The boom in biometric technology also informed this expansion, as features such as "leaderboards" that enabled real-time competition meant even group fitness could be marketed as an arena for individualistic competition and technological mastery, historically reliable strategies for selling men everything from couches to cookware.[4]

MAMILs—"middle-aged men in Lycra"—were becoming more common sights, and not only at the British cycling races that first inspired the acronym. "It's the biggest surprise of my career," a longtime technical-apparel designer at Nike told me. When he had begun working at the Beaverton campus in the late 1990s, "the baggier, the better" was the rule for men's activewear, but by the late aughts, men who weren't track athletes were beginning to jog in tights, and to layer looser shorts over spandex to attend fitness classes with the women in their lives, or even on their own. It was "luon," however, the four-way-stretch fabric devised by Canadian retailer Lululemon Athletica that made activewear, increasingly named "athleisure" for its utility beyond the gym, a hallmark of early twenty-first-century American fashion. Established in 1998 in Vancouver by Chip Wilson, a former swimmer and snowboard-apparel designer who swore by Ayn Rand and the tough-love self-help juggernaut Landmark Forum, Lululemon did more than any other entity to recast a "yoga lifestyle" as a luxury pursuit as likely to be found at a high-end shopping center as an incense-tinged New Age bookstore. Charcoal-black pants with brightly colored waistbands, curved seams, and a no-shine weave that made "everyone's butt look good" pushed one hundred dollars per pair and became the brand's calling card.

Elastic-knit imports shot up in these years, and by 2016, such "stretchy pants"—no longer considered only appropriate for yoga—outsold blue jeans.[5] Unlike sweatpants, famously disdained by fashion designer Karl Lagerfeld as the uniform of a woman who has given up on life, yoga pants communicated control, flexibility, discipline, and sexiness. A woman swathed in spandex telegraphed that she was always ready to exercise, and that she already had achieved a body she was proud to display. A woman with money to spend on expensive yoga pants, but liberated from the corporate get-up of a power suit and heels—or the blue-collar one of a postal worker or restaurant server—communicated that she had achieved *balance*. She—Lululemon specifically named this imaginary ideal woman "Ocean"—was a poster girl of the then-vaunted gig economy: curled up with her laptop, sipping a matcha latte, lines between work and play blissfully blurred in a moment when merchandise bearing slogans such as "If you do what you love, you'll never work a day in your life" and "Health is wealth" were unironically hawked on new platforms such as Etsy, which invited "makers" to turn every hobby into hustle.

Self-fashioning had always been intrinsic to American exercise culture, but in the early 2000s, it took on newly explicit form. Instructors and trainers often recounted having "fallen into" to their profession, and even the most successful were often still asked when they were "going to get a real job." But as the figure of the fitness professional came to be perceived as guru, sex symbol, fashion icon, and therapist, the career path became a more deliberate, and respected, choice. Exultant stories of individuals leaving behind careers of "the long hours, mega-stressed variety" to pursue their calling in careers in health and fitness proliferated. So many office workers were having "firsthand, lifechanging experiences" that inspired them to leave their desks to become yoga instructors, the *Los Angeles Times* reported in 2003, that they were causing a glut in some markets. The tone was one of renunciation and religious conversion: movie executives giving up a big house and a milieu where "everyone wants to have sex with bimbos and drive Ferraris" for a small apartment and a life "making a contribution to the world" through teaching yoga. Even one formerly "big, fat lawyer" who became a yoga teacher and then returned to law when his son's college bills loomed, shared that his experience teaching yoga burnished his reputation; clients would say, "You're not just some bloodsucking leech."[6]

24

Eat, Pray, Buy

Eat, Pray, Love, Elizabeth Gilbert's breathless memoir of abandoning her conventional existence for an international adventure in introspection—or what one critic called "neoliberal self-regulation"—became a bestseller in 2006, and its commercial success made such reinvention narratives more common, and increasingly understood as potentially lucrative.[1] Leaving behind a corporate job to pursue "wellness" no longer meant sacrificing wealth, but could mean capitalizing on the profits to be found in a frothy green juice, the hug of high-end athleisure, a candlelit spin class, a weekend yoga retreat. These new "creators" were often women who had often enjoyed these pursuits as consumers and realized a market opportunity for products and experiences that promised health, beauty, and happiness through the more culturally acceptable language of "wellness" rather than weight loss. As such ventures proved profitable, male founders and investors became more common, but women such as the Hollywood agent who co-founded SoulCycle and the Brown University economics major who conceived of 305 Fitness, a dance workout that approximated a Miami dance club, were crucial in putting this market on the map.

Still, the savvy professionals who seized these entrepreneurial opportunities remained a relatively niche group. Most who gravitated to this field did so more modestly by becoming an instructor or trainer, a path that ironically attracted a group with ever more professional options, but that was enabled by the scant credentials required. By 2022, it has become unremarkable for instructors to offhandedly refer to day jobs or even "former lives" as lawyers, traders, or—in the case of one Peloton instructor—a Buddhist monk.[2] Enrollment in physical-education programs has only continued to fall, and while exercise science was the fastest-growing major in the United States in 2018, such degrees are not a prerequisite for success as a fitness instructor or entrepreneur.[3] Despite the maturity of the fitness industry—gyms and health clubs alone were valued at thirty billion dollars in 2002, which swelled to forty before the pandemic hit in 2020—many brands would hire instructors with an ACE (American Council on Exercise) or AFAA (Athletics and Fitness Association of America) certification earned through a single exam, or even only a commitment to complete proprietary training.[4]

SoulCycle actually preferred untrained "talent," who were easily moldable into personas that appealed to the carefully defined audience segments who flocked to their studios: a pink-haired vegan mom with a six-pack, a muscled Chippendales type, and a tattooed club kid each embodied a particular appeal. Instagram launched in 2010, and as the photo-sharing app became a fixture of the fitness world, a large social-media following, as much as charisma and a sculpted physique, could stand in for expertise. Online "influencers" amassed millions of followers by sharing carefully curated images and exercise advice often based primarily on their own "journey" and in the idiom that suited their "personal brand." A significant following could lead to online opportunities to sell exercise-adjacent products from flat-belly tea to corset trainers to personally branded resistance bands and mats, or—in the brick-and-mortar world—could make the difference in getting a job offer or plum class assignments.

Notably, there was no golden age when expertise was as important as charisma Lavinia Errico remembered that in the early days, the main criterion for an instructor was "Can they pack a room?" It was actually "a B instructor" who tended to come in and say, "I'm ACE certified and in this and that and I have done all these workshops . . . and then you have them do their thing, and they're really good technicians but might not have that magic."[5] Increasingly, the endgame for fitness professionals is to stay—and grow—online, where an apparently endless supply of students and the entirely unregulated ether allow a scale of influence unimaginable in any IRL format.

Celebrity has accordingly permeated the fitness world, and vice versa. Notably, when yoga instructor Hilaria Baldwin—whose renown comes in part from her marriage to actor Alec Baldwin—came under fire in 2020 for lying about her Spanish citizenship, she insisted she simply hadn't bothered to fact-check stories that perpetuated these parts of her biography. Couldn't the world just leave her alone, she pled in the *New York Times*, "to talk about health and fitness and being a mom" to her hundreds of thousand Instagram followers—an entreaty revealing that a commitment to evidence, let alone expertise, is far from considered a prerequisite of authority in the fit nation.[6]

Social media didn't just create fitness celebrities, it transformed ideas about how stars should share themselves, ratcheting up expectations introduced by reality television that fans deserved access to their "real," if not "private," lives. Fitness was the ideal realm to afford such not-quite-unfiltered access. Long before most Americans felt pressure to hit the gym, those whose livelihood depended on their appearance had exercised regularly, even religiously. But especially for stars with painstakingly managed public profiles, exercise had been a behind-the-scenes, even embarrassing, endeavor. Social media, however, encouraged offering a glimpse into even unglamorous aspects of one's life, in service of seeming approachable. Sharing experiences of exercise projected an appealing mix of apparent intimacy and socially approved behavior. Seeing Gwyneth Paltrow stride out of a dance workout with trainer Tracy Anderson gave fans the impression that she had to put in the work to achieve her willowy figure, while witnessing Lena Dunham share a post-workout photo in a sports bra assured the public that, for all her unapologetic public nudity, she was not above working on herself, or perhaps being affected by cruel comments about her appearance. (Of course, looking *too* unfiltered—whether too fat, thin, unhappy, self-satisfied, or angry—could backfire, especially for women.)

Celebrity trainers benefited from this "stars . . . they're just like us!" ethos, but the boutique fitness segment, which became the fastest-growing category in the industry during the 2010s, especially profited from this opportunity to link fitness with a luxurious lifestyle. It is hard to imagine that high-end fitness would have become such a class marker without this medium. The aesthetics of boutique fitness, be it SoulCycle's citrus-yellow hues or the sexy red lights at Barry's Bootcamp, seem deliberately designed to increase online brand recognition, especially that shared organically by participants proud to perform their commitment publicly. Such deliberate hypervisibility extended beyond the high end; one budget gym chain installed a diptych selfie wall, one panel of which was a mirror in which to pose for pictures, the other a screen on which these images—and any others with the club's dedicated hashtag— were immediately projected to motivate others in the gym and online.

But for all of this virtual activity, it was just as meaningful for fitness culture that the real-world economy crashed in 2008. Millions of Americans lost their jobs and homes, widening the gap between rich and poor that had been intensifying since the early 1980s. The fact that working-class and poor families faced foreclosure while financial institutions that had caused the crisis were bailed out by the federal government made the most explicit forms of material consumption seem distasteful, and even immoral. The ostentatious lifestyle that shows such as *Sex and the City* had popularized—all expensive handbags and fancy cocktails—suddenly felt downright offensive, rather than a harmless frivolity. Exercise, however, and its growing assortment of luxury accoutrements, stood in as a socially acceptable, even virtuous form of conspicuous consumption. Sociologist Rachel Sherman has chronicled how the affluent make peace with inequality by reassuring themselves of the virtuousness of their own big spending in realms like education, and even recasting lavish tropical vacations as rare indulgences in service of laudable self-care.[7] A sweaty selfie of a woman drinking a twelve-dollar green juice, wearing hundred-dollar leggings, and emerging from a workout class that cost nearly a dollar a minute projects precisely this sort of affluence: spending that is culturally sanctified because it is expended in the vigorous pursuit of health. These expenses added up, but were small enough to be ephemerally accessible: even if you could never afford an Hermès Birkin bag or a Lamborghini, a premium sports bra or a five-pack of indoor-cycling classes are relatively attainable. And it cost nothing to stage the perfect selfie.

This peculiar and at times perverse logic meant that the financial crash that left millions indigent abetted a boom in the most elite realm of the exercise industry. Less intuitively, the far more socioeconomically diverse realm of group fitness, which fueled the growth in boutique studios but also anchored the programming in many gyms and community centers, also thrived. No one was more surprised than Beto Perez, Alberto Perlman, and Alberto Aghion, the cofounders of Zumba Fitness, the Latin-dance-inspired exercise program they had launched in Miami in 2001. In Bogotá in the 1980s, Perez, a nightclub dancer, had never taught aerobics, but bought a used copy of Jane Fonda's *Workout* book to get up to speed when he was asked to sub an exercise class as a last-minute favor. He was good at it, but one day he forgot his cassettes and popped in salsa and merengue music instead. The class was a hit. Soon, with Perlman, an unemployed tech professional whose mother had been attending Perez's class, Perez launched "Zumba," since "rumba" was already trademarked. Latina women, who had never been targeted as significant fitness consumers, loved it. And white people, it turned out, enjoyed working up a sweat to merengue as well. Ominous news reports about the "Hispanic takeover" of the country were commonplace, but what Steve Stoute calls the "tanning of America"—the broad appeal of nonthreatening versions of minority cultural products—proved more powerful than xenophobia, at least at the gym.[8]

After middling experiments with infomercials and DVD giveaways in Special K cereal boxes, Perlman, Perez, and Aghiar realized that elaborating their existing instructor trainings would be key to the brand's expansion. It was 2006, early days for social media—Facebook had only just expanded beyond educational institutions—so they established a rudimentary online network on which, for forty dollars a month, instructors could share choreography, music, promotional images, and most importantly, their love of Zumba. The idea took, providing a necessary income infusion for their struggling company: in six years, instructors numbered close to one hundred thousand, across more than one hundred countries. Perlman saw the expanded training and network as the perfect way to broaden the Zumba experience beyond exercise: "The new business model helped consumers because they are getting their fitness and therapy in one class. For the instructors, it gives them income and purpose, and they work out while they do what they love. The gyms get new members." But when the financial crisis hit, just as the company had moved into larger offices, the trio was sure their luck had run out. Especially given that Zumba's more working-class clientele and instructor base were most likely to be adversely affected by the economic downturn, it felt as if fitness were a frill people would be quick to cut as they inevitably tightened budgets.

But the business thrived. "Every time we posted an instructor training, it sold out, and people said their classes were packed," Perlman remembered.[9] An instructor certification, it turned out, provided extra income, and an affordable, sweaty dance party—especially the kind that featured simple choreography and that took place at the gym rather than a nightclub—was precisely the sort of small pleasure that felt justifiable, even in a recession. Investing in these fitness spaces could create meaningful community. In the predominantly Latino El Monte neighborhood of Los Angeles, for example, ethnographer Caribbean Fragoza describes Zumba classes held in "pretty much any public or semi-public space," where "booty-shaking ladies" challenged the punitive, competitive nature of programs such as CrossFit as well as the often dangerous machismo of street life. Zumba specifically enables a "barrio feminism," Fragoza argues, but this regenerative, totalizing experience of exercise could be as integral to an expensive Upper East Side boutique studio spinning class as to the "safe spaces" of El Monte Zumba classes, and to many such spaces in between: a transgressive bootcamp where formerly incarcerated men train mostly white, female participants in a "prison workout," or a disco dance-cardio class during which a flamboyant, nonbinary instructor intersperses cues with comments about sexual liberation.[10]

Notably, more Americans than ever sought out these distinct social experiences forged through fitness, inside and outside the studio. When disabled people complained in 2006 that fitness clubs didn't even try to comply with federal Americans with Disabilities Act, a representative of the leading professional association explained that gyms were only just beginning to examine their long-standing, but increasingly outdated, assumption that "people in wheelchairs or with visual impairments didn't want to work out."[11] A year later, the Fitbit launched, making fitness at once more accessible, intimate, and impersonal, as "the gym" could be understood to denote not only a multiplying number of places to go but also a way of life, originating with a wristband that connected you in competition with family, friends, and colleagues who might be far-flung, but who were more likely than ever to be exercising.

25

The Limits of "Let's Move"

Such enthusiasm meant that the early years of the twenty-first century also represented a glimmer of hope for public investment in an inclusive, noncommercial exercise culture. In 2000, while discussing childhood obesity with Larry King, Jack LaLanne had described his personal philosophy in an idiom that revealed an enduring, uninterrogated whiteness of certain aspects of dominant fitness culture: "My body is my slave—that's why I treat it so good!" he proudly announced. Such a statement articulated the power of the imperative to exercise, but was unlikely to appeal to the Black and brown communities least likely to be beneficiaries of the expanding fitness industry. But the administration of Barack Obama, the first Black president, promised a different approach. His predecessor George W. Bush was such a devoted runner that he installed a treadmill on Air Force One, required staffers to exercise, and uncontroversially commented in *Runner's World* that "statistic after statistic is beginning to sink into the consciousness of the American people that exercise is one of the keys to a healthy lifestyle."[1] It was the Obama White House, however, that made the most expansive version of a federal commitment to health and fitness a centerpiece of its administration.

The Obamas arrived in office recognized for their personal commitment to fitness—*Men's Health* called Barack "the fittest president ever," a stealth video of him working out in a Warsaw gym went viral, and Michelle's muscled arms immediately attracted notice. (The Left tended to celebrate her visible strength, while some on the Right criticized her supposed impropriety in explicitly racist terms.) More substantively, democratizing access to "healthy lifestyles" and "well-being"—a deliberate word choice—became a major focus of First Lady Michelle Obama's agenda. Echoing JFK's calls to elevate fitness to civic duty—but crucially, to make it *fun*—the Let's Move campaign she launched in 2010 featured events such as Beyoncé surprising children in a Harlem school gym with an impromptu workout. Unlike Kennedy-era programs, Let's Move decentered athletics, militarism, and bodily measurement, and instead emphasized "active, healthy, lifestyles." Most distinctly, it focused on Black and brown communities—where childhood obesity rates hovered around 40 percent—rather than the affluent, white suburbanites who had been the target of JFK's efforts. Weight gain was no longer primarily associated with the affluent, but the working poor, whose constrained access to exercise—and equally importantly, to nutritious food—was defined as more likely to yield bodies perceived as unhealthily over, rather than under, weight.

As uncontroversial as the promotion of exercise had become, the First Lady drew intense criticism for Let's Move. On the Left, critiques centered on the individualization of a structural public-health issue, and on the initiative's relationships with the food and beverage industry. Obama's willingness to work with the very industry that had helped create the public-health crisis, critics charged, allowed these companies to evade their own responsibility, and the administration to overemphasize exercise—rather than limiting consumption of the products these companies marketed to children—in solving it.[2] More pointedly, a growing chorus of social scientists denied the "obesity epidemic" altogether, defining it as a moral panic enabled by an intensely fat-hating society that especially pathologized Black and brown bodies, rather than a veritable public health crisis. To them, Let's Move gave such stigma the imprimatur of the White House, codifying concern-trolling at the highest reaches of government, while further marginalizing the very groups it purported to help.[3]

The loudest critique came from conservatives and took predictable form: the Obamas were inappropriately deploying the "nanny state" to mandate jumping jacks and snatch birthday cupcakes from children's mouths. Donald J. Trump, who successfully won the presidency in 2016 on his exploitation of anti-Obama animus, skillfully went further to transform the relatively uncontroversial promotion of exercise into a culture-wars issue, framing fitness as an affectation of out-of-touch coastal elites. Painting himself as a luxuriant fat cat who ordered double servings of ice cream and skipped the workouts that were an expected activity of his social peers, Trump announced that followed no diet or exercise regime on the campaign trail, and that "all his friends who work out all the time . . . they're a disaster." In fact, he warned one of his casino executives training for an Ironman triathlon, "You're going to die because of this."[4] As millions of Americans felt increasing pressure to exercise for physical and mental wellness, Trump proudly subscribed to a discredited nineteenth-century theory that argued the opposite: humans are born with a finite amount of energy, which is dangerously depleted by vigorous exercise.

Women, however, got no reprieve, for Trump believed they should labor at the gym for weight loss and beauty. As owner of the Miss Universe pageant, he had humiliated a winner whom he deemed overweight, and he regularly disparaged women who displeased him as fat or ugly. The masculine realm of sports, however, Trump celebrated. In 2018, he changed the name of the presidential body associated with these matters to the Presidential Council on Sports, Fitness, and Nutrition. A seemingly minor change—swapping "fitness" and "sports"—on a council with only advisory power, it nevertheless signified a deliberate elevation of competitive, masculine athletics over recreational, inclusive fitness. His most prominent appointment was Bill Belichick, the coach of the New England Patriots football team (and outspoken Trump supporter). These were pointed digs at Michelle Obama, who in 2010 had taken pains to explain that "not every kid is an athlete," and that the aim of the council and the administration was to support the many ways all Americans could become active and fit. (The Trump base fanned this backlash with a viral meme: a photograph of the progressive January 2017 Women's March overlaid with the words, "In one day, Donald Trump got more fat women out walking than Michelle Obama did in 8 years.")[5] As historian Rachel Louise Moran wrote, Trump's name change of the council did little to shift policy, but signaled loud and clear to conservatives anxious about "participation trophies" and the creeping interventionist effeminacy of the "nanny state" that "it is not Michelle Obama's council, and it imagines fitness as a competitive endeavor."[6]

Let's Move unquestionably defined health and fitness as a social-justice issue, and it reinvigorated the idea that the state had a responsibility to protect what the Obama White House defined as a right, rather than a lifestyle pastime of affluent white people. Trump managed to inflame reactionary opposition to this project, but his crude comments about women's appearance, boasts of sexual assault, and the broader "GOP War on Women" just as intensely inspired many fitness personas and publications to become newly outspoken about the importance of practicing self-care and cultivating bodily strength as a progressive political project. Registrations in women's self-defense classes surged after the 2016 election. I conducted an "Exercise Your Power" workshop after Trump's inauguration, in which we yelled positive affirmations as we punched and kicked during an hourlong intenSati workout class, and then gathered, sweaty and invigorated, for an hourlong conversation on politics and collective action. Many fitness businesses once nervous about alienating consumers by "getting political" increasingly eschewed vague invitations to escapism and instead articulated exercise—and "wellness" and "self-care" more broadly—as forms of political empowerment. Prominent yoga instructor Hala Khouri advised that the conventional advice heard in yoga classes to "stay away from negative thoughts and feelings" actually served to "discount the reality and marginalize even further" those who lacked the privilege of such escapism.[7]

The proof that even a defiantly unfit president was no match for a deeply ingrained national fitness culture is that right-wing animus *also* found expression at the gym. Forgoing fitness—or engaging in long Reddit threads degrading women in yoga pants as symbols of the tragic erosion of traditional gender roles—might be a show of political fealty to Trump, but so could working out. The alt-right *Radix Journal* advised founding a co-op gym to cultivate a masculine "honor culture." Like a "pre-commercial health club" or "CrossFit box," such gyms prize exclusivity over profit to train like-minded "gangs of men" in body and mind—invoking the animating ideal of the fit nation—for a coming revolution.[8] Common to such subcultures—and far from exclusive to those condoned by a neofascist journal—is an attempt to masculinize wellness culture rather than to wholly reject it. Back in 2014, in an exploration of "how the other half lifts," a newcomer to weight lifting discovers his glee at his newly bulging muscles, the community of men he found at the gym, and his sense of superiority over male marathoners who possessed bodies more commonly associated with his white-collar professional class: "They looked gaunt and weak. I could have squashed them."[9] In the twenty-first-century fitness "bro culture" disseminated in weight rooms, in jujitsu studios, and through supplement-sponsored YouTube channels, fellow historian and gym rat Patrick Wyman writes, men celebrate pain, might, and brawn as they figure out "what it means to be a guy."[10]

But as politics have grown more acrimonious, fitness culture can reflect this fractiousness. As characterized by Wyman, this masculinist fitness ethos can link reactionary politics with physical and national renewal to the tune of "Racism isn't real, bro; just fire up the barbecue, grab a kettlebell, put in the work, and watch the game. America is already great, we're making it great again, and fuck any weakling who says otherwise."[11] Expressly right-wing wellness cultures do not always promote conventional machismo or germinate through mixed martial arts or powerlifting; two rioters who stormed the US Capitol on January 6, 2021, to contest the election of Joe Biden were respected local yoga teachers, partially radicalized by online wellness communities. Beliefs about the supremacy of "natural" or "pure" health and individual wisdom, when adopted as ideology, can easily translate into deeply conservative and conspiracist beliefs, especially about identity, government, and expertise. Republican congresswoman Marjorie Taylor Greene posted a video of her pull-ups and clean-and-press and invoked her past as the owner of a CrossFit box as evidence that a rigorous individual fitness regimen, not Democratic-imposed lockdowns or vaccines, was key to crushing the coronavirus.[12] Exercise can still enable escape from the exhausting crush of politics, but—like so much else—it is increasingly of the world, not apart from it.

A real public commitment to wellness felt possible in the Obama years, though the promise proved fleeting. When I would visit New York City public schools in 2011 and 2012 to pitch Healthclass2.0, my experiential wellness program, I sometimes felt bad taking up the time of educators and administrators I knew were overworked. But their eyes would often light up as we talked about the power of exercise not only to affect our physical bodies but to inspire our whole approach to life, and more than one person shared that they personally couldn't live without their Zumba, yoga, or bootcamp classes, and were glad our program would engage their students in such experiences, which rarely existed within schoolhouse doors. Inaccessible as it was to many, the fitness industry—and the many adherents who glommed onto its mind-body-soul messaging—had successfully made "wellness" a household word, to the point that many came to understand it as not only a covetable consumer product, but a worthy policy priority. The Obama administration seized on this sea change and embarked on a public campaign to promote exercise as intrinsic to a full life, a move unprecedented since the Eisenhower/Kennedy years. For all this enthusiasm, privatization of the fit nation only intensified. The Obama administration failed to unmake fitness inequality or to meaningfully resolve the high incidence of childhood obesity that it had presented as its core challenge; obesity remained overrepresented at all ages among working-class people of color.

In 2020, on Michelle Obama's birthday, the Trump administration moved to roll back the school nutrition standards that were at the heart of Let's Move, a move many doubted was a coincidence.[13] Trump's gleeful rejection of a public (or personal) commitment to health and fitness was unprecedented, but his tacit abdication of this responsibility only continued a decades-long, bipartisan tradition of leaving Americans to figure out how to get fit on their own.

26

The Pandemic and the Peloton

As pandemic life established new norms for exercise and everything else, a cliché of the era became the remote worker who acquired "a puppy and a Peloton" to cope with the solitude and sedentariness of confinement. Peloton, the sleek, digitally connected stationary bike that first sold in 2014 for about $1,500, had ever since been a punchline to mock a certain sort of spoiled striver. A 2019 Peloton commercial featured a slim white woman who receives the bike (by then, closer to $2500) as a holiday gift from her husband and, with the wild-eyed look of a hostage, proceeds to make a video about her yearlong "journey" from timid, lonesome exerciser to fearless (virtual) road warrior who rides relentlessly, regardless of whatever family or work obstacle hurls itself in her path. The ad was easy fodder for an internet culture that thrilled in skewering examples of privileged oblivion: a husband so rude and rich that he throws away thousands on a torture device for his already slim wife! A woman who has so internalized patriarchy and productivity culture that she thinks she needs the bike, and is even grateful for this new responsibility! Peloton founder John Foley had never been apologetic about his company's air of elitism, and had pointedly always distinguished Peloton from a lowly fitness company as a loftier "tech startup." More recently, he had taken to calling it the "the Netflix of wellness," intimating the bingeworthiness of its catalog of highly produced programming featuring instructors whose outsized personas—cultivated on-screen, on social media, and in traditional media such as a Super Bowl commercial or a *People* magazine spread—made them unqualified celebrities.

But in 2020, Peloton became a lifeline—albeit an expensive one—to the lost world of sweaty, communal group fitness led by a charismatic instructor, and the gym in general. The machine remained outside the reach of most Americans, but in a moment marked by limited opportunities for both exercise and indulgence—and often overwhelming trauma and uncertainty—Peloton's waiting lists soon swelled to months. And it wasn't only the superrich lining up to pedal their way to wellness. Peloton user groups had long been full of people who financed their bikes or split their subscriptions among multiple family members—some whose rural location or jobs as nurses or firefighters required hours that made getting to the gym challenging—but the commentary on its popularity, and its own messaging, often seemed to deliberately ignore this variety.[1]

Not that this diversity necessarily challenged the diet discourse in many of these online communities; journalist Virginia Sole-Smith asked Peloton to connect her with a fat rider, who turned out to be most effusive about the weight she had lost.[2] After the infamous commercial Peloton insisted "was created to celebrate that wellness and fitness journey," Ruth Zukerman, co-founder of SoulCycle and its less froufrou offshoot, Flywheel, went on CNBC to discuss, and mostly dismiss, the controversy. Zukerman spent most of the segment insisting that the model's thinness was irrelevant, and only proved that a "spin journey" was not centrally about weight loss. Passingly, they also discussed the unapologetic affluence on display. "There will always be luxury brands and items," Zukerman said, arguing that no one mocked Tiffany for selling expensive jewelry, or Lexus for depicting a wife receiving a luxury car with a bow on top. In focusing on the body-image issue that was familiar terrain in the fitness world, Zukerman and the hosts failed to acknowledge that at least some of the anger about the luxury-fitness sector surely derived from a deeply held sense that access to exercise—unlike diamond baubles or fancy cars—*shouldn't* be restricted to the rich.[3]

As the pandemic raged on, such class resentment only sharpened, and it converged with fresh outrage over the police murder of an unarmed Black man named George Floyd. Such attention to inequality would not seem to bode well for Peloton. But a combination of skill and luck allowed Peloton not only to shed its primary image as a punchline about privilege, but also to establish itself as a leader among the growing chorus of entrepreneurs, activists, and influencers who had abandoned the idea that politics should be left at the gym door, braiding together progressivism and at-home exercise. First of all, home fitness leveled up from a convenience or luxury to a symbol of virtue, in that heading to a gym, or even for an outdoor jog, had almost overnight transformed from a sign of morality to one of selfishness. Pelotons were still expensive, but ownership suddenly presented more as a form of respect for public health than as an individual extravagance. Sales not only of bikes but of Peloton-branded apparel also shot up, as riders displayed their logo tees in pictures taken at home or wore the gear to signal belonging in this pack of bikers on trips to the supermarket or walks around the block. Such strutting starkly contrasted with gyms that began operating like speakeasies, sharing keys with select clients and, in a reversal from the days when social-media pictures burnished the image of the exerciser and brought in new business, forbidding them from posting online for fear of public shaming or municipal crackdowns.

Curiously, Peloton instructors almost never mentioned the pandemic even as it helped balloon its community to nearly three million riders, but the brand took a uniquely bold stand on Black Lives Matter. Peloton had always been "a force of good in the world," CEO John Foley wrote in June 2020, but conceded that he had just become aware of what "a privilege it was to have been satisfied with that belief." Unlike many brands that issued vague statements of solidarity, or—showing still less commitment—only posted a black square on social media, Peloton issued a statement of solidarity with Black civil-rights struggles and committed $100 million to raise wages across the company; do internal diversity, equity, and inclusion work; pledge half a million dollars to the NAACP; and democratize access to Peloton programs.[4]

The bad behavior of other fitness companies helped burnish the Peloton brand, at least among liberal-left consumers. In-person gyms didn't just operate surreptitiously but had become sites of anti-lockdown defiance, with MAGA-hat-wearing protestors doing burpees in the parking lots of shuttered gyms, while other gym owners openly flaunted closure and masking orders in shows of toughness they trumpeted online. Two weeks before Foley's statement, CrossFit CEO Greg Glassman had tweeted dismissively about "FLOYD-19," disparaging the seriousness of both the pandemic and systemic racism. The yoga world, long skeptical of conventional medicine, government regulation, and vaccination, became a hotbed of Covid denialism that morphed into a feminized "conspirituality" that came to be known as "pastel QAnon." In this fraught moment when in-person exercise was for many a guilty secret, and a significant swath of an industry founded on health promotion seemed to be undermining it, any frisson of guilt people might have felt about investing in fancy exercise equipment was supplanted by a sense of righteousness over stopping the spread of the virus, supporting a company with defensible politics, and, of course, engaging in the sanctified ritual of working out.

Beyond the bizarre political culture of pandemic-era America, Peloton is the most palpable example of the undeniably digital new direction of fitness. Similar products such as the Mirror, which with the flick of a switch replaces your reflection with streaming exercise classes (and is majority owned by Lululemon), and Tonal, a high-tech simulation of the most old-school workout of all, weight lifting, also boomed in the pandemic. What was once a wild west of individual influencers who mastered social-media algorithms and amassed huge followings before the glow of ring lights in their living rooms became more formalized and corporatized on these and other platforms, and at all price points. Myx Fitness, a lower-cost alternative to Peloton, was acquired by Beachbody, a multi-level marketing firm launched in 1999 that, via sales representatives called "coaches," distributes weight-loss and muscle-building supplements along with exercise programming. In June 2021, Beachbody went public, its CEO touting the brand as the "Disney Plus of fitness." As rituals from reading to religion to retail had increasingly come online in the past decade and a half, "the gym," broadly construed, had often been likened to church or the town square, a last holdout where IRL experience was worth the inconvenience. Big-box gyms were last resorts as "anchor tenants" that might bring foot traffic to dying malls where department stores once stood. In summer 2020, however, nearly 60 percent of former gymgoers held that they would never return to the gym, especially now that they had invested in new equipment and apps and acclimated themselves to new routines.[5]

But a convenient calorie burn—even if achieved alongside a more abundant pack of virtual exercisers than could ever fit in the gym, whose output and biodata are perfectly synced to yours, and at the behest of a gorgeous instructor who seems to effortlessly embody authenticity and attractiveness—is far from all that exercise can deliver. Indeed, as the pandemic entered its fifteenth month and vaccination rates climbed, sales of gym memberships rebounded to nearly their January 2020 levels. The experiences were not identical to those before the world shut down, but despite the inconvenience of innovations such as vaccine-verification QR codes and pre-booking limited-capacity time slots—and the ambient stress of participating in any public gathering—exercisers craving human contact began to rediscover joys of this third space that once again made leaving the house worth it.

Rick Stollmeyer, founder and then-CEO of MindBody, the biggest online booking system for wellness businesses like gyms, physical therapists, and salons, had watched his business "disappear overnight" in March 2020, but a year later, he was convinced the sector would come back stronger than ever, appealing to more than the affluent consumers who had been his base. The pandemic, he told me, had proven that preventative wellness is no luxury perk, but an essential, even lifesaving, expense. In 2017, a consumer-spending study had suggested as much, showing that people were scrimping on essentials such as gas, rather than luxurious extras such as vacations or high fashion, in order to spend on boutique fitness. But there was now an incontrovertible link between severe experiences of coronavirus and comorbidities that could be at least somewhat mitigated by individual "wellness" pursuits such as exercise—a shift that Stollmeyer surmised would especially resonate with the working-class communities hardest hit by the pandemic, and who were often *still* presumed to be uninterested in wellness. In 1997, when budget-chain-gym impresario Lucille Roberts claimed that only the wealthy were seeking well-being as opposed to "wanting to fit into tight jeans," she likely didn't envision her own clubs would later market memberships using these very buzzwords.

Post-pandemic fitness culture remains in flux. But Peloton's share price has plateaued, and online searches for at-home fitness equipment have tumbled with each passing month, suggesting the future will not be online-only.[6] Amanda Freeman, the founder of boutique fitness studio SLT, mused that those who discovered the convenience of at-home workouts might venture out only for longer experiences, which she is considering revising her schedule to offer. Several middle-market chains, including Gold's Gym and 24 Hour Fitness, went bankrupt before this modest recovery commenced, and Equinox is one of a few major players having a hard time luring members back in numbers. Emma Barry, a boutique-fitness consultant, explained a correlation between consumers' quest for community and their search for exercise explains the struggle of such large clubs; those clubs "never knew you anyway," she said, since they had little idea of how clients were using the facilities once they got past the front desk. Small studios—if they were able to hold on through the shutdowns—had stayed connected to clients through social media, and had long made a priority of fostering the community many now craved acutely.

27

Broken Equipment

Except for a few superstars who are paid accordingly, the instructors and trainers indispensable to the fitness boom have always been economically precarious, as their ability to claim bedrock labor protections such as health insurance and sick pay are compromised by the pressure to project an image of "living their best life." In 2013, more than half of trainers and instructors, whose job is health promotion, lacked health insurance. The overrepresentation of women in the most visible but vulnerable independent-contractor roles in the industry means that despite the proclamations of empowerment that are crucial to cultivating a following, they are often misunderstood to be working "just for fun" or for "extra cash." Such assumptions have long undermined women's economic power and obscure the fact that many spend hours traveling to work in neighborhoods where they cannot afford to live, preparing programming and playlists, seeking further certifications, and promoting themselves and their employers on social media. That a fetishization with individual self-fashioning is core to fitness culture—and that for years, exercise *had* been an accidental career for some—has also forestalled organization. But in the last several years, a robust conversation about economic inequality has begun to recognize fitness professionals as part of the precariat, rather than as only an accessory to the wealthy. Yoga teachers, journalist Michelle Goldberg observed after her own instructor showed up to teach on crutches, often bear the brunt of a "brutal economics" that recalls that of adjunct professors: a "grueling" schedule dashing around, travel and prep time unpaid, teaching multiple classes that could be canceled on short notice, and often holding several jobs to supplement what amounts to poverty wages.[1]

At the same time, the fitness industry has only been consolidating, as investors have realized the profitability—and new scalability—of the American obsession with exercise. After Glassman, who had founded CrossFit as a libertarian, anti-elite project, left the company, a Stanford Business School graduate backed with private equity took over, prompting questions about such a fundamental shift in organizational ethos.[2] Since 2017, XPO Fitness has invested substantially in eight boutique studios that offer programs from boxing to barre fitness, and has meaningfully maintained the identity of each brand, an indication that consumer sensibilities have shifted since the days when big-box, one-stop health clubs were in themselves enticing. Sprawling out from the gym even more broadly, Equinox has branched out to invest in not only boutique-fitness brands but also hotels. Lululemon acquired the digital home-fitness device Mirror, has entered the shoe business, and is outfitting Canadian athletes at the 2022 Olympics in Beijing. Women's athleisure retailer Athleta, acquired by Gap Brands in 2008, lured decorated athletes Allyson Felix and Simone Biles away from Nike, signaling not only the profitability of fitness but its rising esteem vis-à-vis sport.

The pandemic only made the position of America's nearly four hundred thousand instructors and trainers more precarious, and new attention to inequality might mean greater sensitivity to the severity of their situation. Making a pittance working for small community studios was one thing, but when yoga and fitness businesses squeezed their employees—while making airy proclamations about karma and unity and securing hefty private-equity investments—it was another. At CorePower, which became the largest yoga chain in the United States after Bikram Choudhury's sexual-abuse scandal pushed many of his affiliates to break ties, instructors filed multiple lawsuits alleging that they were paid less than minimum wage and pressured to sign up for costly trainings and to manipulate others into doing so, despite management knowing they were contributing to a glut of instructors that made employment impossible: In 2016, there were two yoga teachers in training for every one already certified. This oversupply, and new online aggregators that drove down class prices, meant that the gap between the language of abundance and fulfillment instructors professed in class and the anxiety created by their material conditions potentially grew even wider. Even more yawning was the disparity between instructors' material realities and that of CEOs such as CorePower's Travis Tice, who congratulated himself on having created the "Starbucks of yoga." In a lawsuit, Tice maintained that the concepts of "karma" and "authenticity" were mere marketing terms that no one should have taken seriously.[3]

A CorePower instructor who also taught at YogaWorks, by then also private-equity owned, attempted to unionize her colleagues at its four New York City locations. The novel plan to join the International Association of Machinists and Aerospace Workers (IAMAW) was enthusiastically approved by fellow teachers. Incredulous headlines highlighted the hypocrisy of an industry that continued to proclaim its universalism but had become embarrassingly elitist. "The Yoga Instructors vs. the Private Equity Firm," announced the *New York Times*; another outlet saw unionization as the best hope of "healing the wellness industry."[4] Organizing efforts in the fitness industry had been few and halting; one effort by Gold's Gym trainers in 2017 had been scrapped by the trainers themselves; two years later, accounts of unpaid wages and a "Hunger Games" environment among Equinox trainers who often cleared only two hundred dollars a week, though their hourly sessions netted the gym nearly as much, surfaced as part of a labor lawsuit. At an event series I co-organized to cultivate solidarity among women fitness professionals, one popular trainer wondered aloud "why [we] don't have that thing the stagehands have"—a union.

But the Yoga Works effort was inspiring, and instructors at Washington, DC–based Solidcore, another chain of fitness studios hit hard by the pandemic, came together to protest unsafe work conditions— and the unfair layoffs of those who complained about it. In December 2020, they succeeded in gaining recognition as employees rather than independent contractors, a change in status that usually comes with greater job security. It was a modest victory, as Solidcore had laid off 98 percent of its workforce at the start of the pandemic. (YogaWorks, too, shut down all its New York City locations, effectively dissolving the attempted union.) A few months later, Solidcore achieved a much bigger win: a private equity investment to underwrite the opening of thirty additional studios—for a total of one hundred.

Emily Stewart, a Seattle personal trainer and instructor, is aware that even as the pandemic subsides, the challenges that face her colleagues will not unless they take concerted action. She has launched Group Fitness Instructors United, a nascent organization of about six hundred people—who remain anonymous for fear of retaliation—also aligned with the IAMAW. Even with greater attention to inequality in all industries, the road ahead is rough: the lack of required certifications and credentials that makes fitness workers so exploitable also allows an ease of entry to a field that many don't feel is worth sacrificing for labor organization.[5] Plus, the idea that those who teach fitness are "real workers" is far from a consensus position. When one popular SoulCycle instructor shared a vaccine selfie and effused in the caption that she was so glad to be able to serve her elderly riders more safely, the online blowback to "a fucking fitness instructor" getting vaccine priority—as an "educator," it turned out—was so intense that the company issued a statement distancing themselves from her and she locked her account.

However modest such efforts, they chip away at the idea that fitness—even rebranded as wellness—is evidence of moral virtue, and that the only work of exercise worth recognizing is the sweat shed by affluent individuals who pay for the privilege, rather than the often hard labor of those who enable it. One bad-faith deployment of "wellness" at Amazon, and the outrage it inspired, suggests not only how far the ethos of fitness culture has burrowed its way into American life, but also that canny observers are beginning to assess it more critically. The online megacorporation—known for pushing its warehouse employees to work so hard they succumb to workplace accidents at four times the industry rate—released a prescriptive pamphlet encouraging these workers to conceive of themselves as "industrial athletes." The key to succeeding at Amazon, and in life, was taking charge of one's well-being, "like an athlete, training for an event." Sounding like an article that might appear in *Men's Health* or *Shape*, the pamphlet recommended purchasing specialized athletic shoes, hydrating regularly, and following a list of included sleep and exercise tips from personal trainers. The program echoed long-standing advice for white-collar workers to invest in exercise to offset "desk diseases" caused by sedentariness, and to imagine their cerebral work as a heart-pumping athletic contest. But a day's work for these low-paid "industrial athletes" included pushing their physical limits in a way that had little to do with a bootcamp or triathlon: walking up to thirteen miles a day, forgoing meals, and defecating in plastic bags to save time while pursuing quotas. A *Vice* article forced Amazon to acknowledge the ludicrousness of this particular invocation of wellness, one that sought to individualize employees' responsibility for health so obviously compromised by their employer—or at least to claim the pamphlet had been distributed in error.[6]

From any angle, fitness culture remains most accessible to those who can afford to participate in its mostly private forms; but it is nevertheless seeping into every aspect of American life, from "financial fitness" workshops at investment banks to the omnipresence of athleisure far from the gym. Luxury apartments advertise "Peloton nooks," and studio storefronts signal gentrification, but the budget gyms and inexpensive or free online programs at the less mediagenic end of the market are growing fast, and the industry is becoming, haltingly, more demographically diverse.[7] In a notable instance of industry introspection on the topic of identity, in 2020 IHRSA released a decade of statistics on the racial and socioeconomic makeup of gym members: about two-thirds were white, and 12 percent were Black. Over this period, Latino participation grew from 8 to 12 percent, while Asian American participation declined from about 9 to 7 percent. The median household income of a gym member was $81,000—just above the national median of $78,500. Perhaps most strikingly, the percentage of gymgoers who made under $25,000 annually had increased by 40 percent, almost the same jump evident in the group that made over $100,000, though the former still comprised less than 7 percent of health club members.[8] A different survey, measuring physical activity rather than gym membership, tempers any full-throated celebration of this expansion. In the same decade, Americans who earn less than $25,000 actually became *less* physically active, with 46 percent (up from 40 percent) reporting they do not exercise at all. In the next income bracket—those who made between $25,000 and $50,000 annually—the percentage of physically inactive adults also increased slightly to nearly one-third. Only in the highest income brackets—people commanding annual salaries of above $75,000 and $100,000—did Americans become *more* physically active in the 2010s, with only 19 percent and 16 percent of these groups, respectively, defining themselves as inactive.[9]

Gym membership and physical activity metrics don't tell the whole story of the reach of American fitness culture or provide a clear path forward. Equally important to ensuring access to fitness and its subcultures is critical attention to the nature of this ever-expanding project, and the terms on which it engages people and communities. Running, for example, is still mythologized as universally accessible to anyone with sneakers and a sense of discipline, but data have shown that in Baltimore, running correlates with the racial and socioeconomic composition of neighborhoods: in Black communities where there tended to be more crime, fewer runners ventured out. Especially in the wake of the murder of Black runner Ahmaud Arbery in 2020, Black runners spoke of carefully choosing their routes and the time of day for their runs, and of wearing "respectable" clothing as safeguards. White women have long expressed similar sentiments, but when Iowan Mollie Tibbetts was killed while out jogging, one conservative pundit commented that a young woman should not have been outdoors alone anyway, and that women like her should "get a treadmill and watch TV and jog."[10]

The "open" road can be anything but, and solutions lie in resolving thornier problems than the unwillingness of any individual to lace up their shoes. At SoulCycle, where the cost of entry is usually fingered as the biggest problem, the cult of personality around certain popular instructors enabled abusive behavior and its coverup. Instructors were pressured to look so thin they could appear to have a cocaine addiction or an eating disorder, and star teachers were emboldened to coerce young women into sex, to "jokingly" call a Black rider wearing a bandanna "Aunt Jemima," and to generally flex their power in more bizarre ways, such as by hurling an improperly assembled fruit salad across the studio.[11] Students of one yoga community after another have come forward with stories of sexual assault and coercion, some so brazen as to have taken place in rooms full of trainees, captured on camera. Limited accessibility to these sorts of fitness cultures is clearly not the only problem here.

Age is another useful arena in which to consider the mixed legacy of the increasing accessibility of fitness culture. "Boomers" in their seventies go to the gym in a way their parents' generation never did, and adults over fifty-five account for nearly a quarter of members.[12] This trend is unquestionably a sign of progress from the days when books that advanced the earthshaking idea that women over thirty or forty need not resign themselves to being frumpy and physically unfit. The gentle "Silver Sneakers" programs that appeared on health-club schedules in the late 1980s signaled this positive shift but did little to challenge the idea that fitness spaces were centrally for the young, and that the point of working out was to preserve the look of youth as long as possible. Older, more affluent members became a crucial revenue source for health clubs in the 1990s, but businesses such as Equinox—that built their brands around glamour—underscored the fantasy that fitness was primarily a youthful pursuit, in decisions from the slim models in their advertising to the loud pop music pumped through the sound systems. As much of the industry now markets fitness as an avenue to a diffuse "feeling good" for a diverse clientele, the graying of the gym-going demographic is front and center on even the glitziest fitness platforms. Molly Fox, whose career took her from Jane Fonda to owning her own studio to teaching yoga at the first fitness conventions working for Equinox on both coasts, now offers classes on Apple Fitness. Peloton proudly announced it had licensed the rights to the Beatles' music, a testament to the age of a significant segment of its riders, who include the septuagenarian Bidens, though the First Lady apparently favors SoulCycle.

The 2020 Super Bowl halftime performance suggests the promises and the problems of this shift. Jennifer Lopez, fifty, and Shakira, forty-two, headlined the show, singing and dancing in spangled body suits and shiny stockings. The eye-popping performance inspired a viral meme that differentiated "50 today"—represented by taut and toned Lopez—from fifty as recently as the 1980s, evoked by the obviously elderly stars of the *Golden Girls*. Some women cheered how brazenly Lopez and Shakira, both mothers, exploded the idea that middle age meant women could no longer be sexy and athletically formidable. Yet other women in this age group said the performance just made them feel tired and even betrayed: the cold comfort of aging, they had been led to believe, was the alleviation of the lifelong pressure to be sexy and fit. Is this what empowerment looked like? The pressure for older Americans to exercise is not just about maintaining physical appearance, but an almost moral commitment to making longevity a top priority. Retirees today, social critic Barbara Ehrenreich wrote, are often socialized into a new full-time ritual that is the opposite of rest: "You may have imagined a reclining chair or hammock awaiting you after decades of stress and personal exertion. But no, your future more likely holds a treadmill and a lat pull, if you can afford access to these devices.... You have a new job: going to the gym."[13] A related dynamic gives us the twenty-first-century trope of the "supercrip," an athletically accomplished disabled person whose achievement is meant to inspire, but inadvertently fetishizes those who "overcome" their disability and shames those who fail, or refuse, to strive for acceptance in a fitness culture that is becoming more inclusive but which remains individualistic, competitive, and exhausting.[14]

These disparities raise real questions about making such fitness cultures more "accessible" without challenging their disturbing dynamics. The problems can start at the top, with strident ideologues like Greg Glassman of CrossFit or Chip Wilson of Lululemon, whose crass comments make them almost cartoonish villains. But the archetype of the "girlboss" fitness innovator who peddles empowerment in its most individualistic, often white iteration is just as pervasive, and equally problematic. Many entrepreneurs and activists are hard at work, however, deliberately developing programs that reject tired, unattainable images of physical perfection and civilized bodily restraint, instead reimagining what the pursuit of fitness and those who engage in it might look and feel like. Online crusaders against diet culture can take credit for at least nominally banishing the once ubiquitous "bikini body" from mainstream fitness media and making it unacceptable for magazines and catalogs to feature only thin, white models. Unapologetically fat fitness activists such as runner Mirna Valerio, yogi Jessamyn Stanley, and "Fat Kid Dance Party" creator Bevin Branlandingham challenge, in their very physicality and broader work, the notion that fat and fit are incompatible. They speak frankly of the multiple forms that fat discrimination takes in fitness spaces, whether outright disdain, condescension, or acceptance conditional on perpetually performing the pursuit of thinness. Some such efforts are intersectional and institutional, extending beyond individuals to reconfigure fitness spaces: Everybody Gym, a Los Angeles "non-gender-conforming-queer gym," boasts a "fiercely non-competitive" environment, Spanish-language classes, and gender-neutral locker rooms.

IHRSA, the professional organization that expressed surprise in 2006 that disabled people would even *want* access to a gym, is hardly an activist hotbed, but made "all-inclusive" club design and programming for people with disabilities a focus of its 2018 conference.[15] Nike, which once almost exclusively featured slim, white, nondisabled people in its ads, now manufactures shoes for adaptive athletes and hijabs in sweat-wicking fabric, and its superstores feature larger mannequins and sizes. And SHAPE America, the preeminent professional organization of physical educators, is both dedicated to reimagining a profession that had long turned many students *off* physical fitness and to advocating for the importance of its continuing existence and expansion—at a time when 58 percent of fitness and exercise classes in Florida, for example, are taught by uncredentialed teachers.[16]

"You can't out-exercise a bad diet" is a common motivational saw in the fitness world, the kind of well-meaning inspiration to individual action that conveniently ignores all the structures that impede personal and collective fitness. Consider the sorts of catch-phrases that circulate in exercise environments: *If you want it, work for it. This is training for life. Just do it. No pain, no gain.* We are awash in such simplistic pronouncements of the importance of exercise and ubiquitous reminders of its centrality to existence as a fully actualized citizen, consumer, and human being, but we too often continue to consider the expansion of American fitness culture as an unmitigated good, and issues of health as appropriately solved by personal willpower and savvy product development. Borderline absurd examples of our cultural obsession with exercise, from leggings with sewn-in handgun holsters to a boutique studio with a full bar to the existence of groups like the "Pelostoners," who smoke marijuana before their cardio workouts, distract from questions of fitness and justice that have become only more urgent over time. With each public physical-education program cut due to austerity, every basketball hoop removed in the name of public safety, every unexamined juxtaposition of unlit street and shuttered community center with expensive commercial gyms and connected fitness devices, we squander an opportunity to redress a widening fitness gap that divides and defines a polity that largely *agrees* on the value of exercise. Nonprofits have introduced yoga in schools and churches and prisons, running clubs in poor neighborhoods and public parks, and bootcamps in Boys and Girls Clubs, all speaking to the surprisingly widely embraced idea, shared across a polity riven by all sorts of ideological and cultural divisions, that exercise is an intrinsic part of a good life. Yet you can't out-exercise a broken system, and deliberately working out the sorts of fitness cultures we want to build—and evaluating the gains and pains we have made along the way—rather than only uncritically advocating for more "access" to existing, imperfect models, and cultivating the collective will to fight for them—might just enable us to found a truly fit nation, together.

Acknowledgments

I owe an enormous debt to many people who have helped me make sense of the fitness cultures that are at the heart of this book, whether at the gym, on running trails, in the archives, around a seminar table, or, in the last stages of this project, on Zoom. As a scholar, explaining the significance of this research—and of fitness in my own life—has not always been easy. As much as American culture at large enshrines exercise as virtuous, academia is one of the last holdouts where the "life of the mind" is often seen as discrete from, and superior to, bodily pursuits. This meant that for years, I rarely shared with scholarly colleagues the fact that I taught fitness, or I minimized it as "something I started doing on the side" as opposed to a sustaining part of my life. Nonetheless, I have found an incredible community of scholars and writers that has supported this research over the past decade. Foremost, thank you to my editor, Timothy Mennel, and my literary agent, Stephanie Steiker, for seeing the promise in this project and for helping me craft it.

In 2015, historians Neil J. Young and Nicole Hemmer and I launched the *Past Present* podcast, and the weekly doses of brilliance, kindness, and good humor our conversations provided were invaluable in sustaining my confidence that I could finish this book and my energy to keep going. I always knew I wanted to write this book for a general audience, but it has been a privilege to publish portions of this research in three scholarly publications importantly highlighting fitness culture as a rich site for academic inquiry: Thank you to Brenda Frink at *Pacific Historical Review*; Elsa Devienne, Andrew

Diamond, and Guillaume Marche at *Transatlantica*; and Andrew Hartman and Ray Haberski, editors of *American Labyrinth: Intellectual History for Complicated Times.* Conceptualizing fitness as distinct from, but intertwined with, sport has been a central challenge of this work, and I thank historians of sport Andrew McGregor, Anne Blaschke, and Larry Glickman for helping me better understand and articulate these relationships. Several chapters reflect the shrewd feedback of a writing group of historians and journalists: Thank you to David Greenberg, Claire Potter, Jim Traub, Clay Risen, Niki Hemmer, Jim Ledbetter, Dahlia Lithwick, Matthew Connolly, Michael Massing, and Jim Goodman. I am similarly appreciative of the United States Women and Gender History writing group and the Boston University Political History Symposium, each of which offered valuable feedback on individual chapters. Funding from the Heilbroner Center for Capitalism and Faculty Research Fund at the New School were also crucial to the completion of this project. The generous but unsparing feedback of my peer reviewers has surely made this book better; I am grateful to both of them and to be able to thank Michelle Nickerson, whom I have long admired, by name. Several research assistants have provided indispensable support at each stage of research and writing: I can only hope that this experience was similarly useful to Jeremy Witten, Cagla Orpen, Deren Ertas, and Camille McGinnis as they embark upon their own research. Finally, the skills and sensibilities instilled in me by my mentors Estelle Freedman, Al Camarillo, and Jonathan Zimmerman still shape every aspect of my research, writing, and thinking.

The broad sweep of time and space this volume covers—plus the reality that I wrote it while parenting young children and during a pandemic that shuttered many archives—means that much of this book relies on digital collections, and I am grateful to the New School librarians for support in navigating these resources. Writing about topics few have considered worthy of scholarly attention has meant taking advantage of unconventional archives and relying on the efforts of those who also perceive this past as worthy of historical research. Thank you to Beth Comstock for enabling me to access to Nike's collection and to visit its impressive corporate campus. Fitness and yoga trailblazers Leslie Kaminoff, Molly Fox, Judi Sheppard

Missett, and Carol Scott all generously shared materials from their personal archives with me, and historian Jonathan Root allowed me to use the Oral Roberts University newspapers he digitized, which improved my discussion of its "Pounds Off" program immensely. I met Darcy Bingham on a Utah mountaintop where I was speaking about the limits of "strong is the new skinny" messaging, and thanks to her efforts was able to spend time in the archives of the National Intramural and Recreational Sports Association in Oregon, research which complemented the archives of physical-education advocacy organization SHAPE America, to which CEO Stephanie Morris kindly helped me gain access. Finally, Wayne Wilson at the LA84 Foundation helped me understand the centrality of the 1984 Los Angeles Olympics to broader athletic and fitness culture.

I never wrote so much as a blog post based on the research for my first book until after its publication, in part because I had believed the dubious conventional wisdom that "public-facing stuff" must wait and is mere promotional icing on the cake of a finished scholarly monograph. But public engagement has become one of my core intellectual and civic commitments, and this book evolved out of articles and podcasts and public conversations about the place of fitness in our past and present. I am especially grateful for the attention of several editors who have introduced me to new audiences, refined my writing, and been advocates for taking fitness—and its history—seriously. Claire Potter has been a mentor to me since we first met at the Schlesinger Library, but her invitation to write about the precariousness of "fitpro labor" in *Public Seminar* sharpened my economic analysis and, as importantly, resonated with instructors and trainers who left me voicemails and direct messages about how they grapple with being depicted as "living the dream" while barely being able to make financial ends meet. Melisse Gelula, co-founder of *Well + Good*, first suggested that I write a column about fitness history and pushed me to engage wellness-focused readers who were not automatically inclined to read history. Lindsay Crouse at the *New York Times* has been indefatigable in expanding the realm of sports commentary to encompass fitness and in trusting me to make bold arguments about its place in political culture. At the *Atlantic*,

Lenika Cruz accepted my cold pitch about the cultural significance of Jazzercise and helped me craft an essay on the centrality of fitness to late twentieth-century consumer culture and the insufficiency of dominant definitions of feminism to explain its appeal. In 2016, David Wescott at the *Chronicle of Higher Education* invited me to write about reconciling my pursuits of body and mind, a difficult but important assignment that shaped my approach to this research and has apparently influenced junior scholars. When journalist Danielle Friedman first interviewed me for *Harper's Bazaar* on the history of women's fitness, I was apprehensive that such an astute writer and I had overlapping interests. Today I am grateful to be able to engage with such an insightful mind on topics few know as deeply as we do—and to call her a dear friend.

I was exercising before I was analyzing it, and this book would not exist without the many fitness professionals and participants whose presence first planted the idea that these experiences would be an exciting—or possible—realm of study. I am grateful especially to Patricia Moreno for embodying the transformative potential of fitness, and in inviting me to turn from the front row of her class to become an instructor, a moment that taught me to challenge conventions that are as limiting in scholarship as in the studio. May she rest in peace and her memory be a blessing to all of us, especially her widow Kellen Mori and their daughters, Olivia, Sophie, and Stella.

My children Toby and Lucy don't remember a time when I *wasn't* working on this book, and my desire to have a new answer to their understandable "Are you done yet?" inquiries has fueled me to finish this book that I hope will make them proud. So too have I been motivated to persevere by the love and example set by my husband Michal, whose discipline and passion in sport and life is unmatched. My parents are the antithesis of gym rats, but they are both accomplished scholars who inspired me from an early age to ask tough questions and instilled in me the confidence to pursue their answers. Lastly, without caregiver Gratiana Peter, this book would not be possible. For all this support, any errors in this manuscript are my responsibility alone.

NMP

New York City, February 2022

Notes

Author's Note

1. Caley Horan, *Insurance Era: Risk, Governance, and the Privatization of Security in Postwar America* (Chicago: University of Chicago Press, 2021); Matthew Desmond, *Evicted: Poverty and Profit in the American City* (New York: Crown Books, 2016); Priya Fielding-Singh, *How the Other Half Eats: The Untold Story of Food and Inequality in America* (New York: Little, Brown, 2021).
2. "NY Gym Owners File Class-Action Suit Against Governor Cuomo," *Fox and Friends*, aired October 19, 2020, on Fox News, https://video.foxnews.com/v /6202454284001#sp=show-clips; Melissa Rodriguez, "Fitness Industry Still Feels Covid's Negative Impact," *IHRSA Today*, June 3, 2021, https://www.ihrsa .org/improve-your-club/fitness-industry-still-feels-covids-negative-impact/.

Introduction

1. For background on neoliberalism, see David Harvey, *A Brief History of Neoliberalism* (New York: Oxford University Press, 2007); for more on "responsibilization," see Alison Fleming and Jenny Wakefield, eds., *The SAGE Dictionary of Policing*, s.v. "responsibilization," accessed February 22, 2022, https:// sk.sagepub.com/reference/the-sage-dictionary-of-policing/n111.xml.
2. Jürgen Martschukat, *The Age of Fitness: How the Body Came to Symbolize Success and Achievement* (London: Polity, 2021).
3. "The Problem with 'Wellness' as a Virtue," letters, *Chronicle Review*, June 12, 2016, https://www.chronicle.com/article/the-problem-with-wellness-as-a-virtue/.

Part One

1. In Marguerite Martyn, "'The Lady Hercules' Tells Marguerite Martyn," *St. Louis Post-Dispatch*, June 4, 1911.

2. David Waller, *The Perfect Man: The Muscular Life and Times of Eugen Sandow, Victorian Strongman* (New York: Victorian Secrets, 2011): 93.

3. Whitfield B. East, *A Historical Review and Analysis of Military Training and Assessment* (Fort Leavenworth, KS: Combat Studies Institute Press, 2013): 39.

Chapter One

1. Daniel Kunitz, *LIFT: Fitness Culture, from Naked Greeks and Acrobats to Jazzercise and Ninja Warriors* (New York: Harper Wave, 2017): 28–29.

2. Harvey Green, *Fit for America: Health, Fitness, Sport, and American Society* (Baltimore, MD: Johns Hopkins University Press, 1986): 84.

3. Green, *Fit for America*, 85–87.

4. Ava Purkiss, *Fit Citizens: A History of Black Women's Exercise from Post-Reconstruction to Postwar America* (Chapel Hill: University of North Carolina Press, forthcoming).

5. Herbert Manchester, *Four Centuries of Sport in America, 1490–1890* (1931; repr., New York: Derrydale Press, 1991): 135.

6. R. Marie Griffith, *Born Again Bodies: Flesh and Spirit in American Christianity* (Berkeley: University of California Press, 2004): 58.

7. Karen Abbott, "Score One for Roosevelt," *Smithsonian*, September 20, 2011, https://www.smithsonianmag.com/history/score-one-for-roosevelt-83762245/.

8. Green, *Fit for America*, 91, 89.

9. Eugen Sandow, *Strength and How to Obtain It* (New York: Gale and Polden, 1897): 104. https://www.google.com/books/edition/Strength_and_how_to_Obtain_it /BTyeEqAIpuEC?hl=en&gbpv=1&printsec=frontcover.

10. Sandow, 9.

11. Sandow, 123.

12. Sandow, 125.

13. Jonathan Black, "Charles Atlas: Muscle Man," *Smithsonian Magazine*, August 2009.

14. Jan Todd, "Katie Sandwina and the Construction of Celebrity," *Bandwagon* 56, no. 2 (March 2012): 28–35.

15. Todd, "Katie Sandwina and the Construction of Celebrity," 9.

16. Marguerite Martyn, "'The Lady Hercules' Tells Marguerite Martyn," *St. Louis Post-Dispatch*, June 4, 1911.

17. Kate Carew, "Barnum and Bailey's 'Strong Woman' Tells Kate Carew—This Young Goddess of the Tan Bark, Who Tosses Her Husband About as She Would a Feather, Explains How She Came By Her Strength," *New York American*, April 16, 1911: 2-M.

18. Wendy L. Rouse, *Her Own Hero: The Origins of the Women's Self-Defense Movement* (New York: New York University Press, 2017): 24, 35.

19. Martyn, "'The Lady Hercules' Tells Marguerite Martyn."

20. Tessa Hulls, "The Great Sandwina, Circus Strongwoman and Restaurateur," *Atlas Obscura*, December 26, 2017, https://www.atlasobscura.com/articles /the-great-sandwina.

21. Martyn, "'The Lady Hercules' Tells Marguerite Martyn."

22. Martyn.

23. "Enlist Suffragists for a Circus Holiday: Baby Giraffe Named 'Miss Suffrage' at a 'Votes for Women' Rally," *New York Times*, April 1, 1912.

24. Untitled, *Beauty and Health* 6 (March 1903): 21.

25. Hulls, "The Great Sandwina, Circus Strongwoman and Restaurateur."

26. David L. Chapman and Patricia Vertinsky, *Venus with Biceps: A Pictorial History of Muscular Women* (Vancouver: Arsenal Pulp Press, 2011): 23.

27. Bernarr MacFadden, *The Power and Beauty of Superb Womanhood* (New York: Physical Culture, 1901): 21.

28. Micah Childress, "Life beyond the Big Top: African American and Female Circusfolk, 1860–1920," *Journal of the Gilded Age and Progressive Era* 15, no. 2 (April 2016): 176–96.

29. Todd, "Katie Sandwina and the Construction of Celebrity," 17.

30. Childress, "Life beyond the Big Top," 176.

31. Lawrence J. Epstein, *At the Edge of a Dream: The Story of Immigrants on New York's Lower East Side* (New York: Wiley, 2007): 248.

32. Sharon Gillerman, "Samson in Vienna: The Theatrics of Jewish Masculinity," *Jewish Social Studies*, New Series 9, no. 2 (Winter 2003): 65–98, https://www .jstor.org/stable/4467648.

33. Mel Gordon, "Step Right Up and Meet the World's Mightiest Human—a Jewish Strongman from Poland Who Some Say Inspired the Creation of Superman," *Reform Judaism Online* (Summer 2011).

Chapter Two

1. Christopher Forth, *Fat: A Cultural History of the Stuff of Life* (London: Reaktion Books, 2019): 14.

2. Amy Erdman Farrell, *Fat Shame: Stigma and the Fat Body in American Culture* (New York: New York University Press, 2011).

3. Farrell, 27.

4. "New England Fat Men's Outing," *Boston Globe*, October 9, 1904: 6, https:// www.newspapers.com/clip/96165527/the-boston-globe/.

5. "The Apotheosis of Corpulence," *New York Times*, June 27, 1870: 4.

6. Bernarr MacFadden, *The Power and Beauty of Superb Womanhood* (New York: Physical Culture, 1901): 5.

7. "Turns Back Girl Bathers: Is Troubled by Folk Who Say They Hate Clothes," *New York Times*, August 27, 1915.

8. "Beefsteak Eaters Beat Vegetarians," *New York Times*, November 15, 1907.

9. "Graphic Publisher is Hailed to Court," *New York Times*, February 5, 1927.

10. "Auxiliary Fat Men," *New York Times*, February 24, 1877.

11. Anne Hollander, "When Fat Was in Fashion," *New York Times*, October 23, 1977.

12. Lulu Hunt Peters, *Diet and Health—With Key to the Calories* (Chicago: Reilly and Lee, 1918): 65.

13. Michael Zakim, *Accounting for Capitalism: The World the Clerk Made* (Chicago: University of Chicago Press, 2018).

14. Nikil Saval, *Cubed: The Secret History of the Workplace* (New York: Doubleday, 2014): 9.

15. Saval, 14.

16. G. Stanley Hall, *Adolescence* (New York: D. Appleton and Company, 1904): 410–11, https://archive.org/details/adolescenceitsp01hallgoog/page/n422.

17. Karen Abbott, "Score One for Roosevelt," *Smithsonian*, September 20, 2011, https://www.smithsonianmag.com/history/score-one-for-roosevelt-83762245/.

18. NIRSA: Leaders in Collegiate Recreation, "Centennial of Collegiate Recreation: 1913-2013," organizational video based on holdings at NIRSA Archive, Corvallis, OR, posted on YouTube March 13, 2013, 11:04, https://www.youtube.com/watch?v=OmeefD0o-Bs.

19. Elmer D. Mitchell, *Intramural Athletics* (New York: A. S. Barnes and Company, 1934): 10.

20. Mitchell, 70.

21. Wendy L. Rouse, *Her Own Hero: The Origins of the Women's Self-Defense Movement* (New York: New York University Press, 2017): 31.

22. Margaret Coffey, "The Sportswoman—Then and Now," *Journal of Health, Physical Education, and Recreation* 36, no. 2 (February 1965): 38–41, at 38.

23. Coffey, 41.

24. Milton Cantor, "Education and the Nineteenth-Century Working Class," in *Work, Recreation, and Culture: Essays in American Labor History*, ed. Martin H. Blatt and Martha K. Norkunas (New York: Routledge, 1996): 125–62, at 144–45.

25. John Dewey, *Democracy and Education* (New York: Macmillan, 1916; Project Gutenberg, 2008), chap. 9, chap. 11, https://www.gutenberg.org/files/852/852-h/852-h.htm.

26. Martha Verbrugge, *Active Bodies: A History of Women's Physical Education in Twentieth-Century America* (New York: Oxford University Press, 2012).

27. Hall, *Adolescence*, 638, 581.

28. Hall, 428, 431, 523.

29. James Clarke, *Challenge and Change: A History of the Development of the National Intramural-Recreational Sports Association, 1950–1976* (West Point, NY: Leisure Press, 1978): chapter 1.

Chapter Three

1. Eleanor Nangle, "Through the Looking Glass: Silhouette Treatments at a Local Salon Offer Perfect Contours," *Chicago Daily Tribune*, June 7, 1936: D5.

2. Rachel Louise Moran, *Governing Bodies: American Politics and the Shaping of the Modern Physique* (Philadelphia: University of Pennsylvania Press, 2018): 46.

3. Philip E. Wagner, "Musculinity: A Critical Visual Investigation of Male Body Culture" (PhD diss., University of Kansas, 2015), https://kuscholarworks .ku.edu/handle/1808/19558.

4. Margaret Coffey, "The Sportswoman—Then and Now," *Journal of Health, Physical Education, and Recreation* 36, no. 2 (February 1965): 38–41, at 41.

5. Moran, *Governing Bodies*, 4.

6. Josep Armegnol, "Gendering the Great Depression: Rethinking the Male Body in 1930s American Culture and Literature," *Journal of Gender Studies* 23, no. 1 (2014): 59–68, at 65. Depending which lore you believe, the painting was transferred from the PWA to the Navy, where it was banished to either Henry Latrobe Roosevelt's home or the Secretary of the Navy's bathroom, until being transferred to the private, all-male Alibi Club a year later. Not until 1980 did the Navy retake possession and allow it to be publicly displayed a year later, for the first time in nearly half a century.

7. Armegnol, 65–66.

8. "Fireworks Group is Cited on Pricing," *New York Times*, January 28, 1938.

9. Alan Latham, "The History of a Habit: Jogging as a Palliative to Sedentariness in 1960s America," *Cultural Geographies* 22, no. 1 (January 2015): 103–26.

10. David K. Johnson, "Physique Pioneers: The Politics of 1960s Gay Consumer Culture," *Journal of Social History* 43, no. 4 (July 2010): 867–92; George F. Chauncey, *Gay New York: Gender, Urban Culture, and the Making of the Gay Male World, 1890–1940* (New York: Basic Books, 1994): 331.

11. Charles T. Trevor, *Muscular Manhood: Pictorial Studies of the Athletic Male* (Kenton: C. T. Trevor, 1943).

12. Chauncey, *Gay New York*, 116.

13. Erick Alvarez, *Muscle Boys: Gay Gym Culture* (New York: Routledge, 2010): 43.

14. Simon D. Kehoe, *Indian Clubs and How to Use Them* (New York: Peck and Snyder, 1866): 10.

15. Chauncey, *Gay New York*, 179; Kehoe, *Indian Clubs and How to Use Them*, 9.

16. Charles Atlas, "You Get Proof the First 7 Days—I Can Make This NEW MAN of You," advertisement, 1930, https://www.charlesatlas.com/classicads.html.

17. Catherine Beecher, *Miss Beecher's Housekeeper and Healthkeeper* (New York: Harper & Brothers, 1873): 243, 250.

18. Bernarr MacFadden, *The Power and Beauty of Superb Womanhood* (New York: Physical Culture, 1901): 80–81.

19. Ava Purkiss, "'Beauty Secrets: Fight Fat': Black Women's Aesthetics, Exercise, and Fat Stigma, 1900–1930s," *Journal of Women's History* 29, no. 2 (Summer 2017): 14–37, at 27.

20. Marie J. Clifford, "Helena Rubinstein's Beauty Salons, Fashion, and Modernist Display," *Winterthur Portfolio*, 38, no. 2/3 (Summer/Autumn 2003): 83–108.

21. Clifford, "Helena Rubinstein's Beauty Salons, Fashion, and Modernist Display."

22. "Those Reducing Salons: Do They Really Slim a Lady Down?," *Changing Times: The Kiplinger Magazine* 11, no. 3 (March 1957): 13–14, at 13, https://books .google.com/books?id=nwAEAAAAMBAJ&printsec=frontcover&rview=1&lr =#v=onepage&q&f=false.

23. Nangle, "Through the Looking Glass."

24. "Those Reducing Salons," 1413.

25. "Exercise for Beauty's Sake," *Vogue*, November 13, 1926.

26. "West Point Exercises," advertisement, *Chicago Daily Tribune*, August 25, 1939: 19.

27. "Women Reducing Waist," advertisement, *Philadelphia Inquirer*, February 5, 1956.

28. Helen McKenna, "What Dancing Did for Me," *Dance Magazine*, November 1942: 25–27.

29. Nangle, "Through the Looking Glass," D5.

30. "Battle of the Bulges," *British Pathé*, January 13, 1941, MP4 video, 51:00, https://www.britishpathe.com/video/battle-of-the-bulges.

31. Winzola McLendon, "Got a Weighty Problem? Then Take It Lying Down," *Washington Post and Times-Herald*, August 22, 1957.

Chapter Four

1. Marla Matzer Rose, *Muscle Beach: Where the Best Bodies in the World Started a Fitness Revolution* (New York: LA Weekly Books, 2001).

2. Steve Harvey, "Mussel or Muscle? Whatever You Call It, It's a Beach That's Not Forgotten by Many Devotees," *Los Angeles Times*, March 30, 1986.

3. Rose, *Muscle Beach*, 10–11.

4. *California's Gold*, episode 1007, "Muscle Beach," produced by Huell Howser and KCET Los Angeles, aired January 8, 1999, on California Public Television, https://blogs.chapman.edu/huell-howser-archives/1999/01/08 /muscle-beach-californias-gold-1007/.

5. Bob Myers, "Musclemen Undisturbed over Financial Careers," *Los Angeles Times*, May 17, 1948.

6. Jan Todd, "The Legacy of Pudgy Stockton," *Iron Game History* 2, no. 1 (January 1992): 5–7.

7. Josephine Murphey, "Muscle Minded," *Nashville Tennessean*, December 28, 1947: 51.

8. "Man, Drowned, Found After Swimming Party," *Los Angeles Times*, September 6, 1949: 2.

9. Jan and Terry Todd, "The Last Interview," *Iron Game History* 6, no. 4 (December 2000): 1–14, https://starkcenter.org/igh/igh-v6/igh-v6-n4 /igh0604a.pdf.

10. "And No Spinach . . . ," *Los Angeles Times*, August 9, 1942: F16; Marla Matzer, "The Venus of Muscle Beach," *Los Angeles Times*, February 22, 1998.

11. Elsa Devienne, "The Life, Death, and Rebirth of Muscle Beach: Reassessing the Muscular Physique in Postwar America, 1940s–1980s," *Southern California Quarterly* 100, no. 3 (Fall 2018): 324–67, at 336.

12. Devienne, 325.

13. Broderick Chow, "Idle Training: Scenes of Pleasure at Muscle Beach, 1934–1958" (talk presented at the Brunel Performance Research Seminar, Brunel University, London, UK, October 31, 2018), YouTube video, 42:17, https://youtu .be/-uEBvxx8iKI; "Muscle Beach Doomed," *Los Angeles Times*, December 17, 1958.

14. "Morals Case Brings Muscle Beach Closing," *Los Angeles Times*, December 16, 1958.

15. "The Bar Bells Toll Sadly," *Los Angeles Times*, December 21, 1958.

Part Two

1. Douglas Martin, "Bonnie Prudden, 97, Dies; Promoted Fitness for TV Generation," *New York Times*, December 18, 2011.

2. Dorothy Stull, "Go Happy, Go Healthy, with Bonnie," *Sports Illustrated*, July 16, 1956.

Chapter Five

1. Richard Nixon and Nikita Khrushchev, "The Kitchen Debate," transcript, US Embassy, Moscow, Soviet Union, July 24, 1959, https://www.cia.gov/reading room/docs/1959-07-24.pdf.

2. Hans Kraus and Ruth P. Hirschland, "Minimum Muscular Fitness Tests in School Children," *Research Quarterly* 25, no. 2 (May 1954): 178–88.

3. Robert H. Boyle, "The Report That Shocked the President," *Sports Illustrated*, August 15, 1955.

4. Boyle, "The Report That Shocked the President."

5. W. B. J. Drakeley, "Physical Fitness," *Marine Corps Gazette* 40, no. 9 (September 1956): 16–20.

6. Julie Sturgeon and Janet Meer, "The First Fifty Years: The Presidential Council on Physical Fitness Revisits its Roots and Charts Its Future," in *President's Council on Physical Fitness and Sports: The First 50 Years: 1956–2006*, ed. Janet Meer (Washington, DC: US Department of Health and Human Services, 2006): 40–63, at 43.

7. "Fact Sheets: President's Conference on the Fitness of American Youth" (Annapolis, MD: US Naval Academy, June 18–19, 1956), American Council on Education papers, box 278, folder 7, Hoover Institution, Stanford University, Stanford, CA.

8. Arthur S. Adams to Katherine McBride, June 29, 1956, American Council on Education papers, box 278, folder 7, Hoover Institution, Stanford University, Stanford, CA.

9. "Fact Sheets: President's Conference on the Fitness of American Youth."

10. "Fact Sheets: President's Conference on the Fitness of American Youth."

11. "Fact Sheets: President's Conference on the Fitness of American Youth"; "Recreation: A New Profession for Our Time," illustrated leaflet, American Association for Health, Physical Education, and Recreation, Washington, DC, 1955.

12. "The President's Conference on the Fitness of American Youth," *Journal of Health, Physical Education, and Recreation* 27, no. 6 (1956): 8–31.

13. Sturgeon and Meer, "The First Fifty Years," 43.

14. Exec. Order No. 10673, 21 FR 5341 (July 18, 1956).

15. Sturgeon and Meer, "The First Fifty Years," 44.

16. Clay Barrow, "Physically Fit," *Leatherneck* 42, no. 11 (November 1959): 38–47.

17. D. D. Chaplain, letter to the editor, *Marine Corps Gazette* 44, no. 5 (May 1960): 4, 6.

18. Drakeley, "Physical Fitness," 19.

19. Drakeley, "Physical Fitness," 19.

20. Dorothy Stull, "Go Happy, Go Healthy, with Bonnie," *Sports Illustrated*, July 16, 1956.

21. David K. Johnson, *The Lavender Scare: The Cold War Persecution of Gays and Lesbians in the Federal Government* (Chicago: University of Chicago Press, 2004): 119.

22. Mrs. Lyndon B. Johnson, "Help Your Husband Guard His Heart," *Baltimore Sun*, February 12, 1956.

23. Boyle, "The Report That Shocked the President."

24. Exec. Order No. 10830, 24 FR 5985, 3 CFR (1959–63).

25. Diane Ravitch, *The Troubled Crusade: American Education, 1945–1980* (New York: Basic Books, 1983): 58.

26. *Control Your Emotions* (Glenview, IL: Coronet Films, 1950), 13:07, https://archive.org/details/ControlY1950.

27. President's Council on Youth Fitness, "A Community Project: Youth Fitness, What A Community Can Do for Fitness" (Washington, DC: President's Council on Youth Fitness, 1959): 18.

28. President's Council on Youth Fitness, "Focus on Fitness," pamphlet (Washington, DC: President's Council on Youth Fitness, 1960): 8.

29. Rear Admiral Thomas J. Hamilton, "Review of Group Summaries," published proceedings of the Sports for Fitness Forum, President's Council on Youth Fitness, April 13, 1960, Chicago, IL: 14.

Chapter Six

1. Richard Hofstadter, *Anti-intellectualism in American Life* (New York: Knopf, 1963): 365.

2. Shane MacCarthy, Executive Director, President's Council on Youth Fitness, keynote presentation, published proceedings of the Sports for Fitness Forum, President's Council on Youth Fitness, April 13, 1960, Chicago, IL: 33.

3. Shane MacCarthy, keynote presentation, 33.

4. President's Council on Youth Fitness, "Recreation: Workshop Report 1" (Washington, DC: President's Council on Youth Fitness November 23, 1959): 5.

5. President's Council on Youth Fitness, "Focus on Fitness," pamphlet (Washington, DC: President's Council on Youth Fitness, 1960): 10.

6. "Henry T. Heald: NYU's Ten-Year Program to Extend Its Educational and Physical Facilities," WNYC radio broadcast, New York, November 18, 1952, 13:25, NYC Municipal Archives WNYC Collection, WNYC archive ID no. 68617, https://www.wnyc.org/story/henry-t-heald-nyus-ten-year-program-to -extend-its-educational-and-physical-facilities/.

7. Leonard Engel, "Research Attacks the 'Coronary Plague,'" *New York Times*, November 25, 1956.

8. "Heart Disease and the Whole Man," *Pope Speaks*, September 3, 1956: 189.

9. "Heart Disease and the Whole Man," 186.

10. Paul Dudley White, "Rx for Health: Exercise: If Summer Prompts Us to Get Out and Use Our Legs, Dr. White Approves," *New York Times*, June 23, 1957.

11. "It's Time for Americans to Get Back on Our Feet," American Dairy Association announcement, *Broadcasting*, October 2, 1961: 96.

12. *Vogue* editors, "Your Heart's Blood," *Vogue*, January 1, 1959: 116.

13. White, "Rx for Health."

14. Shane MacCarthy, in President's Council on Youth Fitness, "Focus on Fitness," pamphlet (Washington, DC: President's Council on Youth Fitness, 1960): 2.

15. John F. Kennedy and Jacqueline Bouvier *Pose on the Tennis Court at the Joseph P. Kennedy Residence during the "Engagement Weekend,"* June 26–28, 1953, Hyannis Port, MA, photographer unknown, accession no. KFC3049P, John F. Kennedy Presidential Library and Museum, Boston, MA, https://www.jfklibrary .org/learn/about-jfk/media-gallery/sports-and-recreation; Cecil Stoughton, *President John F. Kennedy Swims with His Daughter, Caroline (Right), and Niece, Maria Shriver (Center), near Hyannis Port, Massachusetts,* July 28, 1963, White House photographs, color, 35mm, accession no. ST-C250-15-63, John F. Kennedy Presidential Library and Museum, Boston, MA, https://www.jfklibrary .org/learn/about-jfk/media-gallery/sports-and-recreation.

16. Douglas Jones, *Robert, John, and Edward Kennedy in the Surf at Palm Beach, Florida, April 1957,* April 1957, photograph for *LOOK* magazine, accession no. PX 65-105:165, John F. Kennedy Presidential Library and Museum, Boston, MA, https://www.jfklibrary.org/learn/about-jfk/media-gallery /sports-and-recreation.

17. Philip J. Kelly, *How to Grow Old Rebelliously* (New York: Fleet Pub. Corp, 1963): 28.

18. George A. Silver, "Fits over Fitness," *Nation*, June 9, 1962.

19. Missy McNatt, "Child's Letter to President John F. Kennedy about Physical Education," *Social Education* 73, no. 1 (January/February 2009): 10–14, https://www.socialstudies.org/system/files/publications/articles/se_730110.pdf.

20. James Reston, "Exercise Haters Win in a Walk," *Atlanta Constitution*, February 19, 1963: 4; also quoted in "Beauty Bulletin: Fifty-Mile Hike in Diet Thinking," *VOGUE*, April 1, 1963: 139.

21. "With Vigah," *New Castle News*, February 13, 1963.

22. Ann Burnside Love, "Pain is the Price in a 50-Mile Hike," *Baltimore Sun*, March 25, 1973: H1.

23. Merriman Smith, "Cracks in Mirror Image Irritate Kennedy Fans," *Nation's Business*, April 1963: 52.

24. Joshua Roberts, "Sports and the New Frontier," *Town and Country*, April 1963: 117.

25. "Find Own Fitness Way!," *Austin Statesman*, February 13, 1963: A25.

26. Eugene Rutkowski, letter to the editor, *Simpson's Leader-Times*, March 9, 1963: 6.

27. "Let's Get the Kinks out of the Kids," Presidential Council on Youth Fitness advertisement, *New York Times*, February 5, 1962.

28. Richard A. Meckel, *Classrooms and Clinics: Urban Schools and the Protection and Promotion of Child Health, 1870–1930* (New Brunswick, NJ: Rutgers University Press, 2013).

29. Cited in Missy McNatt, "Child's Letter to President John F. Kennedy about Physical Education," 12.

30. President's Council on Youth Fitness, "Focus on Fitness," 5.

31. Bonnie Prudden, "Fitness from the Cradle," *Sports Illustrated*, May 1, 1960.

32. "Keep Your Child Fit from Birth to Six," print advertisement, *New York Times*, June 21, 1964.

33. "Nobody Asked You!," Presidential Council on Youth Fitness advertisement, *New York Times*, January 8, 1962.

34. Marguerite and Bernarr Adolphus MacFadden, *Physical Culture for Babies* (New York: Physical Culture., 1904): 209.

35. McNatt, "Child's Letter to President John F. Kennedy about Physical Education."

36. "Spend Ten Minutes a Day and Be Fit as a Marine," Presidential Council on Fitness advertisement, *New York Times*, November 10, 1963.

37. "What's Your Child's Physical I.Q.?," Presidential Council on Fitness advertisement, *New York Times*, March 26, 1962.

38. "Jack Be Nimble, Jack Be Quick," Presidential Council on Fitness advertisement, *New York Times*, February 12, 1962.

39. Bonnie Prudden, *How to Keep Slender and Fit after Thirty*, (New York: Random House, 1961): 13, 17.

40. Prudden, 16.

41. George J. Hecht, "Do Our Children Need Toughening Up?," *Parents*, September 1956: 129.

Part Three

1. Norman Vincent Peale, *The Power of Positive Thinking: A Practical Guide to Mastering the Problems of Everyday Living* (New York: Touchstone, 1952): 55–57.

Chapter Seven

1. "Our Children Pioneers?," Presidential Council on Fitness advertisement, *Parents Magazine and Better Homemaking*, July 1965.
2. Stan Musial, "Dramatic Gains in Youth Fitness," *Parents Magazine and Better Homemaking*, August 1966: 41, 8.
3. Fran R. New, "We May Be Sitting Ourselves to Death," American Dairy Association advertisement, *Broadcasting*, February 5, 1962: 15–18.
4. "No Fitness in Schools," editorial, *Milwaukee Star*, June 5, 1968.
5. Michael Zakim, *Accounting for Capitalism: The World the Clerk Made* (Chicago: University of Chicago Press, 2018).
6. C. Ward Crampton, *The Daily Health Builder* (New York: Knickerbocker Press, 1928): 12, 16.
7. Eva Moskowitz, *In Therapy We Trust: America's Obsession with Self-Fulfillment* (Baltimore, MD: Johns Hopkins University Press, 2001): 122.
8. Avner Offer, *The Challenge of Affluence: Self-Control and Well-Being in the United States and Britain since 1950* (New York: Oxford University Press, 2006).
9. *Snap Out of It! (Emotional Balance)* (Glenview, IL: Coronet Films, 1951), 11:24, https://archive.org/details/SnapOuto1951; Diane Ravitch, *The Troubled Crusade: American Education, 1945–1980* (New York: Basic Books, 1983).
10. Diane Whitmore Schanzenbach, Ryan Nunn, and Lauren Bauer, *The Changing Landscape of American Life Expectancy*, Washington, DC: The Hamilton Project, Brookings Institution, June 2016, https://www.hamiltonproject.org/assets/files/changing_landscape_american_life_expectancy.pdf.
11. Eva Moskowitz, *In Therapy We Trust*; Elizabeth Lunbeck, *The Americanization of Narcissism* (Cambridge, MA: Harvard University Press, 2014); *Snap Out of It! (Emotional Balance)*.
12. New, "We May Be Sitting Ourselves to Death," 16.
13. Bill Hettler, co-founder of the National Wellness Institute, developed this definition in 1977. See "Six Dimensions of Wellness," National Wellness Institute website, accessed February 24, 2022, https://nationalwellness.org/resources/six-dimensions-of-wellness; "No Patients in Well Medicine," *Garden City Telegram*, July 3, 1976: 7.
14. Philip J. Kelly, *How to Grow Old Rebelliously* (New York: Fleet Pub. Corp, 1963).

15. Eleanor Chappell and Kathryn Huss, *Your Good Health: Physical and Emotional* (Garden City, NY: Nelson Doubleday, 1966): 4.

Chapter Eight

1. Michelle Goldberg, *The Goddess Pose: The Audacious Life of Indra Devi, the Woman Who Helped Bring Yoga to the West.* (New York: Penguin Random House, 2015); "Books in Review," *Tyler Courier-Times*, June 28, 1959: 33.
2. Indra Devi, *Forever Young, Forever Healthy* advertisement, *Chicago Tribune*, October 3, 1954: 190.
3. "Balzer's Yoga Teacher Tells of Buddhism Plan," *Los Angeles Times*, March 16, 1956: 16.
4. Frank Eleazar, "We Must Learn to Lie Down on Job, Indra Devi Says," *Bend Bulletin*, November 6, 1959: 8.
5. "Indra Devi Introduced Yoga to Russian People," *Times Record*, May 5, 1964: 11.
6. Ida Jean Kain, "Relaxing Exercises Help Relieve Nervous Tension," *Saint Louis Globe-Democrat*, June 16, 1955: 26.
7. "Indra Devi Introduced Yoga to Russian People," 11.
8. "Registration for Yoga Class is Still Open," *Corpus Christi Caller-Times*, May 18, 1966: 30.
9. "Group Offer Yoga Lecture," *Arizona Republic*, March 11, 1959: 24.
10. H. C. Neal, "Yoga at the YMCA," *Daily Oklahoman*, November 17, 1968: 16, 140.
11. "Heart to Heart" advice column, *Dayton Daily News*, July 3, 1968: 24.
12. "YMCA Features Trimnastics Class," *Milwaukee Star*, September 9, 1968.
13. Event announcement, *Honolulu Star-Bulletin*, June 7, 1961: 23.
14. Michael B. Coakley, "An Ancient Art," *Courier-Post*, October 22, 1966.
15. Dodi Schultz, *Slimming with Yoga* (New York: Bantam, 1968).
16. Alexander Bohlander and Verena Geweniger, *Pilates—A Teacher's Manual* (New York: Springer, 2014): 6.
17. Rosalind Gray Davis, "Romana Kryzanowska: Pilates Living Legend: An Interview with the World-Renowned Protegee of Joseph Pilates," *IDEA Fitness Journal* 4, no. 10 (November/December 2007).
18. "Malbin's Muscles," *Philadelphia Inquirer*, November 3, 1957: 208.
19. Roberta Peters, "Problems of a Coloratura Soprano," *Music Journal*, September 1959: 9.
20. Elisabeth Halfpapp, interview with author, October 2, 2015.
21. Natalia Mehlman Petrzela, "How Joseph Pilates Started Today's Mind-Body Boutique Craze Nearly 100 Years Ago," *Well + Good*, October 15, 2015, https://www.wellandgood.com/how-joseph-pilates-started-todays-mind-body-boutique-craze-nearly-100-years-ago/.
22. Gully Wells and Nancy Serano, "Pilates Body," *Vogue*, October 1, 1998: 274–82.

23. Davis, "Romana Kryzanowska: Pilates Living Legend.".

24. Wells and Serano, "Pilates Body."

25. Erma Bombeck, "All Manner of Phobias," *Kenosha News* (syndicated), August 19, 1982: 18.

26. Cal Pozo, interview with author, August 31, 2015.

27. "What's in a Name?," *Joe Weider's Shape* 17, no. 3 (November 1997): 104.

Chapter Nine

1. Marla Matzer Rose, *Muscle Beach: Where the Best Bodies in the World Started a Fitness Revolution* (New York: LA Weekly Books, 2001): 126.

2. Rose, 59–60.

3. Peter Bunzel, "The Health Kick's High Priest," *LIFE*, September 29, 1958: 74.

4. Bill Morem, "Fitness Guru Jack LaLanne, 96, Dies at Morro Bay Home," *San Luis Obispo (CA) Tribune*, January 23, 2011.

5. Shelly McKenzie, *Getting Physical: The Rise of Fitness Culture in America* (Lawrence: University Press of Kansas, 2013); Jonathan Black, *Making the American Body: The Remarkable Saga of the Men and Women Whose Feuds, Feats, and Passions Shaped Fitness History* (Lincoln: University of Nebraska Press, 2013).

6. Robert Alden, "Advertising: Hard Sell for Muscle Flexing," *New York Times*, June 5, 1960: F12.

7. New, "We May Be Sitting Ourselves to Death," 16.

8. George A. Silver, "Fits over Fitness," *Nation*, June 9, 1962: 516.

9. Bunzel, "The Health Kick's High Priest," 71.

10. Vic Tanny advertisement, *Baltimore Sun*, April 16, 1957.

11. Anne Laskey, *Jack LaLanne's European Health Spa, Wilshire Boulevard*, 1978, Marlene and Anne Laskey Wilshire Boulevard Collection, Los Angeles Photographers Collection, Digital Collections of the Los Angeles Public Library, https://tessa.lapl.org/cdm/ref/collection/photos/id/121567.

12. "Club in Scarsdale Donates its Cub to New Texas Zoo," *New York Times*, October 7, 1971: 49.

13. "Mr. Alex Health Club Now Open in Boston," *Jewish Advocate*, April 6, 1961.

14. LaLanne European Health Spa advertisement, *Kansas City Times*, April 28, 1969: 42.

15. Richard Tyler, *The West Coast Bodybuilding Scene: The Golden Era* (Santa Cruz, CA: On Target, 2004).

16. Marla Matzer, "The Venus of Muscle Beach," *Los Angeles Times*, February 22, 1998.

17. Rose, *Muscle Beach*, 117.

18. Rose, *Muscle Beach*, 132.

19. Silver, "Fits over Fitness," 517.

20. Super Speed System advertisement, Sinkram, Inc., 1962, in "More Headlines Continued," Iron League website, accessed February 26, 2022, https://www

.ironleague.com/public/programs/archives.cfm?StartRow=101&show=yes &sort=date&ddesc=all.

21. "In the Matter of Sinkram Incorporated, et al.," in *Federal Trade Commission Decisions*, vol. 64 (Washington, DC: US Government Printing Office, 1964): 1243–73, https://www.ftc.gov/sites/default/files/documents/commission_deci sion_volumes/volume-64/ftcd-vol64january-march1964pages1150-1273.pdf.

22. *Success Story* episode, "Stauffer Motorized Couches and Posture-Rest," directed by Bob Hiestand, sponsored by Richfield Motor Oil, c. 1957, 29:18, Periscope Film LLC archive, https://www.youtube.com /watch?v=Q3VRs02llq8.

23. "In the Matter of Stauffer Laboratories, Inc., et al.," in *Federal Trade Commission Decisions*, vol. 64 (Washington, DC: US Government Printing Office, 1964): 651, https://www.ftc.gov/sites/default/files/documents/commission _decision_volumes/volume-64/ftcd-vol64january-march1964pages629-715.pdf.

24. "In the Matter of Stauffer Laboratories, Inc., et al.," 646–47.

25. Vic Tanny advertisement, *Los Angeles Times*, October 2, 1956.

26. Natalia Mehlman Petrzela, "Slenderizing Spas, Reducing Machines, and Other Hot Fitness Crazes of 75 Years Ago," *Well + Good*, September 1, 2015, https://www.wellandgood.com/weight-loss-salons-reducing-machines/.

27. Bunzel, "The Health Kick's High Priest."

Chapter Ten

1. Edwin D. Goldfield, ed., *Statistical Abstract of the United States: 1960* (Washington, DC: US Government Printing Office, 1960), https://www.census.gov /library/publications/1960/compendia/statab/81ed.html.

2. Tracy D. Morgan, "Pages of Whiteness: Race, Physique Magazines, and the Emergence of Public Gay Culture," in *Queer Studies: A Lesbian, Gay, Bisexual, and Transgender Anthology*, ed. Brett Beemyn and Mickey Eliason (New York: NYU Press, 1996): 280–98.

3. Robert Cochrane, "You Should Know Jack: A Qualitative Study of the Jack LaLanne Show" (MA thesis, University of Nevada, Las Vegas, 2012), https:// digitalscholarship.unlv.edu/thesesdissertations/1548/.

4. Cochrane, 6.

5. Cochrane, 21, 12.

6. Jack LaLanne Show advertisement, WSIX-TV Nashville, *Nashville Tennessean*, September 25, 1960: 32.

7. Robert Lloyd, "Jack LaLanne Offered Perfect Fit for TV," *Paducah Sun*, January 30, 2011: C7.

8. "Amazing Skin Cream Fades Horrid Age Spots Fast," ESOTÉRICA advertisement, *Charlotte Observer*, October 28, 1956: 63.

9. Cochrane, "You Should Know Jack," 34.

10. Excerpt from *The Jack LaLanne Show*, ca. mid-1950s, via Jacklalanneofficial, "Jack LaLanne Fan Mail Cards, Letters and Advice. Facial Exercise," posted

September 17, 2017, YouTube video, 5:17, https://www.youtube.com/watch?v =FGSeminZqhg.

11. "How to Keep Trim—Debbie Drake Column Starts Monday," *Shreveport Journal*, January 6, 1962: 1.

12. "The Debbie Drake Show," n.d., via Midcentury Fashion, "An 11-Minute Episode of Debbie Drake's Exercise Television Show from the 1960s," posted June 9, 2021, Facebook video, 11:33, https://www.facebook.com /watch/?v=2613299585642192.

13. "How to Keep Trim—Debbie Drake Column Starts Monday," *Shreveport Journal*, January 6, 1962: 1.

14. Lulu Hunt Peters, *Diet and Health—With Key to the Calories* (Chicago: Reilly and Lee, 1918): 19.

15. "Debbie Drake, Girl with Beautiful Lines, to Pay Visit," *Birmingham News*, January 16, 1962: 6.

16. Shelly McKenzie, *Getting Physical: The Rise of Fitness Culture in America* (Lawrence: University Press of Kansas, 2013): 77.

17. Dick Kleiner, "Why Would Any Man Like to Watch Debbie Drake Do the Army Dozen?," *Kenosha News*, July 13, 1962: 15.

18. Eleanor Chappell and Kathryn Huss, *Your Good Health: Physical and Emotional* (Garden City, NY: Nelson Doubleday, 1966): 8.

19. "They'll See Yoga Display," *Miami Herald*, August 22, 1958: 79.

20. Connie Gee, "What Hath this Hatha Yoga?," *Miami News*, February 15, 1959: 46.

21. Richard Hittleman, "Everybody's Doing It: Yoga for Health," *Detroit Free Press*, June 26, 1960.

22. Joe Hyams, "Hittleman's Taking Yoga to the Ladies," *Washington Post*, August 7, 1961.

23. *Jack Benny Program*, season 11, episode 16, "Jack Goes to a Gym," February 5, 1961, https://www.youtube.com/watch?v=nOaGizGNqvU.

24. David K. Johnson, *The Lavender Scare: The Cold War Persecution of Gays and Lesbians in the Federal Government* (Chicago: University of Chicago Press, 2004).

25. L. K. White, Central Intelligence Agency Deputy Director for Support, "Physical Fitness Room," memo, January 1, 1964, General CIA Records, National Security Internet Archive, Central Intelligence Agency, https:// archive.org/details/CIA-RDP85-00375R000400110097-1.

26. David K. Johnson, *Buying Gay: How Physique Entrepreneurs Sparked a Movement* (New York: Columbia University Press, 2019): 117–19.

27. "NAACP Accuses Health Club of Discrimination," *Afro-American*, July 1961: 17.

28. Peter Bunzel, "The Health Kick's High Priest," *LIFE*, September 29, 1958: 71.

29. Chappell and Huss, *Your Good Health*, 35.

30. Trimway advertisement, *Bulletin*, November 6, 1968.

31. "New Exerciser Proves Effective for Both Young and Elderly," *Crusader*, February 14, 1969.

32. Robert McAdam, "Changes in Secondary School Boys' Physical Education Programs," *Physical Educator* 18, no. 2 (May 1, 1961): 64; Thomas D. Snyder, ed., *120 Years of American Education: A Statistical Portrait*, report, National Center for Education Statistics, January 1993: 59, https://nces.ed.gov/pubs93/93442.pdf.

33. Charles A. Bucher, "Parents Are Urged to Make Yule Toys 'Active,'" *Milwaukee Star*, December 21, 1972.

Part Four

1. Duston Harvey, "Audience Participation Movie Stresses Touching and Trusting," syndicated column, *Simpson's Leader-Times*, January 25, 1972: 19.

2. Harvey, "Audience Participation Movie Stresses Touching and Trusting," 19.

3. Harvey, "Audience Participation Movie Stresses Touching and Trusting," 19.

4. Frank Jacobs and George Woodbridge, "The Mad Guide to Political Types," *MAD*, October 1972.

5. Jeffrey Kripal, *Esalen: America and the Religion of No Religion* (Chicago: University of Chicago Press, 2007): 105–06.

6. Sam Binkley, *Getting Loose: Lifestyle Consumption in the 1970s* (Durham, NC: Duke University Press, 2007): 231.

Chapter Eleven

1. Pamela Rainbear Portugal, *A Place for Human Beings*, 2nd ed. (San Francisco: Homegrown Books, 1978): 95.

2. Sam Binkley, *Getting Loose: Lifestyle Consumption in the 1970s* (Durham, NC: Duke University Press, 2007): 230–31.

3. Portugal, *A Place for Human Beings*, 73.

4. Jeffrey Kripal, *Esalen: America and the Religion of No Religion* (Chicago: University of Chicago Press, 2007).

5. Kripal, 73.

6. Sharon Nelton, "Esalen Can Be Cold, Frightening," *Miami Herald*, December 22, 1970.

7. Kripal, *Esalen*, 462–63.

8. Jeannine O'Brien Medvin, *Prenatal Yoga and Natural Birth* (Felton, CA: Freestone, 1974): 5–6.20.

9. Medvin, 20.

10. Valerie Wheat et al., eds., "Reviews & Columns," *Booklegger* 2, no. 8 (March/April 1975).

11. *Eros Lib* 1 (Winter 1975), newsletter (San Diego, CA: Sexual Freedom League, 1975).

12. Kerry Thornley, "Reprogram Yourself for Freer Swinging," in *Eros Lib* 2, newsletter (San Diego, CA: Sexual Freedom League, 1975).

13. Judith Guttman, "Bodymind Exploration," *Yoga Journal*, November–December 1977: 49.

14. Diana Alstad, "Interpersonal Yoga," *Yoga Journal*, March 1979: 7.

15. Skip Ferderber, "Topanga Canyon Dwellers Live at Own Happy Pace: Community Reflects," *Los Angeles Times*, July 8, 1973.

16. Sheila Weller, *Girls Like Us: Carole King, Joni Mitchell, Carly Simon and the Journey of a Generation* (New York: Washington Square Press, 2008): 196.

17. Weller, 192, 323.

18. Stanford Women's Center, "A Guide for Stanford Women, 1972" (Stanford, CA: Stanford Women's Center, 1972), Marjorie L. Shuer papers, box 1, folder 11, Department of Special Collections and University Archives, Stanford University Libraries, Stanford, CA.

19. Terrie McDonald, "Dated Facilities Restrict Women," *Stanford Daily*, February 16, 1972.

20. Catherine Kudlick, " 'Save Changes': Telling Stories of Disability Protest," *Nursing Clio*, April 5, 2017, https://nursingclio.org/2017/04/05/save-changes-telling-stories-of-disability-protest/.

21. Alondra Nelson, *Body and Soul: The Black Panther Party and the Fight against Medical Discrimination* (Minneapolis: University of Minnesota Press, 2011).

22. Maryam K. Aziz, "Built with Empty Fists: The Rise and Circulation of Black Power Martial Artistry during the Cold War" (PhD diss., University of Michigan, 2020): 156, https://deepblue.lib.umich.edu/bitstream/handle/2027.42/163044/maryamka_1.pdf.

23. Stephanie Y. Evans, "Black Women's Historical Wellness," *Association of Black Women Historians*, June 21, 2019, http://abwh.org/2019/06/21/black-womens-historical-wellness-history-as-a-tool-in-culturally-competent-mental-health-services/.

24. Aziz, "Built with Empty Fists," 133.

25. Leslie Kaminoff, interview with author, May 31, 2016.

26. Julian Walker, "Enlightenment 2.0: The American Yoga Experiment," in *21st Century Yoga*, ed. Carol Horton and Roseanne Harvey (Chicago: Kleio Books, 2012): 1–26, at 11.

27. Adam Curtis, dir., *The Century of the Self*, documentary series, four episodes, total runtime 240 min., aired 2002 on BBC Two.

28. Aziz, "Built with Empty Fists," 138.

29. Ina Marx, "What Yoga Can Do for You," *Woman's Day*, June 1970: 46–47, 104–05. Jean Pascoe, "A Common Sense Approach to Yoga," *Woman's Day*, June 1970: 44–45, 103–104.

30. Tom Greening and Dick Hobson, "That Sense of Foreboding Must Not Dictate Your Life-Pattern," *Los Angeles Times*, September 18, 1979: H10.

Chapter Twelve

1. Kenneth Cooper, *Aerobics* (Philadelphia: M. Evans/Lippincott, 1968): 9, 4.

2. Cooper, *Aerobics*, 8.

3. Robert Reinhold, "An Interview with Kenneth Cooper," *New York Times*, March 29, 1987.

4. Cooper, *Aerobics*, 4, 11.

5. Cooper, *Aerobics*, introduction.

6. Cooper, *Aerobics*, 53.

7. Kenneth Cooper, *The New Aerobics* (New York: Bantam Books, 1970): 128.

8. Cooper, *The New Aerobics*, 129.

9. Scott Whitaker, dir., *Run Dick, Run Jane!* (Provo, UT: Department of Motion Picture Production, Brigham Young University, 1971), 20:31, https://www.youtube.com/watch?v=Ip07Yndgzzg.

10. Dave Seldon, "New ORU Aerobics Center Called Boost for Fitness," *Daily Oklahoman*, September 30, 1974: 46.

11. "Dr. Cooper Keynote Speaker at Aerobics Center Dedication," *Oracle* (Oral Roberts University student newspaper), September 27, 1974: 1.

12. Jonathan Root, "Pounds Off for Jesus: Oral Roberts University and the Fat Body, 1976-78," *Fat Studies: An Interdisciplinary Journal of Body Weight and Society* 4 (April 8, 2015): 159-77, at 161.

13. Root, 162, 172.

Chapter Thirteen

1. William J. Bowerman and W. E. Harris, M.D., *Jogging* (New York: Grosset and Dunlap, 1967): 1.

2. Bowerman and Harris, 1.

3. Bowerman and Harris, 41, 45, 48.

4. Phil Knight, *Shoe Dog: A Memoir by the Creator of Nike* (New York: Simon and Schuster, 2016).

5. Bowerman and Harris, *Jogging*, 5, 71.

6. Executive Order No. 11562—Developing and Coordinating a National Program for Physical Fitness and Sports, 35 FR 15063 (September 25, 1970); Executive Order No. 11398—Establishing the President's Council on Physical Fitness and Sports, 33 FR 4169 (March 4, 1968); "If Spring Has You Itching to Get Out and Exercise, You'll Be Interested in a Scorecard on the Physical Benefits from Various Activities," *US News and World Report*, April 4, 1977.

7. Mike Tymn, "On Running," *Honolulu Advertiser*, September 7, 1978.

8. Kathrine Switzer, *Marathon Woman* (New York: Da Capo Press, 2009): 77.

9. Tymn, "On Running."

10. Jim Fixx, *The Complete Book of Running* (New York: Random House, 1977): xvii.

11. *Beyond Jogging* workshop in East Burke, Vermont, advertisement, *Burlington Free Press*, August 13, 1978: 25.

12. *The Loneliness of the Long Distance Runner*, directed by Tony Richardson (1962; United Kingdom: Woodfall Film Productions).

13. Vincent Chiappetta, "Profile—Vince Chiappetta Has Been Running for 71 Years," interview, *Lifetime Running*, August 2019, https://www.lifetimerun ning.net/2019/08/august-2019-vincent-chiappetta-co.html.
14. Gerald Eskenazi, "In New York's Marathon, They Also Run Who Only Sit and Wait," *New York Times*, October 2, 1972.
15. Fred Rohe, *The Zen of Running* (New York: Random House, 1974); Valerie Andrews, *The Psychic Power of Running: How the Body Can Illuminate the Mysteries of the Mind* (New York: Rawson Wade, 1978).
16. "Jogging for Joy," *People*, July 4, 1977.
17. David Butwin, "You Can Get Too Pooped to Ping," *Christian Science Monitor News Service*, January 15, 1978.

Chapter Fourteen

1. Lynda Huey, *A Running Start: An Athlete, A Woman* (New York: Crown, 1976): 35–36.
2. Huey, xiv.
3. Nancy Cott, "What's in a Name? The Limits of Social Feminism; Or, Expanding the Vocabulary of Women's History," *Journal of American History* 76, no. 3 (December 1989): 809–29.
4. Marjorie Shuer, "Title IX: The Spirit of the Times," unpublished notes, n.d., Marjorie L. Shuer Papers (SCO733), box 1, folder 2, Department of Special Collections and University Archives, Stanford University Libraries, Stanford, CA.
5. Margie Shuer, "Swim Team Blues," *Stanford Daily*, February 26, 1974, Box 1, Folder 2, Shuer Papers, Stanford University Special Collections.
6. Louise Mead Tricard, *American Women's Track and Field: A History, 1895–1980*, vol. 1 (New York: McFarland, 1996): 597–98.
7. Cyndy Poor, interview with author, October 6, 2017.
8. Kathrine Switzer, *Marathon Woman* (New York: Da Capo Press, 2009): 12, 17–18.
9. Switzer, 67.
10. Switzer, 116.
11. Bob Sales, "Has Marathon Become Battle of Sexes?," *Boston Globe*, April 20, 1967: 52.
12. Switzer, *Marathon Woman*, 15, 148.
13. Al Harvin, "Fireman is First to Finish in Marathon," *New York Times*, September 14, 1970: 54.
14. Al Harvin, "Husband-Wife Teams Entered in Marathon Run Here Today," *New York Times*, September 13, 1970: S25.
15. Vincent Chiappetta, interview by Roger Robinson, *Gotta Run with Will*, episode 378, "Vincent Chiappetta," released June 20, 2019, on Manhattan Neighborhood Network, YouTube video, 43:18, https://www.youtube.com /watch?v=7ttfyVAiopg&t=1074s.

16. Judd Ehrlich, dir., *Run for Your Life: The Fred Lebow Story*, documentary, 2008, Brooklyn, NY: Flatbush Pictures.

17. Chris Ballard, "Running in the Age of Coronavirus," *Sports Illustrated*, May 21, 2020.

18. Kathy Smith, interview with author, December 9, 2019.

19. Switzer, *Marathon Woman*, 169.

20. Jody Avirgan and Hillary Frank, "Six Who Sat," October 30, 2018, in *30 for 30 Podcasts*, produced by Jody Avirgan and Erin Leyden, ESPN and Transmitter Media, MP3 audio, 46:46, transcript available at https://30for30podcasts .com/episodes/six-who-sat/#transcript.

21. Switzer, *Marathon Woman*, 176.

22. Cat Ariail, "'Who Says It Is Not the Most Feminine Thing a Woman Can Do?': The Feminization of Women's Distance Running," *US Sport History Blog*, October 15, 2015, https://ussporthistory.com/2015/10/15/who-says-it -is-not-the-most-feminine-thing-a-woman-can-do-the-feminization-of -womens-distance-running/.

23. "6-Mile 'Marathon' Slated for Women," *Miami Herald*, May 14, 1972: 5.

24. Ehrlich, *Run for Your Life*.

25. Switzer, *Marathon Woman*, 176.

26. "Meet the Winner of the First Women-Only Road Race," *Runner's World*, June 8, 2012.

27. Gerald Eskenazi, "In New York's Marathon, They Also Run Who Only Sit and Wait," *New York Times*, October 2, 1972.

28. Gordon Bakoulis, "'It Means the World to Me': Why Crazylegs Runners Keep Coming Back to the Mini," *New York Road Runners*, June 8, 2019, https://www .nyrr.org/run/photos-and-stories/2019/mini-10k-crazylegs.

29. Huey, *A Running Start*, 135.

30. Amby Burfoot, "Who Was That Guy Who Attacked Kathrine Switzer 50 Years Ago?," *Runner's World*, April 10, 2017.

31. Ariail, "'Who Says It Is Not the Most Feminine Thing a Woman Can Do?'"

32. Maggie Wilson, "'Fitness Fanatics' Run for Their Lives," *Arizona Republic*, March 8, 1978: 31.

33. Horne's Department Store advertisement, *Pittsburgh Press*, June 10, 1979: 37.

34. Martin Cleary, "Race Has Instant Credibility," *Ottawa Citizen*, May 1, 1980: 31.

35. F. M. Williams, "Women Slate September Race," *Tennessean*, June 11, 1978: 37.

36. Gale B. Robinette, "This Sunday Proclaimed 10-K Race Day," *Tennessean*, September 20, 1979: 62.

37. Switzer, *Marathon Woman*, 23.

38. "Guide to the Jogbra, Inc. Records: Biographical/Historical," Jogbra, Inc. records, Archives Center, National Museum of American History, Smithsonian Institution, Washington, DC, accessed February 25, 2022, https://sova .si.edu/record/NMAH.AC.1315#Biographical%20/%20Historical; "Record and Disclosure of Invention, 'Jock Bra,'" October, 14, 1977, Jogbra, Inc. records, Washington, DC, https://sova.si.edu/details/NMAH.AC.1315#ref273.

39. Jim Fixx, *The Complete Book of Running* (New York: Random House, 1977): 103, 102.

40. Allison Keyes, "How the Sports Bra Got Its Stabilizing Start," *Smithsonian Magazine*, March 18, 2020.

41. Jogbra advertisement, ca. 1980, Jogbra, Inc. records, Promotional and Marketing Materials, Archives Center, National Museum of American History, Smithsonian Institution, Washington, DC, filename AC1315-0000026-02.tif, https://edan.si.edu/slideshow/viewer/?eadrefid=NMAH.AC.1315_ref173.

42. Nicholas King, "The Jog-Alongs," *National Review*, August 17, 1979: 1034.

43. "Put an End to Women's Sufferage," Nike Aurora shoe advertisement, *Runner's World*, 1980, Department of Nike Archives (DNA), Nike Inc., Beaverton, OR.

44. *The Women's Movement*, internal report, May 2012, DNA, Nike Inc., Beaverton, OR: 3.

45. Fixx, *Complete Book of Running*, xv, 9, 19, 14.

46. Ballard, "Running in the Age of Coronavirus."

47. Fixx, *Complete Book of Running*, 38, 11, 27, 31.

48. Fixx, 30, 32, 15.

49. Fixx, 24, 29, 5, 40.

50. Fixx, 15, 17.

51. Matthew Lassiter, *The Silent Majority: Suburban Politics in the Sunbelt South* (Princeton, NJ: Princeton University Press, 2007); Lily Geismer, *Don't Blame Us: Suburban Liberals and the Transformation of the Democratic Party* (Princeton, NJ: Princeton University Press, 2014); N. D. B. Connolly, *A World More Concrete: Real Estate and the Remaking of Jim Crow Florida* (Chicago: University of Chicago Press, 2014).

52. Fixx, *Complete Book of Running*, 15.

53. Frank Litsky, "Ted Corbitt, A Pioneer in American Distance Running, Dies at 88," *New York Times*, December 13, 2007.

54. "Reach Out and Touch Someone," Bell System advertisement, *Ebony*, June 1982.

55. Joan Benoit Samuelson, Nike Odyssey sneaker advertisement, ca. early 1980s, DNA, Nike Inc., Beaverton, OR.

56. Deborah Spray (Nikki Craft), "In Defense of Civil Disobedience," April 2, 1980, Women Against Violence Against Women Collection (box 5, folder 6, "Hillside Strangler"), Special Collections, University of California-Los Angeles, cited in Alyssa Corinne Smith, "The Strangers beside Us: A History of Fear, Fascination, and Spectacle Murder in Late Twentieth-Century America" (PhD diss., University of Chicago, 2021).

57. Switzer, *Marathon Woman*, 55.

58. Catherine Breslin, "The Siren Song of Yoga," *Cosmopolitan*, October 1972: 212–16.

59. Joan Breibart, interview with author, July 7, 2020.

60. Shuer, "Title IX, The Spirit of the Times."

61. Judith Sheppard Missett, interview with author, April 22, 2019.

62. Elizabeth Polk, "When the Parade Goes By, Join It!," *Wichita Times*, April 15, 1976.

63. "A Little Music Does the Trick," *Chicago Metro News*, March 20, 1982.

64. Douglas Martin, "Lucille Roberts, 59, Founder of Gym Chain for Women," *New York Times*, July 18, 2003.

65. Leonard Sloane, "Business People: Elaine Powers Founder Plans Diet Formula," *New York Times*, January 26, 1981.

66. "In the Matter of Stauffer Laboratories, Inc., et al.," in *Federal Trade Commission Decisions*, vol. 64 (Washington, DC: US Government Printing Office, 1964): 646, https://www.ftc.gov/sites/default/files/documents/commission _decision_volumes/volume-64/ftcd-vol64january-march1964pages629-715.pdf.

67. Shirley Conran, "Do You Want a 24 Waist?," *London Observer*, February 4, 1968: 28.

68. Danielle Friedman, "The Secret Sexual History of the Barre Workout," *Cut*, January 19, 2018, https://www.thecut.com/2018/01/barre-workout-sexual -history.html.

69. Friedman.

70. Robert Musel, "She Limbers Up the Rich Jet Set," *South Bend Tribune*, April 20, 1971: 10.

71. Conran, "Do You Want a 24 Waist?," 28.

72. Esther Fairfax, *My Improper Mother and Me* (London: Central Books, 2010); Maggie Savoy, "Hope In-Law with a Sense of Humor," *Los Angeles Times*, March 20, 1970: 121.

73. Musel, "She Limbers Up the Rich Jet Set."

74. Angela Taylor, "From Shimmying to Standing on Your Head," *New York Times*, March 24, 1972.

75. Fred DeVito, interview with author, December 8, 2015.

76. Elisabeth Halfpapp, interview with author, October 2, 2015.

77. Lydia Bach, *The Lotte Berk Method, Formerly Called Awake! Aware! Alive!* (New York: Random House, 1973): introduction, 86.

78. Bach, introduction, 85, 70.

Chapter Fifteen

1. "Musical Fitness: A Sport Contains the Benefits of Jogging with Some Fun," *Los Angeles Times*, October 22, 1981.

2. Jean Nidetch, *Weight Watchers: The Memoir of a Successful Loser* (New York: Signet Classics, 1972): vi, 62.

3. Susie Orbach, *Fat is a Feminist Issue: A Self-Help Guide for Compulsive Eaters* (New York: Paddington Press, 1978): 88–89, 16.

4. Nidetch, *Weight Watchers*, 12.

5. Orbach, *Fat Is a Feminist Issue*, 123, 84.

6. Nidetch, *Weight Watchers*, 159, 35.

7. Nidetch, 174.

8. Orbach, *Fat Is a Feminist Issue*, 112, 193.

9. Jane Fonda, *Jane Fonda's Workout Book* (New York: Simon and Schuster, 1981): 18.

10. Gilda Marx, *Body by Gilda: Redesign Every Line* (New York: G. P. Putnam's Sons, 1984).

11. Jane Fonda, *My Life So Far* (New York: Random House, 2005): 387–91.

12. Marx, *Body by Gilda*, 17,18.

13. Leni Cazden and Jane Fonda, interview by Willa Paskin, "Jane Fonda's Workout, Part 1: Jane and Leni," October 13, 2020, in *Decoder Ring*, produced by Benjamin Frisch, podcast, MP3 audio, 54:32, https://slate.com/podcasts /decoder-ring/2020/10/jane-fonda-leni-cazden.

14. James Spada, *Fonda: Her Life in Pictures* (New York: Doubleday, 1985); Femmy DeLyser, *Jane Fonda's Workout Book for Pregnancy, Birth, and Recovery* (New York: Simon and Schuster, 1982): 19, 164.

15. Gloria Steinem, "In Praise of Women's Bodies," *Ms.*, April 1982.

16. Kathy Smith, interview with author, December 9, 2019.

17. Richard Simmons, *Still Hungry—After All These Years: My Story* (New York: GT, 1999): 173.

18. Simmons, *Still Hungry*, 173.

19. Natalia Petrzela, "Why Everyone is Obsessed with a Fitness Podcast About Richard Simmons," *Well + Good*, March 29, 2017, https://www.wellandgood .com/missing-richard-simmons-podcast-fitness-history/.

20. "Stretch and Salad," *Los Angeles Times*, November 14, 1975.

21. Natalia Mehlman Petrzela, "Working, Out," *Slate*, June 20, 2018, https://slate .com/human-interest/2018/06/crossfit-homophobia-reminds-us-that-gyms -have-always-been-gay.html.

22. Robert Lindsey, "Jane Fonda's Exercise Salons Aiding Her Husband's Candidacy," *New York Times*, May 2, 1982.

23. Christopher Lasch, "The Narcissist Society," *New York Review of Books*, September 30, 1976; Edwin Schur, *The Awareness Trap: Self-Absorption instead of Social Change* (New York: Quadrangle Books, 1976).

24. Joel Kramer, "Oracles of the New Age," *Yoga Journal*, January–February 1980.

25. James Harvey Johnson, ed., "American Patriots Cry Out against Treason Rotten Government, Suppression Of News," *Truth Seeker* 98, no. 7 (July 1971).

26. Lasch, "The Narcissist Society."

27. Charles Gaines, *Stay Hungry* (New York: Doubleday, 1972): 60.

28. *Stay Hungry*, directed by Bob Rafelson (1976; Hollywood, CA: United Artists).

29. *Pumping Iron*, directed by George Butler and Robert Flore (1977; New York: White Mountain Films).

30. Pete Manso, "Arnold Schwarzenegger on the Sex Secrets of Bodybuilders," *OUI*, August 1977.

31. DeLyser, *Jane Fonda's Workout Book for Pregnancy, Birth, and Recovery*, jacket.

Part Five

1. Henry A. Solomon, *The Exercise Myth* (San Diego, CA: Harcourt,1984), excerpted in Darrell Sifford, "Runners Laboring under Myth, Says Doctor," *Cincinnati Enquirer*, December 24, 1984: 9.
2. Robert Reinhold, "Has the Aerobics Movement Peaked?," *New York Times*, March 29, 1987: 14.
3. Reinhold, "Has the Aerobics Movement Peaked?," 14.
4. William A. Nolen, "When Exercise Can Hurt You," *McCall's*, July 1980: 82.
5. William Oscar Johnson, "Marching to Euphoria," *Sports Illustrated*, July 14, 1980: 75.
6. Colman McCarthy, "Ashen, Carter Forced to Quit Road Race," *Washington Post*, September 16, 1979.
7. Jane Gross, "James F. Fixx Dies Jogging; Author on Running Was 52," *New York Times*, July 22, 1984.
8. Marc Stern, "The Fitness Movement and the Fitness Center Industry: 1960–2000," *Business and Economic History On-Line* 6 (2008): 12–13.

Chapter Sixteen

1. "Enjoy Some Free Time," *Central New Jersey Home News*, October 14, 1986.
2. MemoryMuseum, "Cher 1985 Jack LaLanne Commercial," posted October 8, 2014, YouTube video, 0:30, https://www.youtube.com/watch?v=_ljz4omRDHk; Cher News, "Cher—Jack LaLanne Health Spa Commercial (1986)," posted August 27, 2018, YouTube video, 0:30, https://www.youtube.com/watch?v=uq9-1O59pW8.
3. Larry Speakes, press briefing, October 15, 1982, White House Office of the Press Secretary, Washington, DC: 3. Available at the Jon Cohen AIDS Research Collection, University of Michigan, https://quod.lib.umich.edu/c/cohenaids/5571095.0487.001?rgn=main;view=fulltext.
4. "Fast Forward," *Advocate*, January 19, 1988: 35.
5. Marcia Pally, "Laissez-Faire Lesbianism: Prize-Winning French Film Takes Sexual Identity in Stride," *Advocate*, September 29, 1987: 62; Edward Guthmann, "The Gripping Tale of the Boy behind the Mask," *Advocate*, April 16, 1985: 40.
6. Natalia Mehlman Petrzela, "Working, Out," *Slate*, June 20, 2018, https://slate.com/human-interest/2018/06/crossfit-homophobia-reminds-us-that-gyms-have-always-been-gay.html.
7. David Rensin, "20 Questions with Jack LaLanne," *Playboy*, October 1984.
8. *Worn Stories*, season 1, episode 7, "Survival," directed by Ted Passon, released April 1, 2021, on Netflix.
9. Brian Moss, interview with author, November 5, 2020; Kathy Acker, "Against Ordinary Language: The Language of the Body," in *The Last Sex: Feminism*

and *Outlaw Bodies*, ed. Arthur and Marilouise Kroker (London: Palgrave,1993): 20–27.

10. Michael Perron, interview with author, October 20, 2015.

11. Monique Dash, interview with author, February 25, 2021.

12. "New Gym in Montrose," *Montrose Star*, January 24, 1980, http://www.hous tonlgbthistory.org/misc-jims.html.

13. William K. Stevens, "Houston Accepts New Political Force," *New York Times*, November 2, 1981.

14. Pete Diamond, "Jim's Gym Reopens Following Fire," *Montrose Voice*, January 10, 1986, http://www.houstonlgbthistory.org/misc-jims.html.

15. Parkway Athletic Club advertisements, *This Week in Texas*, March 11–17, May 6–12, July 15–21, July 29–August 4, 1988, http://www.houstonlgbthistory .org/misc-jims.html.

16. AIDS.gov, "A Timeline of HIV/AIDS," 2016: 3, https://www.hiv.gov/sites /default/files/aidsgov-timeline.pdf.

17. "Gay Rights Measure Loses Big in Houston," *Human Events*, February 9, 1985: 5.

18. Institute for the Scientific Investigation of Sexuality, *Criminality, Social Disruption, and Homosexuality: Homosexuality Is a Crime against Humanity*, pamphlet, 1985, University of North Texas Digital Collections, https://digital .library.unt.edu/ark:/67531/metadc276206.

19. Aaron Levin, "Early On, the HIV/AIDS Epidemic Was a Voyage into the Unknown," *Psychiatry Online*, December 1, 2014, https://psychnews.psychia tryonline.org/doi/10.1176/appi.pn.2014.12a24.

20. "Parkway Athletic Club's Mark Schmidt and Michael Wilson are Planning Big Things," *Montrose Voice*, October 3, 1986; "Man Ordered to Stop Using Urine to Treat AIDS Patients," *Tyler Courier-Times*, August 18, 1987.

21. Parkway Athletic Club advertisements, *This Week in Texas*, May 6–12, July 15–21, July 29–August 4, 1988.

22. Parkway Athletic Club advertisement, *This Week in Texas*, March 11–17, 1988.

23. *Worn Stories*, directed by Ted Passon.

24. *Desert Migration*, directed by Daniel F. Cardone, produced by the HIV Story Project (2015; Warren, NJ: Passion River Films). First names only used in film.

25. Holly Reich, "What Exercisers Do," *New York Daily News*, November 27, 1989.

26. "Dress for Success in the Fitness Class," *Daily Reporter* (Greenfield, IN), October 17, 1989.

27. Molly Fox, interview with author, November 12, 2015.

28. Jeff Martin, interview with author, March 8, 2021.

29. IDEA survey, cited in Margaret Morse, "Artemis Aging: Exercise and the Female Body on Video," *Discourse* 10, no. 1 (Fall/Winter 1987–1988): 20–53.

30. Judi Sheppard Missett, *Building a Business with a Beat: An Empire Built on Passion, Purpose, and Heart* (New York: McGraw Hill, 2019): 66.

31. Marcia Chatelain, *Franchise: The Golden Arches in Black America* (New York: Liveright, 2020): Introduction.

32. Judith Sheppard Missett, interview with author, August 28, 2015; Michael Schroeder, "Looking for a Bigger Slice," *Detroit News*, September 20, 1985; Judith Berlin, interview with author, October 22, 2015.

33. Pauline Bartel, "Women At Large Builds Self-Esteem," *Journal and Courier* (Lafayette, IN), March 29, 1987; Jenny Ellison, *Being Fat: Women, Weight, and Feminist Activism in Canada* (Toronto: University of Toronto Press, 2020): 116.

34. William E. Geist, "About New York: The Mating Game and Other Exercises at the Vertical Club," *New York Times*, May 19, 1984.

Chapter Seventeen

1. "Low Impact Aerobics Are Easier, Less Demanding on the Body," *Modesto Bee*, May 7, 1986.

2. Monique Dash, interview with author, February 25, 2021.

3. Tamilee Webb, interview with author, September 15, 2015.

4. Rancho la Puerta brochure, 1975, Anspach Travel Bureau Collection of Tourism Literature, 1936–2014, 145 General Files, Baja 1971–1998, John W. Hartman Center, Duke University, Durham, NC.

5. "Time for a 'Fitness Vacation,'" *Chicago Metro News*, June 5, 1982.

6. "How Exxon Helps Its People Exercise," *US News and World Report*, January 28, 1980.

7. President's Council on Physical Fitness and Sports advertisement, *Cosmopolitan*, July 1981.

8. Linda Villarosa, "Firms Find Fitness Plans Pay Out Healthy Dividends," *American Banker*, October 19, 1987.

9. US Department of Commerce, Bureau of the Census, *1980 Census of Population: New York* (Washington, DC: US Government Printing Office, August 1982): 68, https://www2.census.gov/prod2/decennial/documents/1980/1980c ensusofpopu80134unse_bw.pdf; US Department of Commerce, Bureau of the Census, *1990 Census of Population, New York*, section 1 of 2 (Washington, DC: US Government Printing Office, April 1992): 172, https://www2.census .gov/library/publications/decennial/1990/cp-1/cp-1-34-1.pdf; Timothy Pytell, interview with author, June 26, 2020.

10. Natalia Mehlman Petrzela, "Jogging Has Always Excluded Black People," *New York Times*, May 12, 2020.

11. Dylan Gottlieb, *Yuppies: Wall Street and the Remaking of New York* (Cambridge, MA: Harvard University Press, forthcoming).

12. Katy Butler, "Bite by Bite, the Croissant Culture Is Swallowing Up the Ghettos," *Los Angeles Times*, August 24, 1980.

13. "Sniper Suspect Pleads Innocent in Federal Charges," *Daily Spectrum* (St. George, Utah), November 11, 1980.

14. Gary Leonard, *1988 Los Angeles Marathon on Sunset Boulevard*, 1988, photographic print, black and white, 29 × 36 cm, Los Angeles Neighborhoods Collection, Digital Collections of the Los Angeles Public Library, https://tessa.lapl.org/cdm/ref/collection/photos/id/3840.

15. Norman Riley, "Arts," *Crisis*, December 1985: 468.

16. "Wolf Pack's Prey," *New York Daily News*, April 21, 1989: 1.

17. "Running Has Made a Difference in My Life," *Chicago Metro News*, October 6, 1984.

18. "Shaping Up," *Ebony*, June 1982: 54–55; "Reach Out and Touch Someone," Bell System advertisement, *Ebony*, June 1982.

19. Herb Boyd, "Cop Calls McCutchen a 'Do-Gooder,' Not a 'Hero,'" *Amsterdam News*, September 24, 1994.

20. Richard Simmons, *Still Hungry—After All These Years: My Story* (New York, GT, 1999): 222.

21. Timothy Aubry and Trysh Travis, eds., *Rethinking Therapeutic Culture* (Chicago: University of Chicago Press, 2015): introduction.

22. Gilad Janklowicz, interview with author, November 4, 2015.

23. Jason Okundaye, "Tony Britts: Who Was the BBC Fitness Instructor?," *I-D Vice*, April 9, 2020.

24. Bernice Kanner, "Home Movies," *New York*, July 16, 1984: 14.

25. Andrew McKevitt, *Consuming Japan: Popular Culture and the Globalizing of 1980s America* (Chapel Hill: University of North Carolina Press, 2017): 138.

26. Nielsen poll, cited in "What's on Television Tonight? Plenty More with Cable, VCRs," *Camden Courier-Post*, September 10, 1989.

27. McKevitt, *Consuming Japan*, 135, 139.

28. Ellen Bilgore, "Arthur Jones: Physical Fitness Turns Back the Clock for Nautilus' Inventor," *New Body*, May 1982.

29. Jane Fonda, *My Life So Far* (New York: Random House, 2005): 395.

30. "Get Your Exercise," Lorimar Home Video advertisement, *Ladies' Home Journal*, August 1987.

31. Fonda, *My Life So Far*, 392.

32. Fonda, *My Life So Far*, 393–95.

33. Kanner, "Home Movies."

34. Simmons, *Still Hungry*, 237; John G., "Richard Simmons Show 1983," posted March 27, 2018, YouTube video, 29:50,https://www.youtube.com/watch?v=QU6j7vjfbEs.

35. Simmons, *Still Hungry*, 239–40.

36. Lizmcg83, "Everyday with Richard Simmons—Opening Scene at Diner," posted July 2025, 2010, YouTube video, 1:21, https://www.youtube.com/watch?v=4aCdfg0h-Sc.

37. *Richard Simmons: Sweatin' to the Oldies*, directed by E. H. Shipley, home video (1988; Hollywood, CA: Ren-Mar Studios).

38. Simmons, *Still Hungry*, 250. Patrick R. Parsons and Herbert J. Rotfeld, "Informercials and Television Station Clearance Practices," *Journal of Public Policy and Marketing* 9 (1990): 62–72.

39. Simmons, *Still Hungry*, 208, 239, 256.

40. Cal Pozo, interview with author, August 31, 2015.

41. Margaret Morse, "Artemis Aging: Exercise and the Female Body on Video," *Discourse* 10, no. 1 (Fall/Winter 1987–1988): 20–53.

42. Nikki Finke, "All Sides Get Worked Up over Study of Aerobics Videos," *Los Angeles Times*, November 12, 1987.

43. *Do It Debbie's Way*, directed by Kevin Carlisle, home exercise video (1983; Los Angeles, CA: Paul Brownstein Productions).

44. Jenny Ellison, *Being Fat: Women, Weight, and Feminist Activism in Canada* (Toronto: University of Toronto Press, 2020): 113.

45. Jo Griffiths, "Women at Large," *Pittsburgh Post-Gazette*, January 25, 1990.

46. VHS Ark, "Women at Large: Breakout," 1987, posted May 24, 2017, YouTube video, 1:10:16, https://www.youtube.com/watch?v=RK0TAHn3-qs.

47. Robin Gaby, "Senior Fitness, Fonda-Style," *Courier-News* (Bridgewater, NJ), August 14, 1986.

48. Richard Simmons, *Reach for Fitness: A Special Book of Exercises for the Physically Challenged* (New York: Grand Central, 1986).

49. Simmons, *Still Hungry*, 251.

Chapter Eighteen

1. *Muscle Motion*, directed by Nick de Noia (1983; Los Angeles: Media Home Entertainment).

2. "Warm Up to Traci Lords," directed by Stewart Dell (1990; White Nights Productions), MP4 video, 47:02, https://ia801903.us.archive.org/7/items /WarmUpToTraciLordsExerciseVideo1990/Warm%20Up%20to%20Traci%20 Lords%21%20%28Exercise%20Video%201990%29.mp4.

3. Alice Zook, interview by Bryant Gumbel, *TODAY Show*, aired May 31, 1984, on NBC; Alice Zook on *Donahue*, 1985, https://archive.org/details /DonahueHSV71985Incomplete.

4. Cynthia Kirk, "Exotic Male Tape Ousts Teacher," *Variety*, July 31, 1984.

5. Richard Simmons, *Still Hungry—After All These Years: My Story* (New York: GT, 1999): 188, 191.

6. Richard Petosa, "Wellness: An Emerging Opportunity for Health Education," *Health Education* 15, no. 6 (October/November 1984): 37–39; *Bulletin* 58, no. 3 (Winter 1985): 11, Springfield College Archives and Special Collections, https://cdm16122.contentdm.oclc.org/digital/collection/p16122coll3/id/14754 /rec/3.

7. Julie Jacobson, "Chiropractor Also Uses Kinesiology," *Times Herald*, May 17, 1981; Dr. James J. Beno D.C. advertisement, *Petoskey News Review*, August 20, 1985.

8. Bill Fay, "Kinesiology: The System to Save Athletic Careers?," *Tampa Tribune*, February 9, 1982.

9. "CSU Adds Exercise Science Classes," *Chico-Enterprise Record*, November 25, 1984.

10. "What Is Kinesiology?," University of Michigan website, accessed January 31, 2021, https://www.kines.umich.edu/about/what-kinesiology.

11. "Lander Program Offers Concentrations in Athletic Training," *Index-Journal*, August 28, 1988.

12. "UW Chops Kinesiology Program," *Spokesman-Review*, November 15, 1982.

13. Lynda Huey, *A Running Start: An Athlete, A Woman* (New York: Crown, 1976): 43, 49, 61.

14. Carol Scott, interview with author, March 11, 2020.

15. Fred DeVito, interview with author, December 8, 2015.

16. Tamilee Webb, interview with author, September 15, 2015.

17. Carol Scott, interview with author.

18. Peter and Kathie Davis, interview with author, March 9, 2020.

19. Douglas H. Richie Jr., Steven F. Kelson, and Patricia Bellucci, "Aerobic Dance Injuries: A Retrospective Study of Instructors and Participants," *Physician and Sportsmedicine* 13, no. 2 (1985): 130–40.

20. Sandra Lanman, "Aerobic Dance Aims for High Standards, Low Impact," *Central New Jersey Home News*, November 18, 1986.

21. Rebecca Overton, "Certification Program in Aerobics Due," *Indianapolis Star*, November 9, 1985.

22. "Area Instructors Attend Jazzercise Convention," *Dunn County News*, September 15, 1982; Cal Pozo, interview with author, August 31, 2015.

23. US Department of Education, National Center for Education Statistics, *Chartbook of Degrees Conferred, 1969–70 to 1993–94*, NCES 98-071, project officer Thomas D. Snyder (NCES: Washington, DC, 1997): 101–276, https://nces.ed.gov/pubs98/98071.pdf; US Department of Education, National Center for Education Statistics, Integrated Postsecondary Education Data System (IPEDS), "Completions," survey, 2019.

24. "Make Kids Walk, Says Specialist," *Chicago Metro News*, July 12, 1986.

Chapter Nineteen

1. Judi Sheppard Missett, *Building a Business with a Beat: An Empire Built on Passion, Purpose, and Heart* (New York: McGraw Hill, 2019): 111.

2. Britni de la Cretaz, "An Audience of Athletes: The Rise and Fall of Feminist Sports," *Longreads*, May 2019, https://longreads.com/2019/05/22/an-audience-of-athletes-the-rise-and-fall-of-feminist-sports/; Susan Ware, *Game, Set, Match: Billie Jean King and the Revolution in Women's Sports* (Chapel Hill: University of North Carolina Press, 2011).

3. Walter LaFeber, *Michael Jordan and the New Global Capitalism* (New York: Norton, 2002): 54; *How Michael Jordan Jumpstarted Nike*, internal report, October 2014, Department of Nike Archives (DNA), Nike Inc.

4. J. B. Strasser and Laurie Becklund, *Swoosh: The Unauthorized Story of Nike and the Men Who Played There* (New York: Harcourt Brace Jovanovich, 1991): 399.

5. *Catalysts: The Power of Women in Sport*, internal report, March 2014, DNA, Nike Inc., Beaverton, OR: 68; *The Women's Movement*, internal report, May 2012, DNA, Nike Inc., Beaverton, OR; Strasser and Becklund, *Swoosh*, 399.

6. Reebok advertisement, *Great Falls Tribune*, December 16, 1982.

7. *Catalysts*, 78.

8. *The Women's Movement*, 3.

9. *The Women's Movement*, 10.

10. Wendy A. Woloson, *Crap: A History of Cheap Stuff in America* (Chicago: University of Chicago Press, 2020).

11. Natalia Mehlman Petrzela, "The Precarious Labor of the Fitpro: Interrogating the Political Economy of Fitness in American Life," *Public Seminar*, December 16, 2019, https://publicseminar.org/essays/the-precarious -labor-of-the-fitpro/.

12. *Aerobicide* (later renamed *Killer Workout*), directed by David Prior (1987; Hollywood, CA: Shapiro Entertainment); Carol Farley, *The Case of the Haunted Health Club* (New York: Avon Books, 1991).

13. Charles Gaines, *Staying Hard* (New York: Kenan Press, 1980): 15.

14. Bureau of Labor Statistics, as reported in Stephanie Vatz, "Why America Stopped Making Its Own Clothes," *KQED*, May 14, 2013, https://www.kqed .org/lowdown/7939/madeinamerica; Norm Zwail, interview with author, August 18, 2015.

15. Rachel Sibony, interview with author, December 15, 2015.

16. David Rensin, "20 Questions with Jack LaLanne," *Playboy*, October 1984.

17. Gaines, *Staying Hard*, 12.

18. Natalia Mehlman Petrzela, "What You Can Learn from the Surprising History of New Year's Resolutions," *Refinery29*, December 29, 2016, https://www .refinery29.com/en-us/2016/12/134160/fitness-new-year-resolutions-history.

Part Six

1. Donald Katz, "Jack LaLanne Is Still an Animal," *Outside*, November 1995.

2. Jacklalanneofficial, "The Jack LaLanne Full Episode (Hangovers)," ca. mid-1950s, posted January 18, 2016, YouTube video, 24:06, https://www.youtube .com/watch?v=tP40RWwhoRw.

Chapter Twenty

1. David Hollinger, *Postethnic America: Beyond Multiculturalism* (New York: Basic Books, 1995): 7.

2. California Bureau of Publications, *Toward a State of Esteem: The Final Report of the California Task Force to Promote Self-Esteem and Personal and Social*

Responsibility, Sacramento: California State Department of Education, January 1990: 11, https://files.eric.ed.gov/fulltext/ED321170.pdf.

3. Caro Evans, "Stress at Work," letters, *Atlanta Journal*, September 1, 1999; Kathleen Helsing, "Stress Free Zone," two-week series, *Los Angeles Times*, August 17, 1998: 5.

4. John Updike, *Rabbit at Rest* (New York: Random House, 1990).

5. David Brooks, *Bobos in Paradise: The New Upper Class and How They Got There* (New York: Simon and Schuster, 2000): 85.

6. Brooks, 216, 198.

7. April Durett, "Industry Watch: Trends in Fitness," *IDEA Health and Fitness Source*, March 2000.

8. "Yoga Statistics and Demographics," compiled by Trisha Lamb, Prescott, AZ: International Association of Yoga Therapists, 2004, updated 2006.

9. Ann Powers, "American Influences Help Redefine Practice of Yoga," *New York Times* August 1, 2000.

10. Editorial, ," *Yoga Journal*, January–February, 1980; Lilias Folan and Alice Rankin, cited in Joel Kramer, "Oracles of the New Age," *Yoga Journal*, January–February, 1980.

11. Bob Condor, "Fonda Flexes Her Workout Clout with Yoga Tape," *Chicago Tribune*, March 3, 1994.

12. Anne Cushman, "Namaste, Jane," *Yoga Journal*, May–June 1994: 47.

13. Rick Fields, "Only Connect," *Yoga Journal*, May–June 1994: 5.

14. "From Our Readers," *Yoga Journal*, November–December 1994: 6–7.

15. Pamela Pietri, "Helping the Omless," *LA Weekly*, June 2, 1988: 24.

16. "Classical Indian and Chinese Music Ensemble," *LA Weekly*, January 30, 1992; Merrill Markoe, "My Favorite Weekend," *Los Angeles Times*, February 13, 1997.

17. Laura Shin, "Free Market Yoga," *Yoga Journal*, March–April 2005: 77.

18. K. Pattabhi Jois, letter to the editor, *Yoga Journal*, November–December 1995.

19. "YOGA," *Los Angeles Times*, November 20, 1994.

20. "Astroyoga," *Yoga Journal*, January–February 1995.

21. "Teaching Application: Jivamukti Yoga Center, New York City," n.d.: 1–7, Leslie Kaminoff personal archive.

22. "Winter/Spring Events 1992," *Jivamukti Newsletter*1, 3, Leslie Kaminoff personal archive.

23. Daryn Eller, "The New Yoga," *Chicago Tribune*, August 23, 1993.

24. Leslie Kaminoff, interview with author, May 31, 2016.

25. "Yogi Desai Resigns from Kripalu," *Yoga Journal*, January–February 1995: 40.

26. Daniel Bowling to Leslie Kaminoff, May 10, 1995, Leslie Kaminoff personal archive.

27. Billy Cox, "Yoga Master Shares Vision with Brevard," *Florida Today*, January 29, 1999; "Yoga Classes Help You Work Up a Good Sweat," *Arizona Daily Star*, August 20, 1998.

28. Dominic Rushe, "Yoga Guru Bikram Choudhury Accused of Rape in Two New Lawsuits," *Guardian*, May 14, 2013; Paddy Calistro, "Yoga Takes Strain for the Stressed," *Calgary Herald*, May 15, 1992.

29. Blair Sabol, "Yogi to the Stars, Everyman," *Los Angeles Times*, November 29, 1974: 74.

30. Sabol, 75.

31. Allison Fish, "The Commodification and Exchange of Knowledge in the Case of Transnational Commercial Yoga," *International Journal of Cultural Property* 13, no. 2 (2006): 189–206.

32. James Greenberg, "Asana TM," *Yoga Journal*, November–December 2003.

33. Callie Batts Maddox and Robin Cooley, "'The Benares of the West': The Evolution of Yoga in Los Angeles," *Journal of Sport History* 41, no. 1 (Spring 2019): 82–97.

34. Hilary E. MacGregor, "Bikram Goes to the Mat," *Los Angeles Times*, March 21, 2005.

35. Tamara Venit Shelton, *Herbs and Roots: A History of Chinese Medicine in the American Marketplace* (New Haven, CT: Yale University Press, 2019).

36. Penelope Green, "Punching and Kicking All the Way to the Bank," *New York Times*, March 21, 1999.

37. Tae Bo advertisement, *Fort Worth Star Telegram*, March 14, 1999.

38. Vijay Prashad, *Everybody Was Kung Fu Fighting* (New York: Beacon Press, 2001): 146.

39. Maryam K. Aziz, "Built with Empty Fists: The Rise and Circulation of Black Power Martial Artistry during the Cold War" (PhD diss., University of Michigan, 2020): 157, https://deepblue.lib.umich.edu/bitstream/han dle/2027.42/163044/maryamka_1.pdf?sequence=1.

40. Amy McKeever, "The Fitness Gospel of Billy Blanks," *Racked*, September 15, 2016.

41. Green, "Punching and Kicking All the Way to the Bank."

42. Cal Pozo, interview with author, August 31, 2015.

43. Green, "Punching and Kicking All the Way to the Bank"; Paul Harber, "Tae Bo Puts a Kick into Workouts," *Boston Globe*, April 25, 1999; "President's Council on Physical Fitness and Sports: Council Members and Executives, July 1956–May 2006," President's Council on Physical Fitness and Sports, accessed February 26, 2022, https://www.hhs.gov/sites/default/files/fitness /pdfs/list-of-council-leadership.pdf.

44. Eileen Fitzpatrick, "Billy Blanks' Tae Bo Phenom Could Revitalize Fitness Genre," *Billboard*, February 27, 1999.

45. Harber, "Tae Bo Puts a Kick into Workouts."

46. John DiLulio, "The Coming of the Super-Predators," *Weekly Standard*, November 27, 1995, https://www.washingtonexaminer.com/weekly-standard /the-coming-of-the-super-predators.

47. Victoria Felkar, "The Iron Bar: The Modern History of Prison Physical Culture and the Correctional Weightlifting Ban," *Stadion* 40 (2014): 19–37.

48. *All My Children*, episode 5699, Felicia Minei Behr, executive producer, aired January 8, 1992, on ABC, https://archive.org/details/AllMyChildren199201Jan ThruMay16.8Gb.

Chapter Twenty-One

1. National Federation of State High School Associations, *Athletics Participation Survey Totals, 2007–08 Athletics Participation Summary*, report, NFSHA, Elgin, IL, 2008, https://www.nfhs.org/media/1020206/hs_participation_survey_history_1969-2009.pdf.

2. Robert Sullivan, "Goodbye to Heroin Chic, Now It's Sexy to be Strong," *Time*, July 19, 1999.

3. T. Jesse Wilde, "Gender Equity in Athletics: Coming of Age in the 90's," *Marquette Sports Law Review* 4, no.2 (1994): 230; "Percentage of U.S. Population Who Have Completed Four Years of College or More from 1940–2020, by Gender," *Statista*, March 15, 2021, https://www.statista.com/statistics/184272/educational-attainment-of-college-diploma-or-higher-by-gender/.

4. Andrew Gottesman, "Gender Equity Hit by Backlash," *Chicago Tribune*, May 7, 1995.

5. John Leo, "Equality—or Else!," *New York Daily News*, March 14, 1998.

6. Gene Wojciechowski and Andrew Gottesman, "Golden Era for Women," *Chicago Tribune*, August 4, 1996.

7. *The Women's Movement*, internal report, May 2012, Department of Nike Archives, Nike Inc., Beaverton, OR: 7.

8. *The Women's Movement*, 8.

9. *The Women's Movement*, 10.

10. Sullivan, "Goodbye to Heroin Chic."

11. Alissa Lustigman, "Cross Training at the Crossroads," *Sporting Goods Business* 24, no. 10 (October 1991).

12. Patty S. Freedson, "Strength Training for Women," *IDEA Personal Trainer* 11, no. 4 (July 2000).

13. Barbara Lloyd, "On Your Own: Step Up (and Down) to Sharper Workouts," *New York Times*, March 26, 1990, https://www.nytimes.com/1990/03/26/sports/on-your-own-step-up-and-down-to-sharper-workouts.html.

14. Ruth Zukerman, *Riding High: How I Kissed SoulCycle Goodbye, Co-Founded Flywheel, and Built the Life I Always Wanted* (New York: St. Martin's Press, 2018): 72.

15. ECA Fitness Convention brochure, 2000, Carol Scott personal archive.

16. Anne S. Lewis, "Recasting a Workout for the Masses," *New York Times*, October 6, 1996.

17. "Trendy Exercisers Bent on Pilates," *Victoria Advocate*, December 25, 1995.

18. Lou Schuler, "The Best Exercises of All Time," *Men's Health*, July/August 2000: 54–60; Patricia Desa, "Gentle Moves for Firm Muscles," *Prevention*,

December 2000; Valerie Vaz, "The Pilates Principle," *Essence*, September 1996.

19. Vernyce Dannells, "Anita Jackson and the Pilates Method," *Afro Hawaii News*, June 30, 1991.

20. Linda Sievers, "Videos to Sweat By Offer a Convenient Way to Work Out," *Anchorage Daily News*, January 15, 1988.

21. Tamilee Webb, interview with author, September 15, 2015; "Buns Exercise Tapes Heat Up Market by Targeting Body Parts," *Gannett News Service*, March 16, 1993.

22. Susan Campbell, "Working Out for 'Buns of Steel' Called Futile," *Record*, December 28, 1995.

23. Sabrina Strings, *Fearing the Black Body: The Racial Origins of Fatphobia* (New York: NYU Press, 2019): 92.

24. Angela Tate, "Eating Disorders Are for White Girls," *Culture Study*, Substack newsletter, ed. Anne Helen Petersen, June 16, 2021, https://annehelen.sub stack.com/p/eating-disorders-are-for-white-girls.

25. Geraldo Rivera, "Women's Bodybuilding: Sweat, Stigma, and Steroids," *The Geraldo Show*, 1990. Dailymotion video, 43:15, https://www.dailymotion.com /video/x5p0nlf.

26. "Richard Bey," segment from *The Richard Bey Show*, ca. 1990s, via Ischemic Attack, posted January 19, 2012, YouTube video, 4:17, https://www.youtube .com/watch?v=sy8hdyRVUmk.

27. Joan Jacobs Brumberg, *The Body Project: An Intimate History of American Girls* (New York: Random House, 1997): 123.

28. Anne Helen Petersen, "The Millennial Vernacular of Fatphobia," *Culture Study*, Substack newsletter, May 23, 2021.

29. Britni de la Cretaz, "An Audience of Athletes: The Rise and Fall of Feminist Sports," *Longreads*, May 2019, https://longreads.com/2019/05/22/an-audience-of -athletes-the-rise-and-fall-of-feminist-sports/.

30. Brian Pronger, *Body Fascism: Salvation in the Technology of Physical Fitness* (Toronto: University of Toronto Press, 2002): 336.

Chapter Twenty-Two

1. Lavinia Errico, interview with author, April 29, 2021.

2. Lavinia Errico, interview with author.

3. Patricia Moreno, interview with author, September 30, 2015. Moreno, Dash, Martin, and Fox all ended up working at Equinox. One day, Moreno came home to her apartment and found a lock on the door. No one had been paying the rent.

4. Ruth Ryon, "Sports Club/LA: It Shapes Up as the Fitness Taj Mahal," *Los Angeles Times*, August 16, 1987.

5. "The Sports Club Company History," *Funding Universe*, accessed January 6, 2022, http://www.fundinguniverse.com/company-histories/the-sports -club-company-history/.

6. Susan Edelman, "He Took Dumbbells to Court and Won," *New York Post,* January 3, 2001.

7. "The Sports Club Company History."

8. I worked at the front desk of this gym from 1998 to 2000.

9. Jennifer Steinhauer, "For Aerobics Die-Hards, There Are No Substitutes," *New York Times,* February 22, 1995.

10. Juliann Sivulka, *Soap, Sex and Cigarettes: A Cultural History of Advertising* (New York: Cengage Learning, 2011): 311.

11. "Doing It," *New York Daily News,* March 5, 1995.

12. Lavinia Errico, interview with author.

13. Pat Stein, "Personal Trainers," *North County Blade-Citizen,* July 25, 1990.

14. George Sauerberg, "Just Do It! A Personal Trainer Adds the Push You May Need," *Gazette* (Cedar Rapids), January 9, 1994.

15. Jennifer Smith Maguire, *Fit for Consumption: Sociology and the Business of Fitness* (Abingdon, UK: Routledge, 2008): 149.

16. "Spanning the Years," *IDEA Fitness Journal,* July–August 2017: 20–35, https://www.ideafit.com/wp-content/uploads/files/IDEA-35year-timeline-01.pdf

17. Maguire, *Fit for Consumption,* 170.

18. Maguire, 172.

19. Kate Dwyer, "The Way We Worked Out," *New York Times,* February 24, 2021.

20. "IDEA Code of Ethics," *IDEA Personal Trainer,* July 2000: 59.

21. Kathie and Peter Davis, "Stand Out from the Crowd," *IDEA Personal Trainer,* October 1996: 2.

22. Paulo Murillo, "Throwback to the Athletic Club West Hollywood," *Weho Times,* April 5, 2018.

23. Sherry Angel, "Builders Get Exercised over Rooms for Fitness," *Los Angeles Times,* June 23, 1990.

24. Stein, "Personal Trainers."

25. National Association for Sport and Physical Education, Shape of the Nation 1993: A Survey of State Physical Education Requirements, Reston, VA: American Alliance for Health, Physical Education, Recreation and Dance, 1993: 1, 3, 4, https://files.eric.ed.gov/fulltext/ED366554.pdf.

26. National Association for Sport and Physical Education, 2.

27. California Bureau of Publications, *Toward a State of Esteem. The Final Report of the California Task Force to Promote Self-Esteem and Personal and Social Responsibility,* Sacramento: California State Department of Education, January 1990: 37, https://files.eric.ed.gov/fulltext/ED321170.pdf.

28. California Bureau of Publications, 51.

29. Office of the Surgeon General, *The Surgeon General's Call to Action to Prevent Overweight and Obesity,* Washington, DC: Department of Health and Human Services, 2001.

30. "Afro-American Healthcare: Why It's a Crisis," *Afro American Gazette,* September 1, 1991.

31. Jonathan M. Metzl and Anna Kirkland, eds., *Against Health: How Health Became the New Morality* (New York: New York University Press, 2010): 2.

Part Seven

1. Jack LaLanne on *The Larry King Show*, 2000, via Jim Magnet Man, "Larry King Jack Lalanne 2000," posted February 13, 2020, YouTube video, 29:42, https://www.youtube.com/watch?v=VXsntOwj-AA.
2. Jason Kelly, *Sweat Equity: Inside the New Economy of Mind and Body* (New York: Wiley, 2016).

Chapter Twenty-Three

1. Annbeth Eschbach, interview with author, December 17, 2015; Fred Devito, interview with author, December 8, 2015; "Yoga Statistics and Demographics," compiled by Trisha Lamb, Prescott, AZ: International Association of Yoga Therapists, 2004, updated 2006: 2, 5.
2. Brittany Kleyn, "The Girls: Where Are They Now?," *Morning Chalk Up*, August 26, 2019.
3. "Yoga Statistics and Demographics," 11.
4. Bill Osgerby, "The Bachelor Pad as Cultural Icon: Masculinity, Consumption, and Interior Design in American Men's Magazines, 1930–65," *Journal of Design History* 18, no. 1 (Spring 2005): 99–113.
5. US census bureau data cited in David Yanofsky, "US Imports of Women's Pants," *Atlas*, 2018, https://theatlas.com/charts/GmCUr1ngH.
6. Jeannine Stein, "Mid-Career Stretches," *Los Angeles Times*, April 21, 2003.

Chapter Twenty-Four

1. Ethel L. Mickey, "'Eat, Pray, Love' Bullshit: Women's Empowerment through Wellness at an Elite Professional Conference," *Journal of Contemporary Ethnography* 48, no. 1 (2019): 103–27.
2. Sam Yo, "Why I Went from Monk to Motivator," *Peloton Blog*, November 13, 2020, https://blog.onepeloton.com/sam-yo-motivation/.
3. Colleen Flaherty, "The Vanishing History Major," *Inside Higher Education*, November 27, 2018.
4. "Gym, Health, and Fitness Clubs in the U.S.: Market Size, 2002–2027," *IBIS World*, updated October 25, 2021, https://www.ibisworld.com/industry-statistics/market-size/gym-health-fitness-clubs-united-states/.
5. Lavinia Errico, interview with author, April 29, 2021.
6. Katherine Rosman, "The Hilaria Baldwin Story: I'm Living My Life," *New York Times*, December 30, 2020.

7. Rachel Sherman, *Uneasy Street: The Anxieties of Affluence* (Princeton, NJ: Princeton University Press, 2017).

8. Steve Stoute, *The Tanning of America: How Hip-Hop Created a Culture that Rewrote the Rules of the New Economy* (New York: Penguin, 2011).

9. Nancy Dahlberg, "How Zumba Still Rocks the Fitness World," *Miami Herald*, August 26, 2018.

10. Natalia Mehlman Petrzela, "Conbody's Success is Forcing the Fitness World to Confront Some Uncomfortable Truths," *Well + Good*, April 11, 2018, https://www.wellandgood.com/why-conbody-prison-workout-is-so-popular/.

11. Abby Ellin, "Disabled, and Shut Out at the Gym," *New York Times*, February 9, 2006.

Chapter Twenty-Five

1. "Running with President George W. Bush," *Runner's World*, October 1, 2002.

2. Matea Gold and Kathleen Hennessey, "Michelle Obama's Nutrition Campaign Comes with Political Pitfalls," *Los Angeles Times*, July 20, 2013.

3. W. Wayt Gibbs, "Obesity: An Overblown Epidemic?," *Scientific American*, December 1, 2006.

4. Julia Belluz, "Donald Trump Thinks Exercise Will Kill You," *Vox*, May 9, 2017.

5. Natalia Mehlman Petrzela, "Why Donald Trump's Diet is Bad for America's Health," *Washington Post*, June 28, 2017.

6. Rachel Louise Moran, "Change We Need? Why the Name of the President's Fitness Council Matters," *Nursing Clio*, May 8, 2018, https://nursingclio.org/2018/05/08/change-we-need-why-the-name-of-the-presidents-fitness-council-matters/.

7. Natalia Mehlman Petrzela, "Why Wellness Has Always Played an Important Role in Politics and Activism," *Well + Good*, November 18, 2016, https://www.wellandgood.com/wellness-and-politics-post-election-trump/.

8. "How to Start a Gang: The Co-Op Gym," *Radix Journal*, January 6, 2013.

9. Daniel Duane, "How the Other Half Lifts," *Pacific Standard*, July 23, 2014.

10. Patrick Wyman, "Bro Culture, Fitness, Chivalry, and American Identity," *Perspectives: Past, Present, and Future*, Substack newsletter, December 4, 2020, https://patrickwyman.substack.com/p/bro-culture-fitness-chivalry-and.

11. Wyman, "Bro Culture, Fitness, Chivalry, and American Identity."

12. Julia Craven, "How Disturbing Was Marjorie Taylor Greene's Workout Video?," *Slate*, April 1, 2021.

13. Lola Fadhu, "Trump Targets Michelle Obama's School Nutrition Guidelines on Her Birthday," *New York Times*, January 17, 2020.

Chapter Twenty-Six

1. Amanda Mull, "Peloton Doesn't Understand the People Who Love It Most," *Atlantic*, December 5, 2019.

2. Virginia Sole-Smith, "Can The Fitness Industry and Body Positivity Coexist?," *Elemental*, January 15, 2020.
3. CNBC Television, "SoulCycle Co-Founder Ruth Zukerman on Peloton's Holiday Ad Controversy," *Squawk Alley*, aired December 5, 2019, on CNBC, posted December 6, 2019, YouTube video, 4:53, https://www.youtube.com /watch?v=YolYFIliDjg.
4. "A Message from Our CEO and Co-Founder, John Foley," *Output Blog*, June 23, 2020, https://blog.onepeloton.com/peloton-pledge/.
5. Jade Sciponi, "59% of Americans Don't Plan to Renew Their Gym Memberships after Covid-19 Pandemic: Survey," *CNBC*, July 23, 2020, https://www .cnbc.com/2020/07/23/many-dont-plan-to-renew-their-gym-memberships -post-pandemic-survey.html.
6. Lauren Thomas, "Americans are Heading Back to Gyms as Interest in At-Home Workouts Wanes, Jefferies Says," *CNBC*, June 18, 2021, https://www .cnbc.com/2021/06/18/americans-back-to-gyms-interest-in-at-home-workout -wanes-jefferies.html.

Chapter Twenty-Seven

1. Michelle Goldberg, "The Brutal Economics of Being a Yoga Teacher," *Cut*, October 8, 2015, https://www.thecut.com/2015/10/brutal-economics-of-being -a-yoga-teacher.html.
2. Matt Hart, "Does CrossFit Have a Future?," *New Yorker*, July 20, 2021, https:// www.newyorker.com/sports/sporting-scene/does-crossfit-have-a-future.
3. Alice Hines, "Inside Core Power Yoga Teacher Training," *New York Times*, April 6, 2019.
4. Colin Moynihan, "The Yoga Instructors vs. the Private Equity Firm," *New York Times*, September 11, 2019; Sarah Jones, "Yoga Teachers are Unionizing to Heal the Wellness Industry," *Cut*, September 12, 2019, https://www.thecut .com/2019/09/yogaworks-teachers-first-yoga-teacher-union.html.
5. Brett Williams, "Fitness Workers Are Organizing to Flex More Muscles in Their Workplaces," *Men's Health*, December 9, 2020.
6. Edward Ongweso Jr., "Amazon Calls Workers 'Industrial Athletes' in Leaked Wellness Pamphlet," *VICE*, June 1, 2021.
7. Richard Florida and Alistair Boone, "Boutique Fitness is Remaking American Neighborhoods," *Atlantic*, January 5, 2018.
8. Rodney J. Morris and Pamela Kufahl, "Addressing Racism in the Fitness Industry Requires Understanding Its Roots," *Club Industry*, October 7, 2020, https://www.clubindustry.com/leadership-management/addressing -racism-fitness-industry-requires-understanding-its-roots.
9. Morris and Kufahl.
10. Gerard du Cann, "Sick Victim Shaming," *Sun*, August 25, 2018.
11. Alex Abad-Santos, "How SoulCycle Lost its Soul," *Vox*, December 23, 2020.

12. Nicholas Rizzo, "77 Gym Membership Statistics, Facts, and Trends 2020/21," *RunRepeat*, June 4, 2021.

13. Barbara Ehrenreich, *Natural Causes: An Epidemic of Wellness, the Certainty of Dying, and Our Illusion of Control* (New York: Hachette, 2018): 161–62.

14. Lenore Bell, "No Excuses: The Supercrip in Three Snapshots," *Nursing Clio*, May 2, 2017.

15. Shannon Vogler, "Implementing Fitness Programs for People with Disabilities," IHRSA blog, April 26, 2018, https://www.ihrsa.org/improve-your-club /implementing-fitness-programs-for-people-with-disabilities/.

16. SHAPE America/NAKHE, *Joint Position Statement from the Society of Health and Physical Educators and the National Association for Kinesiology in Higher Education—Student Recruitment to Physical Education and Health Education Teacher Education Programs*, Reston, VA: SHAPE America, 2018, https://www .shapeamerica.org/standards/guidelines/upload/SA-NAKHE_Student%20 _Recruitment_Position_Statement.pdf.

Bibliography

Archives

American Council on Education Papers, Hoover Institution, Stanford University, Stanford, CA

Bentley Historical Library, University of Michigan, Ann Arbor, MI

Carol Scott Personal Archive, New York, NY

Department of Nike Archives (DNA), Nike, Inc., Beaverton, OR

H. J. Lutcher Stark Center for Physical Culture and Sports, University of Texas at Austin, Austin, TX

Huell Howser Archives, Chapman University, Orange, CA

Jogbra, Inc. Records, Smithsonian Institution, Washington, DC

John F. Kennedy papers, JFK Presidential Library, Boston, MA

John W. Hartman Center for Sales, Advertising, and Marketing History, Duke University Libraries, Durham, NC

Judi Sheppard Missett Personal Archive, San Diego, CA

LA84 Foundation Archive, Los Angeles, CA

Leslie Kaminoff Personal Archive, New York, NY

Library of Congress Prints and Photographs Division, Washington, DC

Los Angeles Times Photographic Archive, Charles E. Young Research Library, University of California at Los Angeles, Los Angeles, CA

Marjorie L. Shuer Papers, Department of Special Collections and University Archives, Stanford University Libraries, Stanford, CA

Molly Fox Personal Archive, Palo Alto, CA

National Intramural and Recreational Sports Association Archive, Corvallis, OR

SHAPE America Archives, Springfield College Archives and Special Collections, Springfield, MA

University of North Texas Digital Collections, Denton, TX

Valley Times Collection, Los Angeles Public Library, Los Angeles, CA

Interviews

Emma Barry, October 12, 2020

Judith Berlin, October 22, 2015

Joan Breibart, July 7, 2020

Monique Dash, February 25, 2021

Peter and Kathie Davis, March 9, 2020

Fred DeVito, December 8, 2015

Lavinia Errico, April 29, 2021

Annbeth Eschbach, December 17, 2015

Amanda Freeman, October 9, 2020

Molly Fox, November 12, 2015

Elisabeth Halfpapp, October 2, 2015

Gilad Janklowicz, November 4, 2015

Leslie Kaminoff, May 31, 2016

Will Lanier, January 18, 2016

Jeff Martin, March 8, 2021

Melissa McNeese, August 20, 2015

Patricia Moreno, September 30, 2015

Brian Moss, November 5, 2020

Michael Perron, October 20, 2015

Cyndy Poor, October 6, 2017

Cal Pozo, August 31, 2015

Timothy Pytell, June 26, 2020

Carol Scott, March 11, 2020

Judith Sheppard Missett, August 28, 2015, and April 22, 2019

Rachel Sibony, December 15, 2015

Kathy Smith, December 9, 2019

Kira Stokes, October 20, 2015

Rick Stollmeyer, October 9, 2020

Tamilee Webb, September 15, 2015

Norm Zwail, August 18, 2015

Primary Sources

Adams, Arthur S. Arthur S. Adams to Katherine McBride, June 29, 1956. American Council on Education papers, box 278, folder 7, Hoover Institution, Stanford University, Stanford, CA.

AIDS.gov. "A Timeline of HIV/AIDS." 2016. https://www.hiv.gov /sites/default/files/aidsgov-timeline.pdf.

"A Message from our CEO and Co-Founder, John Foley." *Output Blog*, June 23, 2020. https://blog.onepeloton.com /peloton-pledge/.

Andrews, Valerie. *The Psychic Power of Running: How the Body Can Illuminate the Mysteries of the Mind.* New York: Rawson Wade, 1978.

Atlas, Charles. "You Get Proof the First 7 Days—I Can Make This NEW MAN of You." Advertisement, 1930. https://www.charles atlas.com/classicads.html.

Avirgan, Jody, and Hillary Frank. "Six Who Sat." October 30, 2018. In *30 for 30 Podcasts*, produced by Jody Avirgan and Erin Leyden. ESPN and Transmitter Media. MP3 audio, 46:46. Transcript available at https://30for30podcasts.com/episodes /six-who-sat/#transcript.

Bach, Lydia. *The Lotte Berk Method, Formerly Called Awake! Aware! Alive!* New York: Random House, 1973.

"Battle of the Bulges." *British Pathé*, January 13, 1941. MP4 video, 51:00. https://www.britishpathe.com/video/battle-of-the-bulges.

Beecher, Catherine. *Miss Beecher's Housekeeper and Healthkeeper.* New York: Harper & Brothers, 1873.

Behr, Felicia Minei, exec. prod. *All My Children*. Episode 5699. Aired January 8, 1992, on ABC. https://archive.org/details/AllMy Children199201JanThruMay16.8Gb.

Bohlander, Alexander, and Verena Geweniger. *Pilates—A Teacher's Manual*. New York: Springer, 2014.

Bowerman, William J., and W. E. Harris. *Jogging*. New York: Grosset and Dunlap, 1967.

Bowling, Daniel. Letter to Leslie Kaminoff, May 10, 1995. Leslie Kaminoff personal archive.

Bulletin 58, no. 3 (Winter 1985): 11. Springfield College Archives and Special Collections. https://cdm16122.contentdm.oclc.org /digital/collection/p16122coll3/id/14754/rec/3.

Butler, George, and Robert Flore, dirs. *Pumping Iron*. 1977; New York: White Mountain Films.

Butler, Katy. "Bite by Bite, the Croissant Culture Is Swallowing Up the Ghettos." *Los Angeles Times*, August 24, 1980.

California Bureau of Publications. *Toward a State of Esteem: The Final Report of the California Task Force to Promote Self-Esteem and Personal and Social Responsibility*. Sacramento: California State Department of Education, January 1990. https://files.eric .ed.gov/fulltext/ED321170.pdf.

Cardone, Daniel F., dir. *Desert Migration*. Produced by the HIV Story Project. 2015; Warren, NJ: Passion River Films.

Carlisle, Kevin, dir. *Do It Debbie's Way*. Home exercise video. 1983; Los Angeles, CA: Paul Brownstein Productions.

Catalysts: The Power of Women in Sport. Internal report, March 2014. Department of Nike Archives, Nike Inc., Beaverton, OR.

Cazden, Leni, and Jane Fonda. Interview by Willa Paskin. "Jane Fonda's Workout, Part 1: Jane and Leni." October 13, 2020. In *Decoder Ring*, produced by Benjamin Frisch, podcast. MP3 audio, 54:32. https://slate.com/podcasts/decoder-ring/2020/10 /jane-fonda-leni-cazden.

Chaplain, D. D. Letter to the editor. *Marine Corps Gazette* 44, no. 5 (May 1960).

Chappell, Eleanor, and Kathryn Huss. *Your Good Health*. Garden City, NY: Nelson Doubleday, 1966.

Cher News. "Cher—Jack LaLanne Health Spa Commercial (1986)." Posted August 26, 2018. YouTube video, 0:30. https://www.you tube.com/watch?v=uq9-1O59pW8.

Chiappetta, Vincent. Interview by Roger Robinson. *Gotta Run with Will*. Episode 378, "Vincent Chiappetta." Released June 20, 2019, on Manhattan Neighborhood Network. YouTube video, 43:18. https://www.youtube.com/watch?v=7ttfyVAiopg&t=1074s.

Chiappetta, Vincent. "Profile—Vince Chiappetta Has Been Running for 71 Years." Interview. *Lifetime Running*, August 2019. https://www.lifetimerunning.net/2019/08/august-2019-vincent -chiappetta-co.html.

Chow, Broderick. "Idle Training: Scenes of Pleasure at Muscle Beach, 1934–1958." Talk presented at the Brunel Performance Research Seminar, Brunel University, London, UK, October 31, 2018. YouTube video, 42:17. https://youtu.be/-uEBvxx8iKI.

CNBC Television. "SoulCycle Co-Founder Ruth Zukerman on Peloton's Holiday Ad Controversy." *Squawk Alley*, aired December 5, 2019, on CNBC. Posted December 6, 2019. YouTube video, 4:53. https://www.youtube.com/watch?v=YolYFIliDjg.

Control Your Emotions. Glenview, IL: Coronet Films, 1950. 13:07. https://archive.org/details/ControlY1950.

Cooper, Kenneth. *Aerobics*. Philadelphia: M. Evans/Lippincott, 1968.

Cooper, Kenneth. *The New Aerobics*. New York: Bantam Books, 1970.

Crampton, C. Ward. *The Daily Health Builder*. New York: Knickerbocker Press, 1928.

Curtis, Adam, dir. *The Century of the Self*. Documentary series, four episodes, total runtime 240 min. Aired 2002 on BBC Two.

Dell, Stewart, dir. "Warm Up to Traci Lords."1990; White Nights Productions. MP4 video, 47:02. https://ia801903.us.archive.org/7 /items/WarmUpToTraciLordsExerciseVideo1990/Warm%20Up %20to%20Traci%20Lords%21%20%28Exercise%20Video%20 1990%29.mp4.

De Noia, Nick, dir. *Muscle Motion*. 1983; Los Angeles: Media Home Entertainment.

Dewey, John. *Democracy and Education*. New York: Macmillan, 1916; Project Gutenberg, 2008. https://www.gutenberg.org /files/852/852-h/852-h.html.

Drakeley, W. B. J. "Physical Fitness." *Marine Corps Gazette* (Quantico: Marine Corps Association) 40, no. 9 (September 1956):16–20.

ECA Fitness Convention brochure. 2000. Carol Scott personal archive.

Ehrlich, Judd, dir. *Run for Your Life: The Fred Lebow Story*. Documentary. 2008. Brooklyn, NY: Flatbush Pictures.

Elizabeth Arden Salon advertisement. October 1944. Duke University Ad Archives, Durham, NC. https://idn.duke.edu/ark:/87924 /r4mk65w0h.

Executive Order No. 10673—Fitness of American Youth. 21 FR 5341 (July 18, 1956).

Executive Order No. 10830—Establishing a Seal for the President's Council on Physical Fitness and Sports. 24 FR 5985, 3 CFR (1959–63).

Executive Order No. 11398—Establishing the President's Council on Physical Fitness and Sports. 33 FR 4169 (March 4, 1968).

Executive Order No. 11562—Developing and Coordinating a National Program for Physical Fitness and Sports. 35 FR 15063 (September 25, 1970).

"Fact Sheets: President's Conference on the Fitness of American Youth." Annapolis, MD: US Naval Academy, June 18–19, 1956. American Council on Education papers, box 278, folder 7. Hoover Institution, Stanford University, Stanford, CA.

Fixx, Jim. *The Complete Book of Running*. New York: Random House, 1977.

Fonda, Jane. *Jane Fonda's Workout Book*. New York: Simon and Schuster, 1981.

Fonda, Jane. *My Life So Far*. New York: Random House, 2005.

Gaines, Charles. *Stay Hungry*. New York: Doubleday, 1972.

Gaines, Charles. *Staying Hard*. New York: Kenan Press, 1980.

Goldfield, Edwin D., ed. *Statistical Abstract of the United States: 1960*. Washington, DC: US Government Printing Office, 1960. https://www.census.gov/library/publications/1960/compendia /statab/81ed.html.

"Guide to the Jogbra, Inc. Records: Biographical/Historical."
Jogbra, Inc. records, Archives Center, National Museum of
American History, Smithsonian Institution, Washington, DC.
Accessed February 25, 2022. https://sova.si.edu/record/NMAH
.AC.1315#Biographical%20/%20Historical.

"Gym, Health, and Fitness Clubs in the U.S.: Market Size, 2002–
2027." *IBIS World*, updated October 25, 2021. https://www
.ibisworld.com/industry-statistics/market-size/gym-health
-fitness-clubs-united-states/.

Hall, G. Stanley. *Adolescence*. New York: D. Appleton and Company, 1904. https://archive.org/details/adolescenceitsp01
hallgoog/page/410/mode/2up.

Hamilton, Thomas J. "Review of Group Summaries." Published
proceedings of the Sports for Fitness Forum, President's Council on Youth Fitness, April 13, 1960, Chicago, IL.

Heald, Henry T. "NYU's Ten-Year Program to Extend Its Educational and Physical Facilities." WNYC radio broadcast. New
York: November 18, 1952. 13:25. NYC Municipal Archives
WNYC Collection, WNYC archive ID no. 68617. https://www
.wnyc.org/story/henry-t-heald-nyus-ten-year-program-to
-extend-its-educational-and-physical-facilities/.

Helsing, Kathleen. "Stress Free Zone." Two-week series. *Los Angeles Times*, August 17, 1998.

How Michael Jordan Jumpstarted Nike. Internal report, October
2014. Department of Nike Archives, Nike Inc., Beaverton, OR.

Howser, Huell, and KCET Los Angeles, prods. *California's Gold*.
Episode 1007, "Muscle Beach." Aired January 8, 1999, on
California Public Television. https://blogs.chapman.edu/huell
-howser-archives/1999/01/08/muscle-beach-californias
-gold-1007/.

Huey, Lynda. *A Running Start: An Athlete, A Woman*. New York:
Crown, 1976.

Institute for the Scientific Investigation of Sexuality. *Criminality,
Social Disruption, and Homosexuality: Homosexuality Is a Crime
against Humanity*. Pamphlet, 1985. University of North Texas

Digital Collections. https://digital.library.unt.edu/ark:/67531
/metadc276206.

"In the Matter of Stauffer Laboratories, Inc., et al." In *Federal
Trade Commission Decisions*, vol. 64. (Washington, DC: US Government Printing Office, 1964): 629–60. https://www.ftc.gov
/sites/default/files/documents/commission_decision_volumes
/volume-64/ftcd-vol64january-march1964pages629-715.pdf.

"In the Matter of Sinkram Incorporated, et al." In *Federal Trade
Commission Decisions*, vol. 64 (Washington, DC: US Government
Printing Office, 1964): 1243–73. https://www.ftc.gov/sites/default
/files/documents/commission_decision_volumes/volume-64
/ftcd-vol64january-march1964pages1150-1273.pdf.

Ischemic Attack. "Richard Bey," segment from *The Richard Bey
Show*, ca. 1990s, posted January 19, 2012. YouTube video, 4:17.
https://www.youtube.com/watch?v=sy8hdyRVUmk.

"It's Time for Americans to Get Back on Our Feet." American
Dairy Association announcement. *Broadcasting*, October 2,
1961: 96.

"Jack Be Nimble, Jack Be Quick." Presidential Council on Fitness
advertisement. *New York Times*, February 12, 1962.

Jack Benny Program. Season 11, episode 16, "Jack Goes to a Gym."
February 5, 1961. https://www.youtube.com/watch?v
=nOaGizGNqvU.

Jacklalanneofficial. "Jack LaLanne Fan Mail Cards, Letters and
Advice. Facial Exercise." From *The Jack LaLanne Show*, ca. mid-
1950s. Posted September 17, 2017. YouTube video, 5:17. https://
www.youtube.com/watch?v=FGSeminZqhg.

Jacklalanneofficial. "The Jack LaLanne Full Episode (Hangovers)."
Ca. mid-1950s. Posted January 18, 2016. YouTube video, 24:06.
https://www.youtube.com/watch?v=tP40RWwhoRw.

Jack LaLanne Show advertisement. WSIX-TV Nashville. *Nashville
Tennessean*, September 25, 1960.

Jim Magnet Man. "Larry King Jack Lalanne 2000." Posted February 13, 2020. YouTube video, 29:42. https://www.youtube.com
/watch?v=VXsntOwj-AA.

Jogbra advertisement, ca. 1980. Jogbra, Inc. records. Promotional and Marketing Materials, Archives Center, National Museum of American History, Smithsonian Institution, Washington, DC. File name AC1315-0000026-02.tif. https://edan.si.edu/slideshow /viewer/?eadrefid=NMAH.AC.1315_ref173.

John F. Kennedy and Jacqueline Bouvier Pose on the Tennis Court at the Joseph P. Kennedy Residence during the "Engagement Weekend." June 26–28, 1953, Hyannis Port, MA. Photographer unknown. Accession no. KFC3049P, John F. Kennedy Presidential Library and Museum, Boston, MA. https://www.jfklibrary.org/learn /about-jfk/media-gallery/sports-and-recreation.

Jones, Douglas. *Robert, John, and Edward Kennedy in the Surf at Palm Beach, Florida, April 1957.* April 1957. Photograph for *LOOK* magazine. Accession no. PX 65–105:165, John F. Kennedy Presidential Library and Museum, Boston, MA. https://www.jfkli brary.org/learn/about-jfk/media-gallery/sports-and-recreation.

"Keep Your Child Fit from Birth to Six." Print advertisement. *New York Times,* June 21, 1964.

Kehoe, Simon D. *Indian Clubs and How to Use Them.* New York: Peck and Snyder, 1866.

Kelly, Jason. *Sweat Equity: Inside the New Economy of Mind and Body.* New York: Wiley, 2016.

Kelly, Philip J. *How to Grow Old Rebelliously.* New York: Fleet Pub. Corp, 1963.

Laskey, Anne. *Jack LaLanne's European Health Spa, Wilshire Boulevard.* 1978. Photographic color slide, 5 × 5 cm. Marlene and Anne Laskey Wilshire Boulevard Collection, Los Angeles Photographers Collection, Digital Collections of the Los Angeles Public Library. https://tessa.lapl.org/cdm/ref/collection/photos /id/121567.

Leonard, Gary. *1988 Los Angeles Marathon on Sunset Boulevard.* 1988. Photographic print, black and white, 29 × 36 cm. Los Angeles Neighborhoods Collection, Digital Collections of the Los Angeles Public Library. https://tessa.lapl.org/cdm/ref/collection /photos/id/3840.

"Let's Get the Kinks out of the Kids." Presidential Council on Youth Fitness advertisement. *New York Times*, February 5, 1962.

lizmcg83. "*Everyday with Richard Simmons*—Opening Scene at Diner." Posted July 25, 2010. YouTube video, 1:21. https://www.youtube.com/watch?v=4aCdfg0h-Sc.

Lynch, A. "Evaluating School Health Programs." In *Health Services: The Local Perspective*, edited by A. Levin, 89–105. New York: Academy of Political Science, Proceedings of the Academy of Political Science, 1977.

MacCarthy, Shane, Executive Director, President's Council on Youth Fitness. Keynote presentation. Published proceedings of the Sports for Fitness Forum. President's Council on Youth Fitness, April 13, 1960, Chicago, IL.

MacFadden, Marguerite, and Bernarr Adolphus MacFadden. *Physical Culture for Babies*. New York: Physical Culture, 1904.

Martyn, Marguerite. "'The Lady Hercules' Tells Marguerite Martyn." *St. Louis Post-Dispatch*, June 4, 1911.

Marx, Gilda. *Body by Gilda: Redesign Every Line*. New York: G. P. Putnam's Sons, 1984.

McFadden, Bernarr. *The Power and Beauty of Superb Womanhood*. New York: Physical Culture, 1901.

Medvin, Jeannine O'Brien. *Prenatal Yoga and Natural Birth*. Felton, CA: Freestone, 1974.

MemoryMuseum. "Cher 1985 Jack LaLanne Gym Commercial." Posted October 8, 2014. YouTube video, 0:30. https://www.youtube.com/watch?v=_ljz4omRDHk.

Mitchell, Elmer D. *Intramural Athletics*. New York: A. S. Barnes and Company, 1934.

Trevor, Charles T. *Muscular Manhood: Pictorial Studies of the Athletic Male*. Kenton: C. T. Trevor, 1943.

National Association for Sport and Physical Education. *Shape of the Nation 1993: A Survey of State Physical Education Requirements*. Reston, VA: American Alliance for Health, Physical Education, Recreation and Dance, 1993. https://files.eric.ed.gov/fulltext/ED366554.pdf.

Nidetch, Jean. *Weight Watchers: The Memoir of a Successful Loser.* New York: Signet Classics, 1972.

Nixon, Richard, and Nikita Khrushchev. "The Kitchen Debate." Transcript. US Embassy, Moscow, Soviet Union, July 24, 1959. https://www.cia.gov/readingroom/docs/1959-07-24.pdf.

"Nobody Asked You!" Presidential Council on Youth Fitness advertisement. *New York Times*, January 8, 1962.

"No Fitness in Schools." Editorial. *Milwaukee Star*, June 5, 1968.

"NY Gym Owners File Class-Action Suit against Governor Cuomo." *Fox and Friends*. Aired October 19, 2020, on Fox News. https://video.foxnews.com/v/6202454284001#sp=show-clips.

Office of the Surgeon General. *The Surgeon General's Call to Action to Prevent Overweight and Obesity.* Washington, DC: Department of Health and Human Services, 2001.

Orbach, Susie. *Fat is a Feminist Issue: A Self-Help Guide for Compulsive Eaters.* New York: Paddington Press, 1978.

"Our Children Pioneers?" Presidential Council on Fitness advertisement, *Parents Magazine and Better Homemaking*, July 1965.

Parkway Athletic Club advertisements. *This Week in Texas*, March 11–17, May 6–12, July 15–21, July 29–August 4, 1988. http://www.houstonlgbthistory.org/misc-jims.html.

Passon, Ted, dir. *Worn Stories*. Season 1, episode 7, "Survival." Released April 1, 2021, on Netflix.

Peale, Norman Vincent. *The Power of Positive Thinking: A Practical Guide to Mastering the Problems of Everyday Living.* New York: Touchstone, 1952.

Peters, Lulu Hunt. *Diet and Health—With Key to the Calories.* Chicago: Reilly and Lee, 1918.

Portugal, Pamela Rainbear. *A Place for Human Beings.* 2nd ed. San Francisco: Homegrown Books, 1978.

President's Council on Youth Fitness. "A Community Project: Youth Fitness, What A Community Can Do for Fitness." Washington, DC: President's Council on Youth Fitness, 1959.

President's Council on Youth Fitness. "Focus on Fitness." Pamphlet. Washington, DC: President's Council on Youth Fitness, 1960.

President's Council on Youth Fitness. "Recreation: Workshop Report 1." Washington, DC: President's Council on Youth Fitness, November 23, 1959.

Prior, David A., dir. *Aerobicide*. Later renamed *Killer Workout*. 1987; Hollywood, CA: Shapiro Entertainment.

Prudden, Bonnie. *How to Keep Slender and Fit after Thirty*. New York: Random House, 1961.

Rafelson, Bob, dir. *Stay Hungry*. 1976; Hollywood, CA: United Artists.

Rancho la Puerta brochure. 1975. Anspach Travel Bureau Collection of Tourism Literature, 1936–2014, 145 General Files, Baja 1971–1998. John W. Hartman Center, Duke University, Durham, NC.

"Record and Disclosure of Invention, 'Jock Bra.'" October 14, 1977. Jogbra, Inc. records, Archives Center, National Museum of American History, Smithsonian Institution, Washington, DC. https://sova.si.edu/details/NMAH.AC.1315#ref273.

"Recreation: A New Profession for Our Time." Illustrated leaflet. Washington, DC: American Association for Health, Physical Education and Recreation, 1955.

Rivera, Geraldo. *The Geraldo Show*. "Women's Bodybuilding: Sweat, Stigma and Steroids." 1990. Dailymotion video, 43:15. https://www.dailymotion.com/video/x5p0nlf.

Rizzo, Nicholas. "77 Gym Membership Statistics, Facts, and Trends 2020/21." *RunRepeat*, June 4, 2021.

Rodriguez, Melissa. "Fitness Industry Still Feels Covid's Negative Impact." *IHRSA Today*, June 3, 2021. https://www.ihrsa.org /improve-your-club/fitness-industry-still-feels-covids -negative-impact/.

Rohe, Fred. *The Zen of Running*. New York: Random House, 1974.

Sanchez, Will. "Vincent Chiappetta, a Co-Founder of the NYC Marathon, Guest Stars." Posted June 15, 2019. YouTube video, 43:18. https://www.youtube.com/watch?v=7ttfyVAiopg.

Sandow, Eugen. *Strength and How to Obtain It*. New York: Gale and Polden, 1897. https://www.google.com/books/edition/Strength _and_how_to_Obtain_it/BTyeEqAIpuEC?hl=en&gbpv=1&printsec

=frontcover.Schur, Edwin. *The Awareness Trap: Self-Absorption instead of Social Change.* New York: Quadrangle Books, 1976.

Schultz, Dodi. *Slimming with Yoga.* New York: Bantam, 1968.

SHAPE America/NAKHE. *Joint Position Statement from the Society of Health and Physical Educators and the National Association for Kinesiology in Higher Education Regarding Student Recruitment to Physical Education and Health Education Teacher Education Programs.* Reston, VA, 2018. https://www.shapeamerica.org /standards/guidelines/upload/SA-NAKHE_Student%20_Recruit ment_Position_Statement.pdf.

Shuer, Marjorie. "Title IX: The Spirit of the Times." Unpublished notes, n.d. Marjorie L. Shuer Papers (SCO733), box 1, folder 2. Department of Special Collections and University Archives, Stanford University Libraries, Stanford, CA.

Simmons, Richard. *Reach for Fitness: A Special Book of Exercises for the Physically Challenged.* New York: Grand Central, 1986.

Simmons, Richard. *Still Hungry—After All These Years: My Story.* New York: GT, 1999.

"Six Dimensions of Wellness." National Wellness Institute web-site. Accessed February 24, 2022. https://nationalwellness.org /resources/six-dimensions-of-wellness.

Snap Out of It! (Emotional Balance). Glenview, IL: Coronet Films, 1951. 11:24. https://archive.org/details/SnapOuto1951.

Solomon, Henry A. *The Exercise Myth.* San Diego, CA: Harcourt, 1984.

Speakes, Larry. Press briefing. October 15, 1982. White House Office of the Press Secretary, Washington, DC. Available at the Jon Cohen AIDS Research Collection, University of Michigan. https://quod.lib.umich.edu/c/cohenaids/5571095.0487.001?rgn =main;view=fulltext.

"Spend Ten Minutes a Day and Be as Fit as a Marine." Presiden-tial Council on Fitness advertisement. *New York Times*, Novem-ber 10, 1963.

Stanford Women's Center. "A Guide for Stanford Women, 1972." Stanford, CA: Stanford Women's Center, 1972. Marjorie L. Shuer Papers, box 1, folder 11. Department of Special

Collections and University Archives, Stanford University Libraries, Stanford, CA.

Stockton notes. Samuel Stark theater program collection (M1149). Department of Special Collections and University Archives, Stanford University Libraries, Stanford, CA.

Stoughton, Cecil. *President John F. Kennedy Swims with His Daughter, Caroline (Right), and Niece, Maria Shriver (Center), near Hyannis Port, Massachusetts.* July 28, 1963. White House photographs, color, 35mm. Accession no. ST-C250-15-63, John F. Kennedy Presidential Library and Museum, Boston, MA. https://www .jfklibrary.org/learn/about-jfk/media-gallery/sports-and -recreation.

Sturgeon, Julie, and Janet Meer. "The First Fifty Years: The Presidential Council on Physical Fitness Revisits Its Roots and Charts Its Future." In *President's Council on Physical Fitness and Sports: The First 50 Years: 1956–2006,* ed. Janet Meer, 40–63. Washington, DC: US Department of Health and Human Services, 2006.

Success Story episode. "Stauffer Motorized Couches and Posture-Rest." Directed by Bob Hiestand, sponsored by Richfield Motor Oil, ca. 1957. 29:18. Periscope Film LLC archive. https://www .youtube.com/watch?v=Q3VRs02llq8.

Super Speed System advertisement. Sinkram, Inc., 1962. In "More Headlines Continued," Iron League website, accessed February 26, 2022, https://www.ironleague.com/public/programs/archives. cfm?StartRow=101&show=yes&sort=date&ddesc=all.

Tanny, Vic. Advertisement. *Baltimore Sun,* April 16, 1957.

Tanny, Vic. Advertisement. *Los Angeles Times,* October 2, 1956.

"Teaching Application: Jivamukti Yoga Center, New York City." n.d. Leslie Kaminoff personal archive.

"The Apotheosis of Corpulence." *New York Times,* June 27, 1870.

The Women's Movement. Internal report, May 2012. Department of Nike Archives, Nike Inc., Beaverton, OR.

Thomas, Lauren. "Americans Are Heading Back to Gyms as Interest in At-Home Workouts Wanes, Jefferies Says." *CNBC,* June 18, 2021. https://www.cnbc.com/2021/06/18

/americans-back-to-gyms-interest-in-at-home-workout-wanes
-jefferies.html.

Updike, John. *Rabbit at Rest.* New York: Random House,
1990.

US Department of Commerce, Bureau of the Census. *1980 Census of Population: New York.* Washington, DC: US Government Printing Office, August 1982. https://www2.census.gov
/prod2/decennial/documents/1980/1980censusofpopu80134
unse_bw.pdf.

US Department of Commerce, Bureau of the Census. *1990 Census of Population: New York.* Section 1 of 2. Washington, DC: US Government Printing Office, April 1992. https://www2.census
.gov/library/publications/decennial/1990/cp-1/cp-1-34-1.pdf.

US Department of Education, National Center for Education Statistics. *Chartbook of Degrees Conferred, 1969–70 to 1993–94.* NCES 98-071, project officer Thomas D. Snyder. NCES: Washington, DC, 1997: 101–276. https://nces.ed.gov/pubs98/98071.pdf.

US Department of Education. National Center for Education Statistics, Integrated Postsecondary Education Data System (IPEDS). "Completions." Survey. 2019.

VHS Ark. "Women at Large: Breakout," 1987. Posted May 24, 2017. YouTube video, 1:10:16. https://www.youtube.com
/watch?v=RK0TAHn3-qs.

"West Point Exercises." Advertisement. *Chicago Daily Tribune,* August 25, 1939: 19.

"What's Your Child's Physical I.Q.?" Presidential Council on Fitness advertisement. *New York Times,* March 26, 1962.

Wheat, Valerie, Sue Critchfield, Celeste West, and Carole Leita, eds. "Reviews and Columns." *Booklegger* 2 no. 8 (March/April 1975).

"Winter/Spring Events 1992." *Jivamukti Newsletter.* Leslie Kaminoff personal archive.

"Women Reducing Waist." Advertisement. *Philadelphia Inquirer,* February 5, 1956.

Yogananda, Paramahansa. *Autobiography of a Yogi.* New York: Philosophical Library, 1946.

"Yoga Statistics and Demographics." Compiled by Trisha Lamb. Prescott, AZ: International Association of Yoga Therapists, 2004, updated 2006.

Yo, Sam. "Why I Went from Monk to Motivator." *Peloton Blog*, November 13, 2020. https://blog.onepeloton.com/sam-yo -motivation/.

Zook, Alice. On *Donahue*, 1985. https://archive.org/details/Donahue HSV71985Incomplete.

Zook, Alice. Interview by Bryant Gumbel. *TODAY Show*. Aired May 31, 1984, on NBC.

Secondary Sources and Periodicals

"6-Mile 'Marathon' Slated for Women." *Miami Herald*, May 14, 1972.

Abad-Santos, Alex. "How SoulCycle Lost its Soul." *Vox*, December 23, 2020.

Abbott, Karen. "Score One for Roosevelt." *Smithsonian Magazine*, September 20, 2011. https://www.smithsonianmag.com/history /score-one-for-roosevelt-83762245/.

Acker, Kathy. "Against Ordinary Language: The Language of the Body," in *The Last Sex: Feminism and Outlaw Bodies*, edited by Arthur and Marilouise Kroker, 20–27. London: Palgrave, 1993.

"Afro-American Healthcare: Why It's a Crisis." *Afro-American Gazette*, September 1, 1991.

Alden, Robert. "Advertising: Hard Sell for Muscle Flexing." *New York Times*, June 5, 1960: F12.

"A Little Music Does the Trick." *Chicago Metro News*. March 20, 1982.

Alstad, Diana. "Interpersonal Yoga." *Yoga Journal*, March 1979.

Alvarez, Erick. *Muscle Boys: Gay Gym Culture*. New York: Routledge, 2010.

"Amazing Skin Cream Fades Horrid Age Spots Fast." ESOTÉRICA advertisement. *Charlotte Observer*, October 28, 1956.

Angel, Sherry. "Builders Get Exercised over Rooms for Fitness." *Los Angeles Times*, June 23, 1990.

"And No Spinach . . ." *Los Angeles Times*, August 9, 1942.

"Area Instructors Attend Jazzercise Convention." *Dunn County News*, September 15, 1982.

Ariail, Cat. "'Who Says It Is Not the Most Feminine Thing a Woman Can Do?': The Feminization of Women's Distance Running." *US Sport History Blog*, October 15, 2015. https://ussporthistory.com/2015/10/15/who-says-it-is-not-the-most-feminine-thing-a-woman-can-do-the-feminization-of-womens-distance-running/.

Armegnol, Josep. "Gendering the Great Depression: Rethinking the Male Body in 1930s American Culture and Literature." *Journal of Gender Studies* 23, no. 1 (2014): 59–68.

"Astroyoga." *Yoga Journal*, January–February 1995.

Aubry, Timothy, and Trysh Travis, eds. *Rethinking Therapeutic Culture*. Chicago: University of Chicago Press, 2015.

"Auxiliary Fat Men." *New York Times*, February 24, 1877.

Aziz, Maryam K. "Built with Empty Fists: The Rise and Circulation of Black Power Martial Artistry during the Cold War." PhD diss., University of Michigan, 2020. https://deepblue.lib.umich.edu/bitstream/handle/2027.42/163044/maryamka_1.pdf.

Bakoulis, Gordon. "'It Means the World to Me': Why Crazylegs Runners Keep Coming Back to the Mini." *New York Road Runners*, June 8, 2019. https://www.nyrr.org/run/photos-and-stories/2019/mini-10k-crazylegs.

Ballard, Chris. "Running in the Age of Coronavirus." *Sports Illustrated*, May 21, 2020.

"Balzer's Yoga Teacher Tells of Buddhism Plan." *Los Angeles Times*, March 16, 1956.

Barrow, Clay. "Physically Fit." *Leatherneck* 42, no. 11 (November 1959): 38–47.

Bartel, Pauline. "Women At Large Builds Self-Esteem." *Journal and Courier* (Lafayette, IN), March 29, 1987.

"Beauty Bulletin: Fifty-Mile Hike in Diet Thinking." *Vogue*, April 1, 1963.

"Beefsteak Eaters Beat Vegetarians." *New York Times*, November 15, 1907.

Bell, Lenore. "No Excuses: The Supercrip in Three Snapshots." *Nursing Clio*, May 2, 2017.

Belluz, Julia. "Donald Trump Thinks Exercise Will Kill You." *Vox*, May 9, 2017.

Beno, Dr. James J. Advertisement. *Petoskey News Review*, August 20, 1985.

Beyond Jogging workshop in East Burke, Vermont, advertisement. *Burlington Free Press*, August 13, 1978: 25.

Bilgore, Ellen. "Arthur Jones: Physical Fitness Turns Back the Clock for Nautilus' Inventor." *New Body*, May 1982.

Binkley, Sam. *Getting Loose: Lifestyle Consumption in the 1970s*. Durham, NC: Duke University Press, 2007.

Black, Jonathan. "Charles Atlas: Muscle Man." *Smithsonian Magazine*, August 2009.

Black, Jonathan. *Making the American Body: The Remarkable Saga of the Men and Women Whose Feuds, Feats, and Passions Shaped Fitness History*. Lincoln: University of Nebraska Press, 2013.

Blakely, W. B. J. "Physical Fitness." *Marine Corps Gazette* 40, no. 9 (September 1956).

Bombeck, Erma. "All Manner of Phobias." *Kenosha News* (syndicated), August 19, 1982.

"Books in Review." *Tyler Courier-Times*, June 28, 1959.

Boyd, Herb. "Cop Calls McCutchen a 'Do-Gooder,' Not a 'Hero.'" *Amsterdam News*, September 24, 1994.

Boyle, Hal. "Reporter's Whatnot." *York Dispatch*, January 4, 1962.

Boyle, Robert H. "The Report That Shocked the President." *Sports Illustrated*, August 15, 1955.

Breslin, Catherine. "The Siren Song of Yoga." *Cosmopolitan*, October 1972: 212–16.

Brooks, David. *Bobos in Paradise: The New Upper Class and How They Got There*. New York: Simon and Schuster, 2000.

Brumberg, Joan Jacobs. *The Body Project: An Intimate History of American Girls*. New York: Random House, 1997.

Bucher, Charles A. "Parents Are Urged to Make Yule Toys 'Active.'" *Milwaukee Star*, December 21, 1972.

"Buns Exercise Tapes Heat Up Market by Targeting Body Parts." *Gannett News Service*, March 16, 1993.

Bunzel, Peter. "The Health Kick's High Priest." *LIFE*, September 29, 1958.

Burfoot, Amby. "Who Was That Guy Who Attacked Kathrine Switzer 50 Years Ago?" *Runner's World*, April 10, 2017.

Butler, Jonathan. *Awash in a Sea of Faith: Christianizing the American People*. Cambridge, MA: Harvard University Press, 1992.

Butwin, David. "You Can Get Too Pooped to Ping." *Christian Science Monitor News Service*, January 15, 1978.

Calistro, Paddy. "Yoga Takes Strain for the Stressed." *Calgary Herald*, May 15, 1992.

Campbell, Susan. "Working Out for 'Buns of Steel' Called Futile." *Record*, December 28, 1995.

Cantor, Milton. "Education and the Nineteenth-Century Working Class." In *Work, Recreation, and Culture: Essays in American Labor History*, edited by Martin H. Blatt and Martha K. Norkunas, 125–62. New York: Routledge, 1996.

Carew, Kate. "Barnum and Bailey's 'Strong Woman' Tells Kate Carew—This Young Goddess of the Tan Bark, Who Tosses Her Husband About as She Would a Feather, Explains How She Came By Her Strength." *New York American*, April 16, 1911: 2-M.

Chapman, David L., and Patricia Vertinsky. *Venus with Biceps: A Pictorial History of Muscular Women*. Vancouver: Arsenal Pulp Press, 2011.

Chatelain, Marcia. *Franchise: The Golden Arches in Black America*. New York: Liveright, 2020.

Chauncey, George F. *Gay New York: Gender, Urban Culture, and the Making of the Gay Male World, 1890–1940*. New York: Basic Books, 1994.

Childress, Micah. "Life beyond the Big Top: African American and Female Circusfolk, 18601920." *Journal of the Gilded Age and Progressive Era* 15, no. 2 (April 2016): 176–96.

Clarke, James. *Challenge and Change: A History of the Development of the National Intramural-Recreational Sports Association, 1950–1976*. West Point, NY: Leisure Press, 1978.

"Classical Indian and Chinese Music Ensemble." *LA Weekly*, January 30, 1992.

Cleary, Martin. "Race Has Instant Credibility." *Pittsburgh Press*, June 10, 1980.

Clifford, Marie J. "Helena Rubinstein's Beauty Salons, Fashion, and Modernist Display." *Winterthur Portfolio* 38, no. 2/3 (Summer/Autumn 2003): 83–108.

"Club in Scarsdale Donates its Cub to New Texas Zoo." *New York Times*, October 7, 1971.

Coakley, Michael B. "An Ancient Art." *Courier-Post*, October 22, 1966.

Cochrane, Robert. "You Should Know Jack: A Qualitative Study of the Jack LaLanne Show." MA thesis, University of Nevada, Las Vegas, 2012. https://digitalscholarship.unlv.edu/thesesdissertations/1548/.

Coffey, Margaret. "The Sportswoman—Then and Now." *Journal of Health, Physical Education, and Recreation* 36, no. 2 (February 1965): 38–41.

Condor, Bob. "Fonda Flexes Her Workout Clout with Yoga Tape." *Chicago Tribune*, March 3, 1994.

Connolly, N. D. B. *A World More Concrete: Real Estate and the Remaking of Jim Crow Florida* (Chicago: University of Chicago Press, 2014).

Conran, Shirley. "Do You Want a 24 Waist?" *London Observer*, February 4, 1968.

Cott, Nancy. "What's in a Name? The Limits of Social Feminism; Or, Expanding the Vocabulary of Women's History." *Journal of American History* 76, no. 3 (December 1989): 809–29.

Cox, Billy. "Yoga Master Shares Vision with Brevard." *Florida Today*, January 29, 1999.

Craig, Maxine. *Sorry I Don't Dance: Why Men Refuse to Move*. New York: Oxford University Press, 2014.

Craven, Julia. "How Disturbing Was Marjorie Taylor Greene's Workout Video?" *Slate*, April 2, 2021.

"CSU Adds Exercise Science Classes." *Chico-Enterprise Record*, November 25, 1984.

Cushman, Anne. "Namaste, Jane." *Yoga Journal*, May–June 1994.

Dahlberg, Nancy. "How Zumba Still Rocks the Fitness World." *Miami Herald*, August 26, 2018.

Dannells, Vernyce. "Anita Jackson and the Pilates Method." *Afro Hawaii News*, June 30, 1991.

Davis, Kathie and Peter. "Stand Out from the Crowd." *IDEA Personal Trainer*, October 1996.

Davis, Rosalind Gray. "Romana Kryzanowska: Pilates Living Legend: An Interview with the World-Renowned Protegee of Joseph Pilates," *Idea Fitness Journal* 4, no. 10 (November/December 2007).

"Debbie Drake, Girl with Beautiful Lines, to Pay Visit." *Birmingham News*, January 16, 1962.

de la Cretaz, Britni. "An Audience of Athletes: The Rise and Fall of Feminist Sports." *Longreads*, May 2019. https://longreads.com/2019/05/22/an-audience-of-athletes-the-rise-and-fall-of-feminist-sports/.

DeLyser, Femmy. *Jane Fonda's Workout Book for Pregnancy, Birth, and Recovery*. New York: Simon and Schuster, 1982.

Desa, Patricia. "Gentle Moves for Firm Muscles." *Prevention*, December 2000.

Desmond, Matthew. *Evicted: Poverty and Profit in the American City*. New York: Crown Books, 2016.

Devienne, Elsa. "The Life, Death, and Rebirth of Muscle Beach: Reassessing the Muscular Physique in Postwar America, 1940s–1980s." *Southern California Quarterly* 100, no. 3 (Fall 2018): 324–67.

Devi, Indra. *Forever Young, Forever Healthy* advertisement. *Chicago Tribune*, October 3, 1954: 190.

Diamond, Pete. "Jim's Gym Reopens Following Fire." *Montrose Voice*, January 10, 1986. http://www.houstonlgbthistory.org/misc-jims.html.

DiLulio, John. "The Coming of the Super-Predators." *Weekly Standard*, November 27, 1995. https://www.washingtonexaminer.com/weekly-standard/the-coming-of-the-super-predators.

Drakeley, W. B. J. "Physical Fitness." *Marine Corps Gazette* 40, no. 9 (September 1956): 16–20.

"Dr. Cooper Keynote Speaker at Aerobics Center Dedication." *Oracle* (Oral Roberts University student newspaper), September 27, 1974.

"Dress for Success in the Fitness Class." *Daily Reporter* (Greenfield, IN), October 17, 1989.

"Doing It." *New York Daily News*, March 5, 1995.

Duane, Daniel. "How the Other Half Lifts." *Pacific Standard*, July 23, 2014.

du Cann, Gerard. "Sick Victim Shaming." *Sun*, August 25, 2018.

Durett, April. "Industry Watch: Trends in Fitness." *IDEA Health and Fitness Source*, March 2000.

Dwyer, Kate. "The Way We Worked Out." *New York Times*, February 24, 2021.

East, Whitfield B. *A Historical Review and Analysis of Military Training and Assessment*. Fort Leavenworth, KS: Combat Studies Institute Press, 2013.

Edelman, Susan. "He Took Dumbbells to Court and Won." *New York Post*, January 3, 2001.

Editorial. *Yoga Journal*, January–February 1980.

Ehrenreich, Barbara. *Natural Causes: An Epidemic of Wellness, the Certainty of Dying, and Our Illusion of Control*. New York: Hachette, 2018.

Eleazar, Frank. "We Must Learn to Lie Down on Job, Indra Devi Says." *Bend Bulletin*, November 6, 1959.

Eller, Daryn. "The New Yoga." *Chicago Tribune*, August 23, 1993.

Ellin, Abby. "Disabled, and Shut Out at the Gym." *New York Times*, February 9, 2006.

Ellison, Jenny. *Being Fat: Women, Weight, and Feminist Activism in Canada*. Toronto: University of Toronto Press, 2020.

Engel, Leonard. "Research Attacks the 'Coronary Plague.'" *New York Times*, November 25, 1956.

"Enjoy Some Free Time." *Central New Jersey Home News*, October 14, 1986.

"Enlist Suffragists for a Circus Holiday: Baby Giraffe Named 'Miss Suffrage' at 'Votes for Women' Rally." *New York Times*, April 1, 1912.

Epstein, Lawrence J. *At the Edge of a Dream: The Story of Immigrants on New York's Lower East Side*. New York: Wiley, 2007.

Eros Lib 1 (Winter 1975). Newsletter. San Diego, CA: Sexual Freedom League, 1975.

Eskenazi, Gerald. "In New York's Marathon, They Also Run Who Only Sit and Wait." *New York Times*, October 2, 1972.

Evans, Caro. "Stress at Work." Letters. *Atlanta Journal*, September 1, 1999.

Evans, Stephanie Y. "Black Women's Historical Wellness." *Association of Black Women Historians*, June 21, 2019. http://abwh .org/2019/06/21/black-womens-historical-wellness-history-as-a -tool-in-culturally-competent-mental-health-services/.

Event announcement. *Honolulu Star-Bulletin*, June 7, 1961.

"Exercise for Beauty's Sake." *Vogue*, November 13, 1926.

Fadhu, Lola. "Trump Targets Michelle Obama's School Nutrition Guidelines on Her Birthday." *New York Times*, January 17, 2020.

Fairfax, Esther. *My Improper Mother and Me*. London: Central Books, 2010.

Farley, Carol. *The Case of the Haunted Health Club*. New York: Avon Books, 1991.

Farrell, Amy Erdman. *Fat Shame: Stigma and the Fat Body in American Culture*. New York: New York University Press, 2011.

"Fast Forward." *Advocate*, January 19, 1988.

Fay, Bill. "Kinesiology: The System to Save Athletic Careers?" *Tampa Tribune*, February 9, 1982

Felkar, Victoria. "The Iron Bar: The Modern History of Prison Physical Culture and the Correctional Weightlifting Ban." *Stadion* 40 (2014): 19–37.

Ferderber, Skip. "Topanga Canyon Dwellers Live at Own Happy Pace: Community Reflects." *Los Angeles Times*, July 8, 1973.

Fielding-Singh, Priya. *How the Other Half Eats: The Untold Story of Food and Inequality in America*. New York: Little, Brown, 2021.

Fields, Rick. "Only Connect." *Yoga Journal*, May–June 1994.

"Find Own Fitness Way!" *Austin Statesman*, February 13, 1963.

Finke, Nikki. "All Sides Get Worked Up over Study of Aerobics Videos." *Los Angeles Times*, November 12, 1987.

"Fireworks Group Is Cited on Pricing." *New York Times*, January 28, 1938.

Fish, Allison. "The Commodification and Exchange of Knowledge in the Case of Transnational Commercial Yoga." *International Journal of Cultural Property* 13, no. 2 (2006): 189–206.

Fitzpatrick, Eileen. "Billy Blanks' Tae Bo Phenom Could Revitalize Fitness Genre." *Billboard*, February 27, 1999.

Flaherty, Colleen. "The Vanishing History Major." *Inside Higher Education*, November 27, 2018.

Florida, Richard, and Alistair Boone. "Boutique Fitness is Remaking American Neighborhoods." *Atlantic*, January 5, 2018.

Folan, Lilias, and Alice Rankin. In Joel Kramer, "Oracles of the New Age." *Yoga Journal*, January–February, 1980.

Folkart, Burt A. "Vic Tanny, First Big Chain Developer, Dies." *Los Angeles Times*, June 12, 1985.

Forth, Christopher. *Fat: A Cultural History of the Stuff of Life*. London: Reaktion Books, 2019.

Freedson, Patty S. "Strength Training for Women." *IDEA Personal Trainer* 11, no. 4 (July 2000).

Friedman, Danielle. "The Secret Sexual History of the Barre Workout." *Cut*, January 19, 2018. https://www.thecut.com/2018/01/barre-workout-sexual-history.html.

"From Our Readers." *Yoga Journal*, November–December 1994.

Gaby, Robin. "Senior Fitness, Fonda-Style." *Courier-News* (Bridgewater, NJ), August 14, 1986.

"Gay Rights Measure Loses Big in Houston." *Human Events*, February 9, 1985.

Gee, Connie. "What Hath This Hatha Yoga?" *Miami News*, February 15, 1959.

Geismer, Lily. *Don't Blame Us: Suburban Liberals and the Transformation of the Democratic Party*. Princeton, NJ: Princeton University Press, 2014.

Geist, William E. "About New York: The Mating Game and Other Exercises at the Vertical Club." *New York Times*, May 19, 1984.

"Get Your Exercise." Lorimar Home Video advertisement. *Ladies' Home Journal*, August 1987.

Gibbs, W. Wayt. "Obesity: An Overblown Epidemic?" *Scientific American*, December 1, 2006.

Gillerman, Sharon. "Samson in Vienna: The Theatrics of Jewish Masculinity." *Jewish Social Studies* New Series 9, no. 2 (Winter 2003): 65–98. https://www.jstor.org/stable/4467648.

Gillian, Frank, and Lauren Gutterman. "Let's Dance!" October 10, 2019. In *Sexing History*, produced by Saniya Lee Ghanoui. Podcast, MP3 audio, 29:15. https://www.sexinghistory.com /episode-25.

G., John. "Richard Simmons Show 1983." Posted May 27, 2018. YouTube video, 29:50. https://www.youtube.com/watch?v =QU6j7vjfbEs.

Gold, Matea, and Kathleen Hennessey. "Michelle Obama's Nutrition Campaign Comes with Political Pitfalls." *Los Angeles Times*, July 20, 2013.

Goldberg, Michelle. "The Brutal Economics of Being a Yoga Teacher." *Cut*, October 8, 2015. https://www.thecut.com/2015/10 /brutal-economics-of-being-a-yoga-teacher.html.

Goldberg, Michelle. *The Goddess Pose: The Audacious Life of Indra Devi, the Woman Who Helped Bring Yoga to the West*. New York: Penguin Random House, 2015.

Gordon, Mel. "Step Right Up and Meet the World's Mightiest Human—a Jewish Strongman from Poland Who Some Say Inspired the Creation of Superman." *Reform Judaism Online* (Summer 2011).

Gottesman, Andrew. "Gender Equity Hit by Backlash." *Chicago Tribune*, May 7, 1995.

Gottlieb, Dylan. *Yuppies: Wall Street and the Remaking of New York*. Cambridge, MA: Harvard University Press, forthcoming.

"Graphic Publisher Is Hailed to Court." *New York Times*, February 5, 1927.

Green, Harvey. *Fit for America: Health, Fitness, Sport, and American Society*. Baltimore, MD: Johns Hopkins University Press, 1986.

Green, Penelope. "Punching and Kicking All the Way to the Bank." *New York Times*, March 21, 1999.

Greenberg, James. "Asana TM." *Yoga Journal*, November–December 2003.

Greening, Tom, and Dick Hobson. "That Sense of Foreboding Must Not Dictate Your Life-Pattern." *Los Angeles Times*, September 18, 1979.

Griffith, R. Marie. *Born Again Bodies: Flesh and Spirit in American Christianity*. Berkeley: University of California Press, 2004.

Griffiths, Jo. "Women at Large." *Pittsburgh Post-Gazette*, January 25, 1990.

Gross, Jane. "James F. Fixx Dies Jogging; Author on Running Was 52." *New York Times*, July 22, 1984.

"Group Offer Yoga Lecture." *Arizona Republic*, March 11, 1959.

Guthmann, Edward. "The Gripping Tale of the Boy behind the Mask." *Advocate*, April 16, 1985.

Gutterman, Leon. "The Wisdom of Physical Fitness." *Wisdom Magazine*, May 1961.

Guttman, Judith. "Bodymind Exploration." *Yoga Journal*, November–December 1977.

Harber, Paul. "Tae Bo Puts a Kick into Workouts." *Boston Globe*, April 25, 1999.

Hart, Matt. "Does CrossFit Have a Future?" *New Yorker*, July 20, 2021. https://www.newyorker.com/sports/sporting-scene/does-crossfit-have-a-future.

Harvey, Duston. "Audience Participation Movie Stresses Touching and Trusting." Syndicated column. *Simpson's Leader-Times*, January 25, 1972.

Harvey, Steve. "Mussel or Muscle? Whatever You Call It, It's a Beach That's Not Forgotten by Many Devotees." *Los Angeles Times*, March 30, 1986.

Harvin, Al. "Fireman is First to Finish in Marathon." *New York Times*, September 14, 1970.

Harvin, Al. "Husband-Wife Teams Entered in Marathon Run Here Today." *New York Times*, September 13, 1970.

Haynes-Clark, Jennifer Lynn. "American Belly Dance and the Invention of the New Exotic: Orientalism, Feminism, and Popular Culture." MA thesis. Portland State University, 2010.

https://pdxscholar.library.pdx.edu/cgi/viewcontent.cgi
?article=1019&context=open_access_etds.

"Heart Disease and the Whole Man." *Pope Speaks*, September 3, 1956.

"Heart to Heart" advice column. *Dayton Daily News*, July 3, 1968.

Hecht, George J. "Do Our Children Need Toughening Up?" *Parents*, September 1956.

Hines, Alice. "Inside Core Power Yoga Teacher Training." *New York Times*, April 6, 2019.

Hittleman, Richard. "Everybody's Doing It: Yoga for Health." *Detroit Free Press*, June 26, 1960.

Hofstadter, Richard. *Anti-intellectualism in American Life*. New York: Knopf, 1963.

Hollander, Anne. "When Fat Was in Fashion." *New York Times*, October 23, 1977.

Hollinger, David. *Postethnic America: Beyond Multiculturalism*. New York: Basic Books, 1995.

Horan, Caley. *Insurance Era: Risk, Governance, and the Privatization of Security in Postwar America*. Chicago: University of Chicago Press, 2021.

Horne's Department Store advertisement. *Pittsburgh Press*, June 10, 1979.

"How Exxon Helps Its People Exercise." *US News and World Report*, January 28, 1980.

"How to Keep Trim—Debbie Drake Column Starts Monday." *Shreveport Journal*, January 6, 1962: 1.

"How to Start a Gang: The Co-Op Gym." *Radix Journal*, January 6, 2013.

Hulls, Tessa. "The Great Sandwina, Circus Strongwoman and Restaurateur." *Atlas Obscura*, December 26, 2017. https://www.atlasobscura.com/articles/the-great-sandwina.

Hyams, Joe. "Hittleman's Taking Yoga to the Ladies." *Washington Post*, August 7. 1961.

"IDEA Code of Ethics." *IDEA Personal Trainer*, July 2000.

"If Spring Has You Itching to Get Out and Exercise, You'll be Interested in a Scorecard on the Physical Benefits from Various Activities." *US News and World Report*, April 4, 1977.

"Indra Devi Introduced Yoga to Russian People." *Times Record*, May 5, 1964.

Jacobs, Frank, and George Woodbridge. "The Mad Guide to Political Types." *MAD*, October 1972.

Jacobson, Julie. "Chiropractor Also Uses Kinesiology." *Times Herald*, May 17, 1981.

"Jogging for Joy." *People*, July 4, 1977.

Johnson, David K. *Buying Gay: How Physique Entrepreneurs Sparked a Movement*. New York: Columbia University Press, 2019.

Johnson, David K. "Physique Pioneers: The Politics of 1960s Gay Consumer Culture," *Journal of Social History* 43, no. 4 (July 2010): 867–92.

Johnson, David K. *The Lavender Scare: The Cold War Persecution of Gays and Lesbians in the Federal Government*. Chicago: University of Chicago Press, 2004.

Johnson, James Harvey, ed. "American Patriots Cry Out against Treason Rotten Government, Suppression of News." *Truth Seeker* 98, no. 7 (July 1971).

Johnson, Mrs. Lyndon B. "Help Your Husband Guard His Heart." *Baltimore Sun*, February 12, 1956.

Johnson, William Oscar. "Marching to Euphoria." *Sports Illustrated*, July 14, 1980.

Jois, K. Pattabhi. Letter to the editor. *Yoga Journal*, November–December 1995.

Jones, Sarah. "Yoga Teachers are Unionizing to Heal the Wellness Industry." *Cut*, September 12, 2019. https://www.thecut.com/2019/09/yogaworks-teachers-first-yoga-teacher-union.html.

Kain, Ida Jean. "Relaxing Exercises Help Relieve Nervous Tension." *Saint Louis Globe-Democrat*, June 16, 1955.

Kanner, Bernice. "Home Movies." *New York Magazine*, July 16, 1984.

Katz, Donald. "Jack LaLanne Is Still an Animal." *Outside*, November 1995.

Kay, H. D. "Does Milk Cause Heart Disease?" *Country Life*, May 15, 1958.

Kennedy, Michael J. "Houston Will Vote on Civil Rights Measure; Opponents Fear Another S.F." *Los Angeles Times*, January 18, 1985.

Keyes, Allison. "How the Sports Bra Got Its Stabilizing Start." *Smithsonian Magazine*, March 18, 2020.

King, Nicholas. "The Jog-Alongs." *National Review*, August 17, 1979.

Kirk, Cynthia. "Exotic Male Tape Ousts Teacher." *Variety*, July 31, 1984.

Kleiner, Dick. "Why Would Any Man Like to Watch Debbie Drake Do the Army Dozen?" *Kenosha News*, July 13, 1962.

Kleyn, Brittany. "The Girls: Where Are They Now?" *Morning Chalk Up*, August 26, 2019.

Knight, Phil. *Shoe Dog: A Memoir by the Creator of Nike*. New York: Simon and Schuster, 2016.

Kramer, Joel. "Oracles of the New Age." *Yoga Journal*, January–February 1980.

Kraus, Hans, and Ruth P. Hirschland. "Minimum Muscular Fitness Tests in School Children." *Research Quarterly* 25, no. 2 (May 1954): 178–88.

Kripal, Jeffrey. *Esalen: America and the Religion of No Religion*. Chicago: University of Chicago Press, 2007.

Kudlick, Catherine. "'Save Changes': Telling Stories of Disability Protest." *Nursing Clio*, April 5, 2017. https://nursingclio .org/2017/04/05/save-changes-telling-stories-of-disability -protest/.

Kunitz, Daniel. *LIFT: Fitness Culture, from Naked Greeks and Acrobats to Jazzercise and Ninja Warriors*. New York: Harper Wave, 2017.

LaFeber, Walter. *Michael Jordan and the New Global Capitalism*. New York: Norton, 2002.

LaLanne European Health Spa advertisement. *Kansas City Times*, April 28, 1969.

"Lander Program Offers Concentrations in Athletic Training." *Index-Journal*, August 28, 1988.

Lanman, Sandra. "Aerobic Dance Aims for High Standards, Low Impact" *Central New Jersey Home News*, November 18, 1986.

Lasch, Christopher. "The Narcissist Society." *New York Review of Books*, September 30, 1976.

Lassiter, Matthew. *The Silent Majority: Suburban Politics in the Sunbelt South*. Princeton, NJ: Princeton University Press, 2007.

Latham, Alan. "The History of a Habit: Jogging as a Palliative to Sedentariness in 1960s America." *Cultural Geographies* 22, no. 1 (January 2015): 103–26.

Leo, John. "Equality—or Else!" *New York Daily News*, March 14, 1998.

Levin, Aaron. "Early On, the HIV/AIDS Epidemic Was a Voyage into the Unknown." *Psychiatry Online*, December 1, 2014. https://psychnews.psychiatryonline.org/doi/10.1176/appi.pn.2014.12a24.

Lewis, Anne S. "Recasting a Workout for the Masses." *New York Times*, October 6, 1996.

Lindsey, Robert. "Jane Fonda's Exercise Salons Aiding Her Husband's Candidacy." *New York Times*, May 2, 1982.

Litsky, Frank. "Ted Corbitt, A Pioneer in American Distance Running, Dies at 88." *New York Times*, December 13, 2007.

Lloyd, Barbara. "On Your Own: Step Up (and Down) to Sharper Workouts." *New York Times*, March 26, 1990. https://www.nytimes.com/1990/03/26/sports/on-your-own-step-up-and-down-to-sharper-workouts.html.

Lloyd, Robert. "Jack LaLanne Offered Perfect Fit for TV." *Paducah Sun*, January 30, 2011.

Locke, Jeannine. "Health Is Beauty, Baby." *Maclean's*, March 1, 1967.

Love, Ann Burnside. "Pain Is the Price in a 50-Mile Hike." *Baltimore Sun*, March 25, 1973.

Love, Robert. *The Great Oom: The Improbable Birth of Yoga in America*. New York: Viking, 2010.

"Low Impact Aerobics Are Easier, Less Demanding on the Body." *Modesto Bee*, May 7, 1986.

Lunbeck, Elizabeth. *The Americanization of Narcissism*. Cambridge, MA: Harvard University Press, 2014.

Lustigman, Alissa. "Cross Training at the Crossroads." *Sporting Goods Business* 24, no. 10 (October 1991).

MacGregor, Hilary E. "Bikram Goes to the Mat." *Los Angeles Times*, March 21, 2005.

Maddox, Callie Batts, and Robin Cooley. "'The Benares of the West': The Evolution of Yoga in Los Angeles." *Journal of Sport History* 41, no. 1 (Spring 2019): 82–97.

Maguire, Jennifer Smith. *Fit for Consumption: Sociology and the Business of Fitness*. Abingdon, UK: 2008.

"Make Kids Walk, Says Specialist." *Chicago Metro News*, July 12, 1986.

"Malbin's Muscles." *Philadelphia Inquirer*, November 3, 1957.

Manchester, Herbert. *Four Centuries of Sport in America, 1490–1890*. 1931. Reprint, New York: Derrydale Press, 1991.

"Man, Drowned, Found After Swimming Party." *Los Angeles Times*, September 6, 1949.

"Man Ordered to Stop Using Urine to Treat AIDS Patients." *Tyler Courier-Times*, August 18, 1987.

Manso, Peter. "Arnold Schwarzenegger on the Sex Secrets of Bodybuilders." *OUI*, August 1977.

Markoe, Merrill. "My Favorite Weekend." *Los Angeles Times*, February 13, 1997.

Martin, Douglas. "Bonnie Prudden, 97, Dies; Promoted Fitness for TV Generation." *New York Times*, December 18, 2011.

Martin, Douglas. "Lucille Roberts, 59, Founder of Gym Chain for Women." *New York Times*, July 18, 2003.

Martschukat, Jürgen. *The Age of Fitness: How the Body Came to Symbolize Success and Achievement*. London: Polity, 2021.

Matzer, Marla. "The Venus of Muscle Beach." *Los Angeles Times*, February 22, 1998.

Marx, Ina. "What Yoga Can Do for You." *Woman's Day*, June 1970.

McAdam, Robert. "Changes in Secondary School Boys' Physical Education Programs." *Physical Educator* 18, no. 2 (May 1, 1961): 64.

McCarthy, Colman. "Ashen, Carter Forced to Quit Road Race." *Washington Post*, September 16, 1979.

McDonald, Terrie. "Dated Facilities Restrict Women." *Stanford Daily*, February 16, 1972.

McKeever, Amy. "The Fitness Gospel of Billy Blanks." *Racked*, September 15, 2016.

McKenna, Helen. "What Dancing Did for Me." *Dance Magazine*, November 1942: 25–27.

McKenzie, Shelly. *Getting Physical: The Rise of Fitness Culture in America*. Lawrence: University Press of Kansas, 2013.

McKevitt, Andrew. *Consuming Japan: Popular Culture and the Globalizing of 1980s America*. Chapel Hill: University of North Carolina Press, 2017.

McLendon, Winzola. "Got a Weighty Problem? Then Take It Lying Down." *Washington Post and Times-Herald*, August 22, 1957.

McNatt, Missy. "Child's Letter to President John F. Kennedy about Physical Education." *Social Education* 73, no. 1 (January/February 2009): 10–14. https://www.socialstudies.org/system/files/publica tions/articles/se_730110.pdf.

Meckel, Richard A. *Classrooms and Clinics: Urban Schools and the Protection and Promotion of Child Health, 1870–1930*. New Bruns- wick, NJ: Rutgers University Press, 2013.

"Meet the Winner of the First Women-Only Road Race." *Runner's World*, June 8, 2012.

Metzl, Jonathan M., and Anna Kirkland, eds. *Against Health: How Health Became the New Morality*. New York: New York Univer- sity Press, 2010.

Mickey, Ethel L. " 'Eat, Pray, Love' Bullshit: Women's Empower- ment Through Wellness at an Elite Professional Conference." *Journal of Contemporary Ethnography* 48, no. 1 (2019): 103–27.

Midcentury Fashion. "An 11-Minute Episode of Debbie Drake's Exercise Television Show from the 1960s." Posted June 9, 2021. Facebook video, 11:33. https://www.facebook.com/watch/?v =2613299585642192.

Missett, Judi Sheppard. *Building a Business with a Beat: An Empire Built on Passion, Purpose and Heart*. New York: McGraw Hill, 2019.

"Morals Case Brings Muscle Beach Closing." *Los Angeles Times*, December 16, 1958.

Moran, Rachel Louise. "Change We Need? Why the Name of the President's Fitness Council Matters." *Nursing Clio*, May 8, 2018. https://nursingclio.org/2018/05/08/change-we-need-why-the -name-of-the-presidents-fitness-council-matters/.

Moran, Rachel Louise. *Governing Bodies: American Politics and the Shaping of the Modern Physique*. Philadelphia: University of Pennsylvania Press, 2018.

Morem, Bill. "Fitness Guru Jack LaLanne, 96, Dies at Morro Bay Home." *San Luis Obispo (CA) Tribune*, January 23, 2011.

Morgan, Tracy D. "Pages of Whiteness: Race, Physique Magazines, and the Emergence of Public Gay Culture." In *Queer Studies: A Lesbian, Gay, Bisexual, and Transgender Anthology*, edited by Brett Beemyn and Mickey Eliason, 280–98. New York: NYU Press, 1966.

Morris, Rodney J., and Pamela Kufahl. "Addressing Racism in the Fitness Industry Requires Understanding Its Roots." *Club Industry*, October 7, 2020. https://www.clubindustry.com/leadership -management/addressing-racism-fitness-industry-requires -understanding-its-roots.

Morse, Margaret. "Artemis Aging: Exercise and the Female Body on Video." *Discourse* 10, no. 1 (Fall/Winter 1987–1988): 20–53.

Moskowitz, Eva. *In Therapy We Trust: America's Obsession with Self-Fulfillment*. Baltimore, MD: Johns Hopkins University Press, 2001.

Moynihan, Colin. "The Yoga Instructors vs. the Private Equity Firm." *New York Times*, September 11, 2019.

Mull, Amanda. "Peloton Doesn't Understand the People Who Love It Most." *Atlantic*, December 5, 2019.

Murillo, Paulo. "Throwback to the Athletic Club West Hollywood." *Weho Times*, April 5, 2018.

Murphey, Josephine. "Muscle Minded." *Nashville Tennessean*, December 28, 1947.

"Muscle Beach Doomed." *Los Angeles Times*, December 17, 1958.

"Muscle Beach Party." Advertisement. *Fort Worth Star-Telegram*, April 10, 1964.

Musel, Robert. "She Limbers Up the Rich Jet Set." *South Bend Tribune*, April 20, 1971.

Musial, Stan. "Dramatic Gains in Youth Fitness." *Parents Magazine and Better Homemaking*, August 1966.

"Musical Fitness: A Sport Contains the Benefits of Jogging with Some Fun." *Los Angeles Times*, October 22, 1981.

"Mr. Alex Health Club Now Open in Boston." *Jewish Advocate*, April 6, 1961.

Myers, Bob. "Musclemen Undisturbed over Financial Careers." *Los Angeles Times*, May 17, 1948.

"NAACP Accuses Health Club of Discrimination." *Afro-American*, July 1961.

Nangle, Eleanor. "Through the Looking Glass: Silhouette Treatments at a Local Salon Offer Perfect Contours." *Chicago Daily Tribune*, June 7, 1936.

National Federation of State High School Associations. *Athletics Participation Survey Totals, 2007–08 Athletics Participation Summary*. Report. NFSHA, Elgin, IL, 2008. https://www.nfhs.org/media/1020206/hs_participation_survey_history_1969-2009.pdf.

Neal, H. C. "Yoga at the YMCA." *Daily Oklahoman*, November 17, 1968.

Nelson, Alondra. *Body and Soul: The Black Panther Party and the Fight against Medical Discrimination*. Minneapolis: University of Minnesota Press, 2011.

Nelton, Sharon. "Esalen Can Be Cold, Frightening." *Miami Herald*, December 22, 1970.

"New England Fat Men's Outing." *Boston Globe*, October 9, 1904: 6. https://www.newspapers.com/clip/96165527/the-boston-globe/.

"New Exerciser Proves Effective for Both Young and Elderly." *Crusader*, February 14, 1969.

New, Fran R. "We May Be Sitting Ourselves to Death." American Dairy Association advertisement. *Broadcasting*, February 5, 1962.

"New Gym in Montrose." *Montrose Star*, January 24, 1980. http://www.houstonlgbthistory.org/misc-jims.html.

Nielsen poll. In "What's on Television Tonight? Plenty More with Cable, VCRs." *Camden Courier-Post*, September 10, 1989.

NIRSA: Leaders in Collegiate Recreation. "Centennial of Collegiate Recreation: 1913–2013." Organizational video based on holdings at NIRSA Archive, Corvallis, OR. Posted on YouTube March 13, 2013. 11:04. https://www.youtube.com/watch?v=OmeefD0o-Bs.

Nolen, William A. "When Exercise Can Hurt You." *McCall's*, July 1980.

"No Patients in Well Medicine." *Garden City Telegram*, July 3, 1976: 7.

"N.Y. Probes Collapse of Flab Empire." *Des Moines Register*, December 11, 1963.

Offer, Avner. *The Challenge of Affluence: Self-Control and Well-Being in the United States and Britain since 1950.* New York: Oxford University Press, 2006.

Okundaye, Jason. "Tony Britts: Who Was the BBC Fitness Instructor?" *I-D Vice*, April 9, 2020.

Ongweso, Edward Jr. "Amazon Calls Workers 'Industrial Athletes' in Leaked Wellness Pamphlet." *Vice*, June 1, 2021.

Osgerby, Bill. "The Bachelor Pad as Cultural Icon: Masculinity, Consumption, and Interior Design in American Men's Magazines, 1930–65." *Journal of Design History* 18, no. 1 (Spring 2005): 99–113.

Overton, Rebecca. "Certification Program in Aerobics Due." *Indianapolis Star*, November 9, 1985.

Pally, Marcia. "Laissez-Faire Lesbianism: Prize-Winning French Film Takes Sexual Identity in Stride." *Advocate*, September 29, 1987.

"Parkway Athletic Club's Mark Schmidt and Michael Wilson are Planning Big Things." *Montrose Voice*, October 3, 1986.

Parsons, Patrick R., and Herbert J. Rotfeld. "Infomercials and Television Station Clearance Practices." *Journal of Public Policy and Marketing* 9 (1990): 62–72.

Pascoe, Jean. "A Common Sense Approach to Yoga." *Woman's Day*, June 1970.

"Percentage of U.S. Population Who Have Completed Four Years of College or More from 1940–2019, by Gender." *Statista*. March 15, 2021. https://www.statista.com/statistics/184272

/educational-attainment-of-college-diploma-or-higher-by
-gender/.

Petersen, Anne Helen. "The Millennial Vernacular of Fatphobia."
Culture Study, Substack newsletter, May 23, 2021.

Peters, Roberta. "Problems of a Coloratura Soprano." *Music Journal*, September 1959.

Petosa, Richard. "Wellness: An Emerging Opportunity for Health
Education." *Health Education* 15, no. 6 (October/November 1984):
37–39.

Petrzela, Natalia Mehlman. "Conbody's Success is Forcing the
Fitness World to Confront Some Uncomfortable Truths."
Well + Good, April 11, 2018. https://www.wellandgood.com
/why-conbody-prison-workout-is-so-popular/.

Petrzela, Natalia Mehlman. "How Joseph Pilates Started Today's
Mind-Body Boutique Craze Nearly 100 Years Ago." *Well + Good*,
October 15, 2015. https://www.wellandgood.com/how-joseph
-pilates-started-todays-mind-body-boutique-craze-nearly-100
-years-ago/.

Petrzela, Natalia Mehlman. "Jogging Has Always Excluded Black
People." *New York Times*, May 12, 2020.

Petrzela, Natalia Mehlman. "Slenderizing Spas, Reducing
Machines, and Other Hot Fitness Crazes of 75 Years Ago."
Well + Good, September 1, 2015. https://www.wellandgood.com
/weight-loss-salons-reducing-machines/.

Petrzela, Natalia Mehlman. "What You Can Learn from the Surprising History of New Year's Resolutions." *Refinery29*, December 29, 2016. https://www.refinery29.com/en-us/2016/12/134160
/fitness-new-year-resolutions-history.

Petrzela, Natalia Mehlman. "Why Donald Trump's Diet is Bad for
America's Health." *Washington Post*, June 28, 2017.

Petrzela, Natalia Mehlman. "Why Everyone is Obsessed with a
Fitness Podcast About Richard Simmons." *Well + Good*,
March 29, 2017. https://www.wellandgood.com/missing-richard
-simmons-podcast-fitness-history/.

Petrzela, Natalia Mehlman. "Why Wellness Has Always Played
an Important Role in Politics and Activism." *Well + Good*,

November 18, 2016. https://www.wellandgood.com/wellness-and
-politics-post-election-trump/.

Petrzela, Natalia Mehlman. "Working, Out." *Slate*, June 20, 2018,
https://slate.com/human-interest/2018/06/crossfit-homophobia
-reminds-us-that-gyms-have-always-been-gay.html.

Petrzela, Natalia Mehlman. "The Precarious Labor of the Fitpro:
Interrogating the Political Economy of Fitness in American
Life." *Public Seminar*, December 16, 2019. https://publicseminar
.org/essays/the-precarious-labor-of-the-fitpro/.

Pietri, Pamela. "Helping the Omless." *LA Weekly*, June 2, 1988.

Polk, Elizabeth. "When the Parade Goes By, Join It!" *Wichita
Times*, April 15, 1976.

Pollack, Ben, and Jan Todd. "American Icarus: Vic Tanny and
America's First Health Club Chain." *Iron Game History* 13–14,
no.1 (December 2016): 17–27.

Powers, Ann. "American Influences Help Redefine Practice of
Yoga." *New York Times*, August 1, 2000.

Prashad, Vijay. *Everybody Was Kung Fu Fighting*. New York: Beacon
Press, 2001.

President's Council on Physical Fitness and Sports advertisement.
Cosmopolitan, July 1981.

"President's Council on Physical Fitness and Sports: Council
Members and Executives, July 1956–May 2006." President's
Council on Physical Fitness and Sports. Accessed February 267,
2022. https://www.hhs.gov/sites/default/files/fitness/pdfs/list-of
-council-leadership.pdf.

Pronger, Brian. *Body Fascism: Salvation in the Technology of Physical
Fitness*. Toronto: University of Toronto Press, 2002.

Prudden, Bonnie. "Fitness from the Cradle." *Sports Illustrated*,
May 1, 1960.

Purkiss, Ava. "'Beauty Secrets: Fight Fat': Black Women's Aesthetics, Exercise, and Fat Stigma, 1900–1930s." *Journal of Women's
History* 29, no. 2 (Summer 2017): 14–37.

Purkiss, Ava. *Fit Citizens: A History of Black Women's Exercise from
Post-Reconstruction to Postwar America*. Chapel Hill: University
of North Carolina Press, forthcoming.

"Put an End to Women's Suffrage." Nike Aurora shoe advertisement. *Runner's World*, 1980. Department of Nike Archives, Nike Inc., Beaverton, OR.

Ravitch, Diane. *The Troubled Crusade: American Edition, 1945–1980*. New York: Basic Books, 1983.

"Reach Out and Touch Someone." Bell System advertisement. *Ebony*, June 1982.

Reebok advertisement. *Great Falls Tribune*, December 16, 1982.

"Registration for Yoga Class is Still Open." *Corpus Christi Caller-Times*, May 18, 1961.

Reich, Holly. "What Exercisers Do." *New York Daily News*, November 27, 1989.

Reinhold, Robert. "An Interview with Kenneth Cooper." *New York Times*, March 29, 1987.

Reinhold, Robert. "Has the Aerobics Movement Peaked?" *New York Times*, March 29, 1987.

Rensin, David. "20 Questions with Jack LaLanne." *Playboy*, October 1984.

Reston, James. "Exercise Haters Win in a Walk." *Atlanta Constitution*, February 16, 1963: 4.

Richardson, Tony, dir. *The Loneliness of the Long Distance Runner*. 1962; United Kingdom: Woodfall Film Productions.

Richie, Douglas H., Jr., Steven F. Kelson, and Patricia Bellucci. "Aerobic Dance Injuries: A Retrospective Study of Instructors and Participants." *Physician and Sportsmedicine* 13, no. 2 (1985): 130–40.

Riley, Norman. "Arts." *Crisis*, December 1985.

Roberts, Joshua. "Sports and the New Frontier." *Town and Country*, April 1963.

Robinette, Gale B. "This Sunday Proclaimed 10-K Race Day." *Tennessean*, September 20, 1979.

Root, Jonathan. "Pounds Off for Jesus: Oral Roberts University and the Fat Body, 1976–78." *Fat Studies: An Interdisciplinary Journal of Body Weight and Society* 4 (April 8, 2015): 159–77.

Rose, Marla Matzer. *Muscle Beach: Where the Best Bodies in the World Started a Fitness Revolution*. New York: LA Weekly Books, 2001.

Rosman, Katherine. "The Hilaria Baldwin Story: I'm Living My Life." *New York Times*, December 30, 2020.

Rouse, Wendy L. *Her Own Hero: The Origins of the Women's Self-Defense Movement.* New York: New York University Press, 2017.

"Running Has Made a Difference in My Life." *Chicago Metro News*, October 6, 1984.

"Running with President George W. Bush." *Runner's World*, October 1, 2002.

Rushe, Dominic. "Yoga Guru Bikram Choudhury Accused of Rape in Two New Lawsuits." *Guardian*, May 14, 2013.

Rutkowski, Eugene. Letter to the editor. *Simpson's Leader-Times*, March 9, 1963.

Ryon, Ruth. "Sports Club/LA: It Shapes Up as the Fitness Taj Mahal." *Los Angeles Times*, August 16, 1987.

Sabol, Blair. "Yogi to the Stars, Everyman." *Los Angeles Times*, November 29, 1974.

Sales, Bob. "Has Marathon Become Battle of the Sexes?" *Boston Globe*, April 20, 1967.

Samuelson, Joan Benoit. Nike Odyssey sneaker advertisement, ca. early 1980s. Department of Nike Archives, Nike Inc., Beaverton, OR.

Sauerberg, George. "Just Do It! A Personal Trainer Adds the Push You May Need." *Gazette* (Cedar Rapids), January 9, 1994.

Saval, Nikil. *Cubed: The Secret History of the Workplace.* New York: Doubleday, 2014.

Savoy, Maggie. "Hope In-Law with a Sense of Humor." *Los Angeles Times*, March 20, 1970.

Schanzenbach, Diane Whitmore, Ryan Nunn, and Lauren Bauer. *The Changing Landscape of American Life Expectancy.* Washington, DC: The Hamilton Project, Brookings Institution, June 2016. https://www.hamiltonproject.org/assets/files/changing _landscape_american_life_expectancy.pdf.

Schmidt, Leigh Eric. *Heaven's Bride: The Unprintable Life of Ida Craddock, American Mystic, Scholar, Sexologist, and Madwoman.* New York: Basic Books, 2010.

Schroeder, Michael. "Looking for a Bigger Slice." *Detroit News*, September 20, 1985.

Schuler, Lou. "The Best Exercises of All Time." *Men's Health*, July/August 2000.

Sciponi, Jade. "59% of Americans Don't Plan to Renew Their Gym Memberships after Covid-19 Pandemic: Survey." *CNBC*, July 23, 2020. https://www.cnbc.com/2020/07/23/many-dont-plan-to-renew-their-gym-memberships-post-pandemic-survey.html.

Seldon, Dave. "New ORU Aerobics Center Called Boost for Fitness." *Daily Oklahoman*, September 30, 1974.

"Shaping Up." *Ebony*, June 1982.

Sherman, Rachel. *Uneasy Street: The Anxieties of Influence*. Princeton, NJ: Princeton University Press, 2017.

Shin, Laura. "Free Market Yoga." *Yoga Journal*, March–April 2005.

Shipley, E. H., dir. *Richard Simmons: Sweatin' to the Oldies*. Home video. 1988; Hollywood, CA: Ren-Mar Studios.

Shuer, Margie. "Swim Team Blues." *Stanford Daily*, February 26, 1974. Marjorie L. Shuer Papers, box 1, folder 2. Department of Special Collections and University Archives, Stanford University Libraries, Stanford, CA.

Sievers, Linda. "Videos to Sweat By Offer a Convenient Way to Work Out." *Anchorage Daily News*, January 15, 1988.

Sifford, Darrell. "Runners Laboring under Myth, Says Doctor." *Cincinnati Enquirer*, December 24, 1984.

Silver, George A. "Fits over Fitness." *Nation*, June 9, 1962.

Sivulka, Juliann. *Soap, Sex and Cigarettes: A Cultural History of Advertising*. New York: Cengage Learning, 2011.

Sloane, Leonard. "Business People: Elaine Powers Founder Plans Diet Formula." *New York Times*, January 26, 1981.

Smith, Alyssa Corinne. "The Strangers beside Us: A History of Fear, Fascination, and Spectacle Murder in Late Twentieth-Century America." PhD diss., University of Chicago, 2021.

Smith, Merriman. "Cracks in Mirror Image Irritate Kennedy Fans." *Nation's Business*, April 1963.

"Sniper Suspect Pleads Innocent in Federal Charges." *Daily Spectrum* (St. George, Utah), November 11, 1980.

Snyder, Thomas D., ed. *120 Years of American Education: A Statistical Portrait*. Report. National Center for Education Statistics, January 1993. https://nces.ed.gov/pubs93/93442.pdf.

Sole-Smith, Virginia. "Can The Fitness Industry and Body Positivity Coexist?" *Elemental*, January 15, 2020.

Spada, James. *Fonda: Her Life in Pictures*. New York: Doubleday, 1985.

"Spanning the Years." *IDEA Fitness Journal*, July–August 2017: 20–35. https://www.ideafit.com/wp-content/uploads/files/IDEA -35year-timeline-01.pdf

Spray, Deborah (Nikki Craft). "In Defense of Civil Disobedience." April 2, 1980. Women Against Violence Against Women Collection (box 5, folder 6, "Hillside Strangler"), Special Collections, University of California-Los Angeles.

Steinhauer, Jennifer. "For Aerobics Die-Hards, There Are No Substitutes." *New York Times*, February 22, 1995.

Stein, Jeannine. "Mid-Career Stretches." *Los Angeles Times*, April 21, 2003.

Stein, Pat. "Personal Trainers." *North County Blade-Citizen*, July 25, 1990.

Steinem, Gloria. "In Praise of Women's Bodies." *Ms.*, April 1982.

Stern, Marc. "The Fitness Movement and the Fitness Center Industry: 1960–2000." *Business and Economic History On-Line* 6 (2008): 12–13.

Stevens, William K. "Houston Accepts New Political Force." *New York Times*, November 2, 1981.

Stoute, Steve. *The Tanning of America: How Hip-Hop Created a Culture that Rewrote the Rules of the New Economy*. New York: Penguin, 2011.

Strasser, J. B., and Laurie Becklund. *Swoosh: The Unauthorized Story of Nike and the Men Who Played There*. New York: Harcourt Brace Jovanovich, 1991.

"Stretch and Salad." *Los Angeles Times*, November 14, 1975.

Strings, Sabrina. *Fearing the Black Body: The Racial Origins of Fatphobia*. New York: NYU Press, 2019.

Stull, Dorothy. "Go Happy, Go Healthy, With Bonnie." *Sports Illustrated*, July 16, 1956.

Sullivan, Robert. "Goodbye to Heroin Chic, Now It's Sexy to be Strong." *Time Magazine*, July 19, 1999.

Switzer, Kathrine. *Marathon Woman*. New York: Da Capo Press, 2009.

Tae Bo advertisement. *Fort Worth Star Telegram*, March 14, 1999.

Tate, Angela. "Eating Disorders Are for White Girls." *Culture Study*, Substack newsletter, edited by Anne Helen Petersen, June 16, 2021. https://annehelen.substack.com/p/eating -disorders-are-for-white-girls.

Taylor, Angela. "From Shimmying to Standing on Your Head." *New York Times*, March 24, 1972.

"The Bar Bells Toll Sadly." *Los Angeles Times*, December 21, 1958.

"The President's Conference on the Fitness of American Youth," *Journal of Health, Physical Education, and Recreation* 27, no. 6 (1956): 8–31.

"The Problem with 'Wellness' as a Virtue." Letters. *Chronicle Review*, June 12, 2016. https://www.chronicle.com/article /the-problem-with-wellness-as-a-virtue/.

"The Sports Club Company History." *Funding Universe*. Accessed January 6, 2022. http://www.fundinguniverse.com /company-histories/the-sports-club-company-history/.

"They'll See Yoga Display." *Miami Herald*, August 22, 1958.

Thornley, Kerry. "Reprogram Yourself For Freer Swinging." *Eros Lib* 2. Newsletter. San Diego, CA: Sexual Freedom League, 1975.

"Those Reducing Salons: Do They Really Slim a Lady Down?" *Changing Times: The Kiplinger Magazine* 11, no. 3 (March 1957): 13–14. https://books.google.com/books?id=nwAEAAAAMBAJ &printsec=frontcover&rview=1&lr=#v=onepage&q&f=false.

"Time for a 'Fitness Vacation.'" *Chicago Metro News*, June 5, 1982.

Todd, Jan. "Katie Sandwina and the Construction of Celebrity." *Bandwagon* 56, no. 2 (March 2012): 28–35.

Todd, Jan. "The Legacy of Pudgy Stockton." *Iron Game History* 2, no. 1 (January 1992): 5–7.

Todd, Jan, and Jerry Todd. "The Last Interview." *Iron Game History* 6, no. 4 (December 2000): 1–14. https://starkcenter.org/igh/igh -v6/igh-v6-n4/igh0604a.pdf.

"Trendy Exercisers Bent on Pilates." *Victoria Advocate*, December 25, 1995.

Tricard, Louise Mead. *American Women's Track and Field: A History, 1895–1989*, Vol. 1. New York: McFarland, 1996.

Trimway advertisement, *Bulletin*, November 6, 1968.

"Turns Back Girl Bathers: Is Troubled by Folks Who Say They Hate Clothes." *New York Times*, August 27, 1915.

Tyler, Richard. *The West Coast Bodybuilding Scene: The Golden Era.* Santa Cruz, CA: On Target Publications, 2004.

Tymn, Mike. "On Running." *Honolulu Advertiser*, September 7, 1978.

Untitled. *Beauty and Health* 6 (March 1903): 21.

"UW Chops Kinesiology Program." *Spokesman-Review*, November 15, 1982.

Van der Veer, Peter. *Imperial Encounters: Religion and Modernity in India and Britain*. Princeton, NJ: Princeton University Press, 2001.

Vatz, Stephanie. "Why America Stopped Making Its Own Clothes." *KQED*, May 14, 2013. https://www.kqed.org/lowdown/7939/madeinamerica.

Vaz, Valerie. "The Pilates Principle." *Essence*, September 1996.

Venit Shelton, Tamara. *Herbs and Roots: A History of Chinese Medicine in the American Marketplace*. New Haven, CT: Yale University Press, 2019.

Verbrugge, Martha. *Active Bodies: A History of Women's Physical Education in Twentieth-Century America*. New York: Oxford University Press, 2012.

Villarosa, Linda. "Firms Find Fitness Plans Pay Out Healthy Dividends." *American Banker*, October 19, 1987.

Vogue editors. "Your Heart's Blood." *Vogue*, January 1, 1959.

Vogler, Shannon. "Implementing Fitness Programs for People with Disabilities." IHRSA blog, April 26, 2018. https://www.ihrsa.org/improve-your-club/implementing-fitness-programs-for-people-with-disabilities/.

Wagner, Philip E. "Musculinity: A Critical Visual Investigation of Male Body Culture." PhD diss., University of Kansas, 2015. https://kuscholarworks.ku.edu/handle/1808/19558.

Walker, Julian. "Enlightenment 2.0: The American Yoga Experiment." In *21st Century Yoga: Culture, Politics and Practice*, edited by Carol Horton and Roseanne Harvey: 1–26. Chicago: Kleio Books, 2012.

Waller, David. *The Perfect Man: The Muscular Life and Times of Eugene Sandow, Victorian Strongman*. New York: Victorian Secrets, 2011.

Ware, Susan. *Game, Set, Match: Billie Jean King and the Revolution in Women's Sports*. Chapel Hill: University of North Carolina Press, 2011.

"Weightlifters Display Talent at Y Tonight." *Los Angeles Times*, December 9, 1949.

Weller, Sheila. *Girls Like Us: Carole King, Joni Mitchell, Carly Simon and the Journey of a Generation*. New York: Washington Square Press, 2008.

Wells, Gully, and Nancy Serano. "Pilates Body." *Vogue*, October 1, 1988: 274–82.

"What Is Kinesiology?" University of Michigan website. Accessed January 31, 2021. https://www.kines.umich.edu/about /what-kinesiology.

"What's in a Name?" *Joe Weider's Shape* 17, no. 3 (November 1997).

Whitaker, Scott, dir. *Run Dick, Run Jane!* Provo, UT: Department of Motion Picture Production, Brigham Young University, 1971. 20:31. https://www.youtube.com/watch?v=Ip07Yndgzzg.

White, David Gordon, ed. *Tantra in Practice*. Princeton, NJ: Princeton University Press, 2000.

White, L. K., Central Intelligence Agency Deputy Director for Support. "Physical Fitness Room." Memo, January 1, 1964. General CIA Records, National Security Internet Archive, Central Intelligence Agency. https://archive.org/details/CIA -RDP85-00375R000400110097-1.

White, Paul Dudley. "Rx for Health: Exercise: If Summer Prompts Us to Get Out and Use Our Legs, Dr. White Approves." *New York Times*, June 23, 1957.

Wilde, T. Jesse. "Gender Equity in Athletics: Coming of Age in the 90's." *Marquette Sports Law Review* 4, no. 2 (1994).

Williams, Brett. "Fitness Workers Are Organizing to Flex More Muscles in Their Workplaces." *Men's Health*, December 9, 2020.

Williams, F. M. "Women Slate September Race." *Tennessean*, June 11, 1978.

Williamson, Lola. *Transcendent in America: Hindu-Inspired Meditation Movements in America*. New York: New York University Press, 2010.

Wilson, Maggie. "'Fitness Fanatics' Run for Their Lives." *Arizona Republic*, March 8, 1978.

"With Vigah." *New Castle News*, February 13, 1963.

Wojciechowski, Gene, and Andrew Gottesman. "Golden Era for Women." *Chicago Tribune*, August 4, 1996.

"Wolf Pack's Prey." *New York Daily News*, April 21, 1989.

Woloson, Wendy A. *Crap: A History of Cheap Stuff in America*. Chicago: University of Chicago Press, 2020.

Wyman, Patrick. "Bro Culture, Fitness, Chivalry, and American Identity." *Perspectives: Past Present and Future*, Substack newsletter, December 4, 2020. https://patrickwyman.substack.com/p/bro-culture-fitness-chivalry-and.

Yanofsky, David. "US Imports of Women's Pants." *Atlas*, 2018. https://theatlas.com/charts/GmCUr1ngH.

"YMCA Features Trimnastics Class." *Milwaukee Star*, September 9, 1968.

"Yoga Classes Help You Work Up a Good Sweat." *Arizona Daily Star*, August 20, 1998.

"YOGA." *Los Angeles Times*, November 20, 1994.

"Yogi Desai Resigns from Kripalu." *Yoga Journal*, January–February 1995.

Zakim, Michael. *Accounting for Capitalism: The World the Clerk Made*. Chicago: University of Chicago Press, 2018.

Zukerman, Ruth. *Riding High: How I Kissed SoulCycle Goodbye, Co-Founded Flywheel, and Built the Life I Always Wanted*. New York: St. Martin's Press, 2018.

Index